American Evangelists and Tuberculosis in Modern Japan

American Evangelists and Tuberculosis in Modern Japan

Elisheva A. Perelman

HKU
PRESS
香港大學出版社

Hong Kong University Press
The University of Hong Kong
Pok Fu Lam Road
Hong Kong
https://hkupress.hku.hk

ISBN 978-988-8528-14-1 (*Hardback*)

British Library Cataloguing-in-Publication Data
A catalogue record for this book is available from the British Library.

Digitally printed

This work would not be possible without the assistance and support of
my editors, Yuet-Sang Leung and Eric Mok at
Hong Kong University Press,
my parents, Seth and Leslie Perelman, and
my husband, Paul Benjamin Cherlin.

I wish to dedicate this monograph to the memory of those whom the tuberculosis epidemic claimed and to those who struggled, in their way, to assist them. Let the work go on.

Love is anterior to life,
Posterior to death,
Initial of creation, and
The exponent of breath.

—Emily Dickinson

Contents

Introduction

The Story of Something That Did Not Happen

This is the story, in large measure, of something that did not happen. Implicitly, it is also the story of what happened instead. It answers the question as to why the nationwide threat of tuberculosis was viewed as not within state purview in Japan in the late nineteenth and early twentieth centuries but was relegated instead to the private sphere, to be struggled against by foreign Protestant evangelists, often to the detriment of the victims of the epidemic. It will accordingly consider the reasons for this dismissal with respect to bureaucratic infighting, to concerns over possible loss of economic progress, and to avoidance of public health expenditures. Conversely, it will analyze both the motivations of the evangelists who would shoulder the burden in place of the government—their desire to find a place in society and their hope for converts. No less significant, it will detail the plight of the tubercular victims, who were primarily young female factory workers, as it was among them that the epidemic began, only to spread to the rest of society.

Tuberculosis ran rampant in Japan during the late Meiji and Taishō years (1880s–1920s) and the government seemed ill disposed to combat it. Perhaps this was not surprising. Politically, this was a time of action. After all, these were the years of nation building in the archipelago, and the creation of a nation takes considerable political effort. Yet inaction is equally the domain of politics, and willful governmental inaction, as much as its actions, shaped Japanese national modernization from the 1880s and 1890s to the 1920s. That politicians overlooked considerable swaths of constituents—suffrage being a conspicuous example—is hardly surprising. What is perhaps surprising is that among those who were overlooked were the new nation's victims of tuberculosis. As the proverbial "modern epidemic" (a disease whose devastation worsened with the accomplishments of modernity),[1] tuberculosis struck the modernizing nation hard. Among its victims were the women (and later, men) populating first the factories and then the villages of Japan's so-called family-state. Their collective existence and their shortened individual lives brought into question the nature of both Japanese society and the Japanese state. How could a nation like Japan, whose medical and scientific achievements were extraordinary, justify inaction in the face of a terrible epidemic? The answer lies

1. See William Johnston's *The Modern Epidemic: A History of Tuberculosis in Japan.*

in a desire not to stall the nation's modernization. From that, therefore, was a fear that the acknowledgment of the cost of this modernization—namely, thousands of lives—would impede the efforts made on behalf of the nation. So long as the victims remained primarily young rural women, a seemingly endless resource, the sacrifice seemed nearly ineluctable. To top this off, bureaucratic infighting plagued the political sphere, and addressing the epidemic was often bogged down by political strife.

This monograph looks at how outsiders attempted to fill gaps in health care, largely without success—yet another version of something that did not happen. The scientists at the forefront of disease research and prevention, here represented by Kitasato Shibasaburō, the mentee and friend of tubercle bacillus isolator Robert Koch, were prone to political backbiting and superciliousness, and proved unable to combat the epidemic effectively. Instead, these outsiders (namely, American Protestant nondenominational evangelists, prominently including those associated with the Young Men's Christian Association (YMCA), the Salvation Army, St. Luke's Hospital, and the Omi Mission) sought to assist in Japan's nation building as a way to garner converts among a land untouched by missionizing for centuries. In this respect, concentration on the years between the 1880s and 1920s is necessary—not solely because this was when the modern Japanese nation was substantially created, but because it was similarly when evangelists were first able to proselytize, with varying degrees of success, in the nascent nation. It was these evangelists, rather than Catholics, Russian Orthodox, and even native Buddhists, who saw the opportunities offered by various lacunae in nation building as a means to an end.

Such a consideration—looking at these lacunae thus—brings up questions of the moral enterprise: How did both the Japanese government, often represented here by politician Ōkuma Shigenobu, and foreign evangelical organizations paint themselves as the more moral party vis-à-vis the Japanese public in relating to each other? How did each convince the public that theirs was the one with the best interests of the Japanese people at heart? How did they paint themselves as moral entrepreneurs? Originally identified by sociologist Howard S. Becker, the moral entrepreneur was one who defined behavior and sought to codify moral rectitude. However, the concept was altered by Jack Nelson, who established a definition whereby the Salvation Army in Japan, by undertaking work on prostitution, sought to alter a nation's moral consideration of an issue. My work is an analogue to Nelson's, in that I argue that the relationship between the Japanese government and the Salvation Army (among other organizations), with regard to its work on tuberculosis, was one of moral entrepreneurship on both sides. This was also the case, with differing levels of success, with respect to the efforts of other foreign evangelical organizations to combat tuberculosis and to the government's interactions with them. In these various cases, each side maneuvered to maintain the appearance of the moral high ground in their presentations of the situation to the other side.[2]

2. Becker, 162; Nelson, 35.

Neither were these relationships solely between evangelical organizations and the Japanese government, as the organizations themselves were constantly maneuvering with each other—the YMCA, the Salvation Army, and, to a lesser extent, St. Luke's Hospital and the Omi Mission. All four were constantly aware of the work of the others, including their respective evangelical shortcomings. This, therefore, created a rather complex web of moral enterprise, yet one that failed adequately to consider a vital component—namely, the tubercular themselves. This was an unfortunate yet obvious oversight that calls into question the validity and utility of the moral enterprise. If those upon whom one's claim to morality is established are considered only as chattel, how moral is this enterprise really?

This consideration, in turn, brings up the question of the soteriological value of potential converts, as well as their suffering, both from the point of view of the Christian organizations and of the sufferers of the disease themselves. What is the worth of a human life, and to whom? The question in analyzing these relationships was, therefore, cui bono? Who benefits and how, as the nature of the work was on some level self-interest, particularly when it involved so little reward for the evangelical organizations, both in terms of influential converts (or any converts at all) and of funds earned through such work. Ostensibly, the tubercular themselves were the beneficiaries, when the work was undertaken, but to what end? Since the disease remained incurable during this time, evangelical organizations could offer little pharmacological medicine. Often claims to assist the tubercular were founded on attention drawn to their plight. Yet this made individuals with a disease into a collective and, in doing so, removed their agency, essentially making them pawns in the constantly evolving chess games between the organizations and the government. At best, of course, those organizations that did attempt to assist the tubercular medically could alter the game, but only to a minimal extent. Even if the infirm were no longer merely pawns, they remained without full agency, reduced to afflicted passivity, even in a place of love and acceptance within which they could convalesce.

Should this moral enterprise be condemned as little more than a farce? Yes and no. Certainly, in this case it seems that moral entrepreneurship more often than not failed those it used to justify itself, but that does not mean that the enterprise itself is wholly bankrupt. After all, the moral enterprise sparked the relationships that allowed for care of the tubercular, although, as we shall see, such care only proved successful after the entanglements of moral entrepreneurship were cast aside.

If the tubercular benefit from these relationships in which they are considered currency only after the entanglements are abandoned, who benefits before then? These relationships benefited the Japanese government writ large, allowing it to maintain that it was dealing with an epidemic at a grassroots level without actually expending resources on it. The Japanese Diet itself, often embodied by the prime minister, likewise benefited through the ties such relationships maintained with the home countries of the evangelists. Similarly, the evangelical organizations benefited, as these relationships allowed them to proselytize in Japan with the complicity of the Japanese government, so long as they proved themselves useful to it.

The nature of these relationships and of the roles of each of the participants in them help to shed light on a variety of topics, including the nature of subjection within an imperial state, albeit expected by both the state itself and its subjects. In addition, it illuminates the value of women within that society as subjects, as workers, and as national resources, and it also limns the American evangelical movements' valuation of both foreign and native women, as the majority of the epidemics' early victims were the young women in the textile mills of the nation (and it is with them that I analyze the costs of both the epidemic and the relationships surrounding it). An analysis of these interactions also involves the role of class in Japanese society in the early twentieth century, both independent of and as related to gender, since most of the early victims of the epidemic, these women, were poor and from rural regions. Finally, with tuberculosis as a nexus within the machinations of a government and a series of both nationally and religiously foreign organizations, the character of a disease can be seen to follow the progression from diagnosis to definition, wherein tuberculosis itself consumes the identity of an individual again and again.

With these themes as its subject, this monograph respectfully follows in the footsteps of such works as *The Modern Epidemic* (William Johnston), *Factory Girls* (E. Patricia Tsurumi), *Kekkaku to Nihonjin* (Tsuneishi Keiichi), *Kekkaku toiu bunka* (Fukuda Mahito), *The Formation of Science in Japan* (James Bartholomew), and *A World of Crisis and Progress* (Jon Thares Davidann). Hopefully, the current work combines various thoughts of each to create a cohesive synthesis. Standing on the shoulders of such giants in medical history, history of science, women's history, and evangelical history permits us to touch on ramifying issues that previous scholars did not address. For instance, this monograph is the first to analyze the work performed by the evangelical groups with regard to ministering to the tubercular and, more important, the desired effects of such missionizing, in terms of the aforementioned questions: To what end the moral enterprise? What is the value of a human life? Who benefits?

This book is divided into eight chapters, an afterword, and a conclusion. The first chapter looks at the history of factory girls in Meiji and Taishō Japan. These individuals proved the backbone of Japan's modernization, as the funds for nation building came directly from coffers of the textile industry. This workforce comprised almost entirely women, many of whom were children. So, too, were these women—living and working, as they did, in insalubrious conditions—the majority of tuberculosis' early victims. As long as the disease remained confined to these girls, mostly from rural communities, the government could devote but scant attention to the scourge.

Chapter 2, in turn, examines the history of the scourge itself during the same period. The cultural baggage of the disease would come to be as victimizing as the disease itself. Yet what about the epidemic? Though attempts like 1911's Factory

Law were passed (though often unenforced, especially for the first five years), how could a nation whose industrial achievements were as extraordinary as Japan's justify action that would result in reduced productivity, much less a work stoppage? Moreover, what really could be done? After all, there was no cure for the disease until the 1920s, and even then it was not until the 1940s that a cure was considered effective. Of course, and with this in mind, if the government could pay lip service to combative efforts, like the Factory Law, it could reap the moral sense of paternalism that such constituent care connoted. Naturally, actually addressing the issue would be to acknowledge problems inherent in the state's effort to modernize along industrial lines. So long as the epidemic remained limited to society's neglected, primarily the young, impoverished female textile workers (upon whose backs the society was built), both the epidemic and its victims could be, and were, written off as a sacrifice the government was willing to sustain, having already saved face with passage of ostensibly ameliorative legislation.

Chapter 3 analyzes the scientific battle against the disease, waged primarily by an eminent bacteriologist and colleague of Robert Koch, Kitasato Shibasaburō. Both a government scientist and an independent researcher, Kitasato was well placed to deal with the disease, and to convince the government to do similarly. Yet Kitasato, a man who refused to suffer fools, gladly or otherwise, including those above him bureaucratically, was also precariously positioned. His political and personal peccadilloes interfered with the nation devoting the necessary attention to its glaring public health lacuna.

This lacuna comes further into focus in Chapter 4, which evaluates the political role of Meiji and Taishō Japan, particularly in light of the leadership of the remarkable Ōkuma Shigenobu, two-time prime minister and member of the nation's political elite. Ōkuma's relationship with foreigners in general and evangelists in particular is analyzed here, as the former's was notoriously complex, but more so, exceedingly politically savvy and adept. To wit, Ōkuma was a man who knew how to be a moral entrepreneur par excellence.

But so, too, were many of his counterparts among the foreign evangelical community. In Chapter 5, an analysis of evangelical work in Japan, summarizes that if politics, in all its actions and inaction, ruled the Japanese politicians, so, too, did it rule the American Protestant evangelists seeking converts in Japan. To them, Japan seemed to be a promising land full of intelligent potential converts. Certainly, they were acting according to a charitable impulse—namely, the salvation of mankind—but both salvation and charity, in practice, required a judiciousness no less and possibly more at home in politics than in philanthropy. After all, unfocused soteriological work was fruitless. So as not to waste energy and resources, evangelism required a targeted approach, to both subject and technique. The American evangelists in Japan were no less aware of the necessity of this approach than they were of the need they perceived for evangelism in Japan.

Most of these evangelists sought to concentrate their evangelism within Japan's cities—not so they could pursue proselytizing work among the urban slums and industrial settings, but so that they might concentrate on the nation's educated elite, particularly those connected politically, intellectually, or economically to the upper echelons of Japanese society. Among these men and, occasionally, women, American evangelists sought to sow the seeds of both faith and support, an act of moral entrepreneurship, wherein gaining funds or access to funds was equally as promising as gaining converts. The emphasis on the former required accepting not necessarily the faith itself or reward in the next world but instead that the work pursued was of use to the nation in this world. This meant that the interaction between the state that permitted their work (particularly since their religion had been banned until barely a decade prior) and the evangelists themselves required finesse. For the latter, proof of utility was in order, and for the former, a constant reconfiguring of the relationship to ensure that the interactions remained wholly utilitarian, and not ones that could be considered pretextual. Often, for the evangelists, utility could be found in education, particularly the teaching of English. But there were many teachers, and restrictions against religious discussion could, as can be seen throughout this work, be pursued on a whim.

Turning to a specific organization, Chapter 6, an examination of the role of the YMCA in Japan, notes that, what first began in teaching and education, quickly sought a niche in war work, particularly with the start of the Russo-Japanese War in 1904. Indeed, like the YMCA, some evangelical organizations, given their personnel and their expertise, endeavored to assist Japan's leadership in other ways. The medical missionary movement had gained strength, although much of the work was done on the Asian mainland, and less on the Japanese archipelago, as most of the evangelical efforts in this sphere were devoted to military medicine, on the battlefield and in the encampments. Ministering to the bodies and souls of the nation's soldiers certainly assisted evangelists' efforts to ingratiate themselves with the nation's government, supporting, as they were, both their own religious missions and Japan's national mission of parity with the rest of the world's great powers. Certainly, Japanese medical science was at the forefront of work on the frontlines, but the ministrations among stable casualties could be time consuming and arduous, and much of this work was easily fobbed off onto grateful foreign Christian women, who were often happy to play a significant role in the evangelical movements that might have otherwise marginalized them.

In Chapter 7, which looks at the workings of the Salvation Army, however, we see another form of the moral enterprise at work. Indeed, among those whose medical missionary work was not concerned with nursing war wounds, a handful of evangelists considered turning their attention to the throngs of subjects suffering from an as yet incurable disease. For many, it seemed an obvious religious choice. Although, unlike leprosy, tuberculosis is not a disease mentioned in the scriptures, its consumption of the body, leaving only the soul, seemed a poetic analogue to

Christianity's emphasis on the valuation of the soul above the body, and the incurability of the disease was a challenge to be met by the power of faith in health. Its afflicted, the victims of stigma as much as of their illness, often desired acceptance and love, a currency Christians felt assured they could offer.

More than its symbolism, however, tuberculosis as an area of medical missionary work in Japan was a political choice. Although the medical missionaries who chose this work were hardly stepping on the toes of Japan's leadership, by emphasizing this area of medical work, whether the concentration was on treatment or hospice, foreign evangelists were choosing to take responsibility for a community on the neglected social periphery. By highlighting, however unintentionally, a deficit within Japan's public health sphere, their efforts to fill this need changed the nature and dynamic of their relationship with the nation's government. Regardless of whether evangelists believed this work was the responsibility of the government and regardless of whether they felt that the state had intentionally neglected it, they sought to address this lacuna, in part, to maintain a mutually beneficial relationship with the Japanese state. They hoped thereby to continue their religious work within the nation. This shaped the interaction between evangelist and nation sufficiently to ensure that it remained one of moral entrepreneurship.

Chapter 8, which analyzes the individual evangelists Rudolf Bolling Teusler (of St. Luke's Hospital) and William Merrell Vories (of the Omi Mission), sees the fruition of evangelical moral entrepreneurial efforts. While these men certainly did not stanch the tide of tuberculosis deaths in the nation, they did seek to answer the question of who benefits. Who benefits is as significant as who fails to benefit, and the victims of tuberculosis were primarily nonbenefactors. Although records are incomplete, to put it mildly, official estimates of tuberculosis mortality—as noted in the *Kekkaku nenpō* (Tuberculosis statistical yearbook), no. 5—reached 5,735,981 during the period from 1900 to 1950. However, this number does not include the casualties from tuberculosis between 1944 and 1946, when the war and its aftermath made record keeping difficult. Nor does it address, as historian William Johnston noted, the numbers who hid their disease or the families who refused to disclose the true cause of death of their relatives. Suffice it to say, Japan's tuberculosis epidemic caused a considerable loss of life and manpower.[3]

The numbers also fail to address the fact that the majority of the victims were young and destitute factory workers, many of whom were female. The nature of gender politics, as much as the importance of Japan's modernizing mission, meant that theirs was already the plight of the periphery. Given an epidemic that reduced its victims physically (by killing them) and politically (by rendering them invalids unable to protect their own interests), these sufferers could easily be forgotten as individuals, even as attempts to quantify them (and thus dehumanize them) were made. Yet Teusler and Vories sought to remember them far more than had both the

3. Johnston 1995, 4, 309.

nation in which they worked and the evangelical organizations under whose auspices they had once tenuously belonged. These men knew that the work of caring for the tubercular in a time without a curative treatment was one first and foremost of love.

The afterword of this monograph briefly examines the work of the evangelical organizations to the end of World War II and the ultimate conquest of the scourge under the occupation of Japan by General Douglas Macarthur's SCAP forces. Thus, the majority of the work concentrates on these American Protestant nondenominational evangelical organizations and individuals who would fill this lacuna of responsibility for the nation's subaltern sick. The men and women populating the ranks of these organizations—namely, the YMCA, the Salvation Army, and additional foreign proselytizing organizations often under the auspices of the previous two, proved willing to accept this burden beyond the fact that it was a Christian mission, but also in exchange for the opportunity to attempt to proselytize in a new religious market.[4]

This would be a near miracle for the evangelists. After all, in order to enter into a new nation that had only just repealed the ban on their religion in 1873, some five years after the Meiji Restoration, evangelists sought to prove their utility and mettle to the leaders of a nation still indisposed to conversion. It was not merely about proving the worth of Christian soldiers; rather, by assisting the nation's leaders, evangelists hoped they could earn new patrons, either as donors or as converts (or better still, both) among the nation's elite. As we shall see, seeking out a niche in a potentially still "heathen" landscape came easier to some groups than others. While work among the subaltern was considered by all four groups discussed in this book—namely, the YMCA, the Salvation Army, Rudolf Teusler's St. Luke's Hospital, and William Vories' Omi Mission (later Omi Brotherhood)—the YMCA would find a more advantageous prospect of assisting Japan's military on the frontlines and the home front, beginning with the Russo-Japanese War of 1904–1905. The Salvation Army, a later entry into the field, would focus more work on the victims of tuberculosis as an avenue for missionizing, but their endeavors were often diverted for work abolishing prostitution and other social ills. The signal efforts made by St. Luke's and the Omi Mission, however, though on a considerably smaller scale, ended up proving a miracle for the few victims of tuberculosis who would attend their sanatoriums, though no medical breakthroughs were yet forthcoming.

But throughout the record that this book traces, it is primarily about something that did not happen. Tuberculosis was not cured by the Japanese government or its scientists or the American evangelists who served at the behest of the former. This imposes a more speculative and, perhaps, challenging task for the author than would a text in which something does, in fact, happen. Yet the study of history often obligates one to such an analysis.

4. Garon 2010, 317.

When seeking the causes of something that happened, one may begin with an occurrence and scrutinize that which is prior and proximate to it. Since the causes of an occurrence must have preceded it in time and must have been proximate to it in time and space, one can start with the event and consider what occurred either shortly before it, culminated in it, or, at least, bore some plausible relation to it. Causality is much more discernible if it depicts a recurrent relationship.

Attempting to explain why something did not happen, however, is more notional and difficult. One must first justify why one might reasonably have expected something to occur that did not occur. Such an analysis, which is necessarily normative, must deftly navigate the twin risks of ethnocentrism and presentism. Accordingly, the normative expectations against which one must judge what did and did not happen should be founded on the values, priorities, and exigencies of the actors in the period studied. Why was tuberculosis neither cured nor addressed in Japan? Why did the government not act in the nation's putative interests? One must set aside one's assumptions and instead consider countervailing factors.

Furthermore, one cannot analyze those things bearing on a known event in time and space. After all, something that did not happen has neither moment nor locus. How can one determine if something preceded anything that did not happen? Nothing was prior to it. How can one determine if something was proximate in space to something with no existence, and hence has no location? Nothing can be proximate to something that does not exist.

In such cases, one has to consider not a moment in time but a period in time when something might have been expected to occur, but did not. One cannot consider those realities in a particular time and place but must examine a wider set of phenomena that might have been expected to lead to something in any of a number of locations, but did not.

Only then may one describe phenomena that arguably could have (and perhaps normatively should have) led to something but ultimately did not. One may then finally account for those factors that, one imagines, operated on the contrary to suppress or prevent it. Hence, we look to the late Meiji period and continue to the start of the Shōwa period.

In this case, those countervailing factors were the decisions of the actors in their calculations attendant on the moral enterprise, especially in the pursuit of perceived benefit, and in the service of soteriological value. Thus, one approaches the analysis from the viewpoint of cui bono. How did the Japanese government and foreign evangelists benefit from the epidemic, and what informed their decisions and actions such that there was a relatively long delay in realizing an effective national response to the tuberculosis epidemic? This book answers that question.

1

"Dead, Shriveled Trees"

Factory Girls in Meiji and Taishō Japan

To many individuals worldwide, Japan's modernization under the Meiji emperor (1868–1912) was nothing short of miraculous. Indeed, Japan's government undertook a myriad of actions to transform Japan from what American businessman and author Carl Crow deemed a "secluded nation of Asiatics" to a nation both "after the European pattern," and so successfully modernized that "she is now able to compete with her teachers."[1] The Meiji period saw not only the overturning of unequal treaties, but also the rehauling of Japan's economic, military, political, and even scientific spheres at the behest of a new government of relatively young politicians-cum-oligarchs acting under an even younger emperor.

These changes were not without their costs. Such costs included the creation of a tuberculosis epidemic where previously the disease had only been endemic. This health crisis proliferated in the textile mills of the new nation, which seemed unprepared or unwilling to combat it, despite the fact that within Japan's textile industry the number of the diseased was certainly high enough to merit government attention. At the request of the Meiji and Taishō Ministries of Agriculture and Commerce in the early twentieth century, multiple reports were filed detailing the extensive connections between Japan's tuberculosis epidemic and the women and girls working in Japan's textile factories. Yet care was expensive, and legislation was not only difficult to pass, but hard to enforce. Furthermore, the textile industry bolstered the rise of modern Japan; it funded all the trappings of Meiji society and undergirded the tremendous growth of the nation's military, trade, international relations, and domestic policies. To curtail it sharply was essentially calling for the cessation of Japanese modernity.[2] Indeed, mere awareness of the issues rampant in industrial society did not necessarily lead to a valuation of such issues above industrialization. As Sidney L. Gulick, evangelist and staunch proponent of positive Japanese and American relations, declared, "The political leaders and the organizers of industrial Japan . . . are men of cosmopolitan education and are well versed in the best and most recent literature of the West on these matters [of industry conditions and their results]." They were not ignorant of the plight of many workers in the

1. French, 15; Crow, 54.
2. Tsurumi 1995, 19; Hunter 1992, 16.

textile industry. But by 1930, although textile workers (who were overwhelmingly female) made up a third of the total workers in Japanese manufacturing (or around 1.6 million people), this number still barely totaled over 2.5 percent of the archipelago's total population.[3]

The number of female textile workers should have been significant enough to merit legislative protection, as these women were deemed the "flowers of the people," those whose work would ensure that Japan would fulfill the mission its government had established for it—the acknowledgment of equality with the Euro-American powers. So important was the work of these "flowers" that the government itself opened and administered a number of textile factories, despite the initial financial losses such mills incurred. Even with the privatization of factories and the initial skepticism of the cotton industry, the Meiji government still recognized the importance of the textile industry as a significant contributor to national wealth, both in terms of economics and morale.[4] After all, the top three highest-earning industries in Japan by 1926, "each with more than 500,000,000 yen were raw silk, cotton spinning, and cotton fabrics." These textile trades bolstered Japanese modernization, as raw silk alone exported annually "for more than 50 years . . . has constituted at least 20 per cent of the total annual value of all national exports and in prosperous years this percentage has risen to more than 40 per cent."[5]

Textile work, whether silk or cotton, had long been the realm of women. Even before the Meiji period, Tokugawa period sericulture was, as Sidney Gulick maintained, woman's work, as "it takes the deft hand and quick eye of a girl to catch the thread in the boiling water, connect it with the wheel, and unroll without breaking the almost invisible thread so wonderfully wound up by the worm." Apparently, such deft hands and quick eyes served regardless of the fabric or thread, as female workers would perform 60 to 90 percent of textile work by 1890.[6]

Even once the Meiji government encouraged privatization of the textile factories, government support and assistance would continue, despite the wealth and power of the new owners. Men like Shibusawa Eiichi, the "father of Japanese modern industries or the father of Japanese capitalism," who embraced the textile industry from which the government had failed to force a profit, became both savvy entrepreneurs and industry saviors, assisted by government contracts and economic incentives, as increasing success and funds were reeled around spool after spool of thread caught on the hands of thousands upon thousands of young girls. But it was to the government, not to the girls that such businessmen were beholden. There was only one government capable of ensuring further success and a sufficient number of young girls upon which to build it. By 1930, after all—and to reiterate—only 2.5 percent of Japan's populace was employed in the textile industry. Out

3. S. Gulick 1915, 158–59; International Labour Office, 4.
4. Faison, 14; Tang, 7.
5. Matsuoka, 29.
6. S. Gulick 1915, 34; Nolte and Hastings, 153.

of the remaining 97.5 percent, surely there were other girls who could replace those at the spindles. As political economist Dorothy J. Orchard noted flippantly, "The individual worker (in Japan's textile mills) is cheap."[7]

Orchard certainly spoke to questions of cui bono; after all, by assessing the price of human lives thus, she created a valuation in a cost-benefit analysis that the nation utilized. Who sacrificed what for the nation was a relevant question, and their sacrifice was a high priority in this new Japan.

Nevertheless, business owners and especially business managers were not wholly flippant with the lives of their workers. There were fewer than one hundred cotton mills in Japan before World War I, the vast majority of those having been built within the twenty-five years leading up to the war. While comparatively few in number, these mills accounted for Japan's ascendancy in the international cotton textile market. Since turnover in the mills reached upwards of 50 percent per annum at the end of the Meiji period, a few managers tried to induce workers to stay, if only to avoid having to train new recruits. Thus, within the confines of cost-effectiveness, there were small ways in which to ensure that, barring illness and death, women would be motivated to continue working. While Sharon Sievers and E. Patricia Tsurumi, among others, point out "the industry's preference for recruiting new labor and using it up, rather than investing in improved working conditions and higher wages," a small, though significant, number of mill owners and managers did come to recognize the cheap improvements, like better ventilation and lighting, that would mildly improve conditions, if not wages.[8] Nevertheless, as labor investigator Dr. Matsuoka Asa noted in 1929, labor improvements, whether legal or otherwise, were "conceived as necessary more for the protection of the interests of the State than those of the individual worker. There was no driving force, sentiment, or motive, religious or humanitarian, which played a chief role in its construction." After all, such improvements at government hands were often delayed, "on the ground that immediate enforcement . . . would cause a great disturbance in national economy. . . . The real answer was that national economy, and not individual health, was the principal point of consideration . . . and the consequence was that the health and welfare of women and children were sacrificed to economic demands."[9]

But how cheap could the price of such improvements be? Unscrupulous businessmen like nothing better than a free lunch, and it was to such a lunch that a few mill owners and managers, to say nothing of government officials, realized they could be treated by the foreign evangelical groups in their country, as will be apparent in the course of this book.

Overwhelmingly female, overwhelmingly from rural areas, and overwhelmingly young, these workers (and those recruited to work) were believed tractable enough to accept the work and conditions without too much fuss. Labor

7. Tsurumi 1990, 9; Tai, 43; Orchard, 222.
8. Saxonhouse, 117, 97; Sievers, 65; "Electric Lighting in Japan," 164.
9. Matsuoka, 67–68.

management consultant Hashimoto Ryūtarō noted that, for work in the spinning mills, only "docile girls should be chosen. . . . In general it can probably be said that girls brought up in the mountains tend to be more docile, calmer, and of a simple and honest discipline."[10]

Yamanouchi Mina, an employee of the Tokyo Muslin Company, would be one of a number of women unaccounted for in Hashimoto's thesis, as she later became a labor organizer at Tōyō Muslin. Nevertheless, she recalled her 1912 arrival at the factory, where fiber "was held in the air," floating into lungs, and workers had twelve-hour shifts, including, of course, night shifts (despite being outlawed by legislation in 1911, although this was clearly unenforced until 1916, if then). A twelve-year-old girl, Yamanouchi was relieved that hers was a factory considered less dangerous, one in which, owing to new machinery, "you could work and feel safe." (Unfortunately, what Yamanouchi did not realize was that new machinery did little to halt the virulence of the tubercle bacillus, and, in the case of the looms at the Toyoda Cotton Spinning and Weaving Company—not to mention the myriad other companies who purchased looms from Toyoda Loom Works—actually exacerbated the spread of the disease, as the shuttle on the loom before 1924 required the operator to blow on it, like a flute, when the thread broke.)[11]

Yamanouchi soon discovered that it was not the machinery she needed to fear. Rather, the physicality of the work proved deadly. "After two or three days at the factory, standing for twelve hours a day, at night when it was time to go to the cafeteria, your legs felt so heavy that you didn't really want your meal." Lack of proper nutrition coupled with physical exhaustion rendered the body of the worker fertile ground for multiple illnesses. As Yamanouchi herself realized, the taxing conditions meant that, despite rest, a worker's "body could not heal its sluggishness." The mandatory breaks, amounting to a total of one hour in twelve, did little to allow the body to repair itself sufficiently. These breaks consisted only of "a fifteen minute break at 9:00 a.m., a thirty minute break for lunch, and another fifteen minute break at 3 in the afternoon." The reference to breaks was actually misleading: "They called them 'breaks' but there were no benches whatsoever," meaning that the women were forced to remain standing for the entire twelve hours.[12]

The work "week" was interrupted by a day off every ten days. Without enough money to leave the factory, Yamanouchi recalled spending her days off with the other girls, either making kimonos, as they had none, or putting on shows, including *Hototogisu*, in which the prettiest girl would play Namiko, the tubercular unfortunate, and the tallest girl her sailor husband. Save for those brief respites, the rest of the time was spent on the factory floor or in the factory dormitories. These dormitories served as the only resting place for many women and girls, sharing bedding that was constantly in use, during the allotted four to five hours of sleep. These

10. Hashimoto, 60–62 (translated by Janet Hunter in "Gendering the Labor Market").
11. Hosoi, 5; Tomida, 65; Yamanouchi, 105; Dore, 438; Mass and Robertson, 5.
12. Yamanouchi, 106.

rooms, some fifteen to twenty-four square feet, would be constantly packed with twenty-three to forty-five women sleeping on their sides, tightly packed because of a lack of room and a lack of heat, and the rooms would quickly become "filthy and suffocating." Every three or four days, the women would be allowed to bathe with some hundred other women in only twenty baths, which were rarely warm. Because they were forced to bathe by hand, the tub got progressively dirtier, and the water colder. The summers were fine, but "winters were cold and the wind blew," so the windows were kept closed.[13]

On the factory floor, the steam from the boilers fueling the machinery intensified the temperature differential between the dormitories and the factory. The girls rapidly became overheated, and, in the middle of the night shift particularly, "your body and extremities become soft and tender, and your head can become dull." To stave off sleep, the women often sang as they worked. Yamanouchi remembered one song in particular:

> At 2 or 3 a.m.
> The grass and trees sleep.
> I'm tired, but I suppose it's impossible.
> If the female spinners are human,
> Then the dead, shriveled trees of the mountain bloom.[14]

The unhealthy life of the factory girl was hardly uncommon knowledge, no matter how hard those who merely bought the fruits of her labor tried to ignore it. And, after a time, it seemed pointless to try to pretend otherwise. After the turn of the century, recruiting agents for Japan's textile mills were finding it increasingly more difficult to do their jobs, as word of the factory working conditions, not to mention the living conditions (assuming one managed to survive), had spread throughout Japan. So, too, had awareness of the passage of Japan's Girls' High School Law of 1900, by which each prefecture had to establish one high school for four years of education specifically for females. In doing so, the government had highlighted further the discrepancy between what was promised by factories' recruiting agents and the real lives of these workers. One such worker, Takai Toshio, future wife of muckraker Hosoi Wakizō, noted that she longed to enjoy the education promised but lived a life dictated by movement from one dirty factory to the next.[15] While recruiters had claimed that work within Japan's mills and factories created a young woman certain to fulfill her national role as a "good wife, wise mother," the actuality seemed far removed. These girls and women were taught the repetitive tasks of modern industry, tasks that would serve no further purpose outside the confines of their insalubrious factory. And, again, that was if they survived the labor—the physical toll of long hours, night shifts, poor nutrition, and the potential dangers of

13. Matsumoto, 53; Yamanouchi, 113, 110; Thompson, 93; Yamanouchi, 108, 112.
14. Yamanouchi, 109.
15. Takai, 46.

the machines themselves. Compared to their peers at the prefectural high school, there was no education to be found in the factory, where they would be "schooled" by strangers, finding little worth pursuing there, save for a paltry wage. The harshness of life in the factory led Jan Oudegeest to denounce Japan's admittance to the International Labour Organization in 1919, "A large amount of sickness prevails in Japan through working women and children over 13 hours a day . . . 120 hours a year overtime, and thus you have conditions in Japan which are absolutely unworthy of human existence. . . . What conditions do we see in Japan? Tuberculosis and general disease and such conditions of poverty that they are really demoralizing for the people." Oudegeest went so far in his diatribe as to assert, "The Japanese people should be protected by us from their own Government that wants to exploit them."[16]

Nevertheless, as historian Barbara Molony pointed out, the women and girls of Japan's factories were not merely passive victims. These women often chose the work they did, even if their parents believed that the education they received in the city was not worth the loss of their daughters' presence and assistance. But these jobs, as horrible as they were, provided opportunities, or the perception of them. True, to an outsider, and indeed, to many insiders, the industry apparently took "industrious and comparatively moral farming class" daughters, and forced them "into intimate relations with the lowest, most dissolute, despised, and really despicable classes" running rampant among the working classes of Japan's cities. Yet, whether paternalistic, patronizing, or protective, such opinions provided the impetus to actually make factory work more appealing, to create more of the opportunities, or at least the perception of these, that brought the workers there in the first place.[17]

Labor laws in Japan were not unheard of. The first labor act was passed in 1875, the "Government Constructional Services Laborers Accident Allowance Regulation," which mandated accident compensation for those in construction, but labor laws that affected the factory girls would remain beyond the pale, despite government efforts, until 1916 permitted the execution of a law debated from 1909 and passed in 1911, much to the chagrin of many factory owners. Even then, the substance of the act was hardly liberal. Child labor was limited to those above twelve years, with those under fifteen allowed to work for twelve hours per day and no restriction on weekly working hours.[18]

Though the industry served the nation, the nation certainly was not reciprocating when owners and managers desired more opportunities for their workers. Truly, governments in Europe and America had not provided such opportunities to these women unprompted, faced with strikes and unions. As Gulick maintained in 1915, though Japan could utilize the example and experiences of industrialization in other countries, "she seems slow to do it." Great Britain had passed legislation on factory employment of children beginning in 1802, and issued its first comprehensive

16. Taira 1997, 281; Hara, 99; Hosoi, 80; Satō and Ōbayashi, 175; League of Nations, 163.
17. Molony, 225; S. Gulick, 1915, 41.
18. "Japan's Factory Law," 1; Nakayama, 2.

factory act in 1833. The United States, led by Massachusetts, saw laws on amelioration of conditions in factories from 1836 to 1867. Even Germany, a recent entrant to both national consolidation and industrialization, had factory laws on the books by 1890.[19]

Despite legislation "feebly" calling for reform, Gulick noted, only "one section of the government [was] seeking to ameliorate social and economic conditions" so as to create the opportunities so many workers pursued, while the vast majority of the government sought to continue industrial work without improving the quality of life within the factories.[20] The factory girls, who numbered over three million by the end of the Taishō period in 1926, had seen factory legislation considered, delayed, and finally passed, but often unenforced. As Dr. Matsuoka Asa reported in 1931, "Efforts to secure factory legislation in Japan date back to 1882," but would have to wait until "the factory act of 1911, the first important law in Japan for the protection of workers. . . . [But] as soon as the act, ordinances, and regulations were promulgated, the experts who had done most to create it demanded a revision of the act. It was pronounced spineless and a deformed child, because of the serious defects." Instead, it was not until the attention brought to global labor with the establishment of the International Labour Organization through the Treaty of Versailles of 1919 that Japan issued the 1923 revision of the labor law, which would not come into effect until 1929. Certainly, no one involved wanted these workers to fall ill, least of all the workers themselves, but the perfect storm of conditions engendered by this industry combined with living conditions suffered by the workers—a relatively weak constitution, overcrowding, a poor diet and a lack of sleep—meant that this would be a national problem. Yet, to quote political economist Dorothy J. Orchard once more, "The individual worker is cheap," worth less than the product she produced.[21]

But truly doing something about the conditions would mean caring about the workers who were often seen as little more than prostitutes, and thus expendable. The permeability of the two careers (and the perception of such permeability) proved to tar each with the brush of the other. Japan's intellectual elite considered the nation's female factory workers hypersexual by nature, a condition exacerbated by "living in small, crowded housing." Even the champion of the female textile factory worker, Hosoi Wakizō, himself dying of tuberculosis, reported on the extreme instances of masturbation purportedly common within the factory dormitories, and the rampant lesbianism, which "includes a wide range of practices ranging from mutual psychological love to extremely lustful activities, which are accompanied by a strong sense of jealousy."[22] Sidney Gulick, yet another contemporary self-proclaimed advocate of women, determined that the wretched conditions in which

19. Grundfossen, 16; Whittesley and Hadley, 7, 10; Birnie, 211.
20. S. Gulick, 1915, 85–86.
21. Matsuoka, 6, 9, 1; Orchard, 222.
22. Frühstück, 72; Hosoi, 369–70.

the factory workers lived were not only "disease-spreading and vermin-breeding" but "immoral boarding-houses, where they were deliberately tempted. Some of the landlords were also brothel keepers." Gulick placed the blame for the sexual indiscretions of the factory workers on the factory owners and managers, thus attacking their paternalism, as well as on the decency of the women, who quickly became involved in "drinking and immoral carousings." They therefore returned home "ruined not only in health but in character."[23]

These ruined women, owing to their perceived promiscuity, were assumed in turn to corrupt the wholesome young men of their villages. From bed to bed, tuberculosis would spread like a venereal disease. This argument, made in Ishihara's report, was the one that affected not only political opinion in Japan's legislature but also the moral opinions of many foreign evangelical groups, as will become clear below. After years of postponed and unenforced legislation purportedly intended to improve the lot of the factory workers, the government now began to consider the prospect of assisting the tubercular. In March 1914, Japan's Sanitary Bureau, represented by its chief, Sugiyama Shigorō, presented the Diet with suggestions for a draft bill to provide partial government support for the building of six sanatoriums. Advocated by Kitajima Ta'ichi of the Infectious Diseases Institute, these sanatoriums would cordon off tuberculosis patients from the rest of society, essentially imprisoning them. As Kitajima pointed out in 1913, 40 percent of deaths in Japan's military and 40 percent of the reasons for physical disability discharge were caused by tuberculosis. These men cost the Japanese government more than 182 million yen per annum, which nearly matched the 199 million yen spent on military expenses that same year. The Diet concurred. Thus, with the 1914 "Law Concerning the Establishment of Pulmonary Tuberculosis Sanatoria and Their National Assistance," the Japanese government was eventually to provide half the construction costs and a quarter of the yearly operating costs of these institutions.[24] Tuberculosis was being recognized, if not ameliorated, as a national problem, albeit only because it was affecting the military.

23. S. Gulick, 1915, 68–69.
24. Maegawa, 120; Johnston 1995, 242–45.

2

"The Snow-White Shawl"

Tuberculosis in Meiji and Taishō Japan

Of course, tuberculosis was neither confined to Japan nor limited to modernity. The history of tuberculosis is the history of humanity, with the earliest evidence of the disease dating from around 5000 BCE, and cases appearing throughout the world.[1] Similarly, the experience of the disease in connection to industrialization was not unique to Japan. Japan was not the only country to suffer from the disease, nor was it the only country to experience the disease as an epidemic. Nevertheless, where other countries were quick to attempt to curtail the association between the epidemic and its industrial conditions, with legislation on the books as early as 1802 in the case of Great Britain and industrializing countries, including Prussia (1839), following suit, Japan remained silent for far longer.[2] The experience of tuberculosis in modern Japan proved unique and devastating, with nearly six million deaths directly attributed to it in the first half of the twentieth century.[3] The disease itself—along with the impact it had on labor, gender relations, scientific research, and politics in Japan—proved as decisive to the national experience as any military or moral victory during that same period. In this chapter, we shall consider the various social ramifications of tuberculosis in Japan.

Despite its ancient origins, tuberculosis has only come to be understood within the last 150 years. The advent of germ theory illuminated the etiology of a previously mysterious disease that seemed paradoxically random and hereditary, all consuming and survivable, and ubiquitous and unseen. A disease of contradictions, the enigma of it fueled both myth and, as Susan Sontag so famously illustrated, metaphor.[4] The mythopoeia surrounding the disease, therefore, fed into the mystery, which, in turn, reinvigorated the mythos—a vicious cycle that proved difficult to break even after Robert Koch had determined the more mundane nature of the disease. Moreover, although the mythopoeia Sontag analyzed was European, the same inventions and stereotypes that plagued the victims as much as the disease itself proved similar in Japan.

1. Ryan, 5.
2. Meikeljohn, 1; Price, 103.
3. Johnston 1995, 4, 309.
4. Sontag, 5.

A young physician and promising bacteriologist, Robert Koch had established both his own merit and that of bacterial etiology with his study of, and subsequent conclusions on, the pathogenesis of the *Bacillus anthracis*, but it was his work on tuberculosis for which he is most famous.[5] It was in working on the etiology of this disease that Koch clarified his postulates for determining the causative relationship between microbe and illness, and, thus, as he proudly reported to The Physiological Society of Berlin,

> On the ground of my abundant observations, I regard it was proved that in all Tubercular affections of men and animals, the Bacteria, designated by me as Tubercle Bacilli, which through their characteristic properties are differentiated from all other micro-organisms, are constantly present.[6]

The growing acceptance of germ theory throughout the medical community worldwide was hardly enough to combat the disease. In the absence of a cure, tuberculosis blossomed in the modern modus vivendi. Cities proved an ideal breeding ground, and, with the industrial revolution, rapid urbanization led to overcrowding in both metropolises and factories; the disease thrived anywhere humans lived and worked in close proximity. Accordingly, regardless of "climate, in the North, and in the South, East and West, however various the conditions under which men live, however much they may differ in race, in diet, and clothing, and in habits of life, wherever human beings are congregated together there is tuberculosis to be found," Dr. Arthur Ransome, Manchester physician and professor, lamented.[7]

The pathogenesis of the *Mycobacterium tuberculosis* bacillus most often involves dissemination through the respiratory system, generally as an inhalation of infected sputum or air droplets. After inhalation, the bacillus catalyzes the development of a Ghon focus, which is the primary lesion in the lung of a previously uninfected organism. (At times, this lesion may then catalyze the development of a similar lesion in the lymph system.) The focus, depending on the robustness of the individual's immune system, often is isolated, essentially walled off, to cavitate, become caseous and necrotic, and/or ossify.[8] Regardless, the bacilli remain latent, though the individual appears asymptomatic. Should the immune system be compromised or a new strain introduced, the disease will advance, and the cavity often permits the bacteria more access to oxygen, thus allowing them to multiply.[9]

That one could carry the bacteria and show no signs of the disease made both detection and prevention exceedingly difficult. It also allowed old wives' tales to propagate faster than the bacillus itself. Doctors debated questions of heredity, psychology, constitution, and sociology as they tried to combat the insidious disease. These questions did not merely stem from ignorance: tuberculosis had presented

5. Salmon, 212.
6. Fukuda 2008, 83; Koch, 649.
7. Otis, 5–6.
8. Dannenberg, 11; Kayne et al., 63, 74.
9. Grosset, 835.

signs that argued for the consideration of all these factors. Though the disease would prove disconnected from genetic heredity, the fact that families often succumbed seemed to suggest otherwise. So, too, did the role of economic and social issues, often creating conditions wherein individuals would appear to be predisposed to the disease. The proximity of family in various economic and social conditions also presented an illusion of heredity—if not of the disease itself, then of constitution.[10] Psychology proved the hardest to disassociate—not because the evidence for a connection between mental illness and tuberculosis was so abundant, but because a diagnosis of tuberculosis so often plunged a patient into a strong depression, since it appeared little more hopeful than a death sentence. This fatalism was not uncommon in Japanese victims when faced with diagnosis, which, in turn, affected how the disease itself was considered throughout the nation both by the burden of secrecy and the acceptance of moral opprobrium.

In addition, since the common perceptions included the belief that the disease was, in fact, hereditary and psychological, the burden of these misconceptions rested upon patients and their families, who rarely doubted the misconceptions themselves. Thus, the disease not only bestowed a death sentence on the tubercular but also tarred the entire lineage and those associated with the family. The responsibility of maintaining the good name of the family proved an added pressure to those seeking to combat their disease. Ultimately, secrecy ruled the day. The patient sought to hide the disease, and the family sought to evade the public's scrutiny for fear of opprobrium.

But psychological markers were difficult to stereotype into one simple category. Not only was tuberculosis a putative mark of insanity, it supposedly also marked genius. As famed microbiologist René Dubos noted, the concept of *spes phthisica*, or the euphoria brought about by tuberculosis, often concomitant with creative intelligence, was considered both a symptom and a complication of the disease.[11] This psychological-physiological connection was not limited to Europe, although it was most commonly associated with the Romantic movement of the nineteenth century. Among artists like Keats and Chopin, tuberculosis became a mark of distinction, of sentimentality.[12] This emphasis proved a particularly appealing feminine stereotype. The disease soon became eroticized, and what was, at its heart, a sign of declination became a badge of a sensual, if still somewhat chaste, life. The appearance brought on by the wasting disease, the wanness, the paleness, and the litheness, all became beautiful, at first subverting concepts of beauty, and then merely defining them. The heroines of popular culture of mid- to late nineteenth-century Europe, including Violetta of *La Traviata* and Mimi of *La Bohème*, became synonymous with the beauty and seductiveness associated with their disease. Although questions of cause

10. Worboys, 82.
11. Dubos and Dubos, 60.
12. Fukuda 2001, 92, 98.

and effect were unanswered (Did the temperament catalyze the disease, or vice versa?), the result remained, as Susan Sontag noted, one of romanticized appeal.[13]

In real life, of course, there was, as biologist Irwin W. Sherman so eloquently stated, nothing romantic about "a painful death by drowning in one's own blood."[14] Yet this eroticism spilled over from popular culture and permeated society. As in the Europe of Puccini's opera, the romantic culture of tuberculosis became a taboo cult of aesthetics. Composer Camille Saint-Saëns recalled in 1913 the earlier obsession with tubercular beauty in nineteenth-century Europe. "Good health was not chic. It was fashionable to be pale and drained." For women especially, these traits became a new standard of beauty, and were not merely appreciated by men but cultivated by women. If not the disease itself, certainly the symptoms had become idealized. "I cough continually!" Tubercular artist and diarist Marie Bashkirtseff wrote in her posthumously popular journal. "But for a wonder, far from making me look ugly, this gives me an air of languor that is very becoming." Bashkirtseff died of her disease in 1884, at the age of 25.[15]

For the tubercular as well, therefore, it proved difficult to distinguish between the mythos of the disease and its actuality. Beyond mere ignorance, the stereotypes surrounding tuberculosis had infected the patients as firmly as the disease itself had. The fear of heredity or psychology settled deeply in the psyche, though the eroticism was more easily shed. Bashkirtseff herself admitted later that, while she took "a sort of pride" in her illness, she was "scarcely pleased at it. It is an ugly death—a very slow one, four, five, ten years perhaps, and one grows so thin, and loses all one's good looks."[16] For the Maries and the Mimis, it was clearly warranted to distance oneself from the myth of the consumptive beauty, not merely because one could see and feel the ravages of the disease, but because beauty itself, unhindered by consumption, was ephemeral—women would age, and youth fade ineluctably. The process, however, seemed faster when tubercular, as the disease seemed to make the fleeting that much more transient. Edgar Allan Poe lauded his "delicately, morbidly angelic" young wife, who, when singing "stopped, clutched her throat and a wave of crimson blood ran down her breast . . . It rendered her even more ethereal!"[17] Yet, for those not suffering from the disease, the erotic cult of the ethereal consumptive beauty was far less transient, and would continue into the next century, and the one after that.

But even in combating self-perceptions of the erotic in the disease, the other stereotypes remained entrenched in tuberculosis patients as firmly as they were in the rest of society, both in Europe and Japan. Franz Kafka, nearly forty years after Koch's evidence of the tubercle bacillus, reported that he was convinced that his

13. Hutcheon and Hutcheon, 38; Barnes, 266; Fukuda 1995, 100–102.
14. Sherman, 275.
15. Sontag, 28; Bashkirtseff, 195; H. Wilson, 506.
16. Bashkirtseff, 220–21.
17. Dormandy, 93–94.

was not a mere case of germ theory: "For secretly," he wrote to sometime-fiancée Felice Bauer, "I don't believe this illness to be tuberculosis, at least not primarily tuberculosis, but rather a sign of my general (moral) bankruptcy."[18] That similar beliefs pervaded Japanese society was not solely a sign of Westernization but also a natural outgrowth of the stereotypes that developed independently in both locales.

In both Euro-America and Japan, physicians, too, saw tuberculosis as evidence of moral failing, either in the patient in particular or in civilization generally. For professor and physician Charles Denison, himself a sufferer of the disease, these same failings would prevent the disease's ultimate elimination. "It is evident that the fundamental obstacle to even an approximate success in the eradication of tuberculosis lies in the constitution of our faulty civilization," he reported to his colleagues. This civilization, "so dwarfed by conventionality and perverted by artificiality, manifest in the lives and homes of the people, that a fruitful soil is provided for degenerative diseases." Chief among the harvest was tuberculosis, which "most naturally springs" from this soil. Indeed, Denison proclaimed, "the punishment of the race for its shortcomings is through this dyscrasic disease, and eradication is possible only through fundamental and radical reform."[19]

Although the erotic mythos of tuberculosis persisted after Koch's discovery, the concept of tuberculosis as punishment for moral failings skyrocketed after the acceptance of germ theory. The hope to eradicate the disease was, save perhaps for Denison, placed in the desire to keep one's surroundings pristine, free of the germs that brought disease. What historian Nancy Tomes influentially deemed the gospel of germs had indeed become a religion of cleanliness aimed to rid society of the "dirty" disease. In his 1909 address on "Preventive Measures against Tuberculosis," Eastern State Penitentiary physician M. V. Ball intoned that each individual, by keeping "this conviction strong in his heart . . . becomes as zealous in the promulgation of what he calls 'the light' as the most devout convert of some new religious truth. The antituberculosis campaign has in it much of the fervor of a new religion."[20]

The zeal of the new proponents of germ theory, particularly with regard to tuberculosis, manifested itself in science as in religion. In America, from which the Protestant evangelists to Japan would come, the doctrine of tuberculosis employed sacral semantics and symbols. Tomes has repeatedly pointed out this rhetoric in the literature of organizations like the Illinois State Board of Health and the New York City Department of Health and the Committee on Prevention of Tuberculosis of the Charity Organization Society at the turn of the twentieth century. The former repeatedly invoked the terms "tract" and "catechism," and deemed its work against tuberculosis a "crusade" in search of "salvation." Germ theory became a byword for kosher concepts—the idea that something polluted or impure is irredeemable.[21]

18. Kafka, 287.
19. Mitman, 98; Denison, 28.
20. Bacon, 134; Tomes 1998, 114.
21. Tomes 1997, 278; Douglas, 134.

Religions often make use of similar dichotomies, juxtaposing the holy and the profane, the pure and the impure, so it is hardly surprising that germ theory, rather than displacing religion, was syncretized with it in Japan. Evangelist and Christian hymnal composer Mitani Tanekichi easily incorporated these concepts into his missionary tracts, referring to the "germs" (*baikin*) of Japan's "spiritual disease" (*reibyō*), and its panacea, Christianity.[22] As elsewhere, the gospel of germs in Japan was indeed used to shame people into adherence, creating and then mandating proper behavior. But this behavior, like those in religious practices, required definition. And for those without that power, as Helen Hardacre established, at least in Japan, "the ancestors (as in Shinto beliefs) are already connected in a world view that is real and intelligible to the individual in a way that germs and germ theory are not."[23] Thus, humans fit new ideas into preexisting slots to categorize and understand them.

Regardless of the nature of acceptance, the stigmas surrounding tuberculosis common in Europe and America were mirrored in Japan. The erotic cult of the disease in Japan was noted particularly, as elsewhere, in its literature. One of the most famous novels from the turn of the century, and certainly the most famous involving tuberculosis as both a plot point and a metaphor, is Tokutomi Roka's *Hototogisu*. The story touched the nation and saturated popular culture. Its protagonist, the romantic heroine Namiko, contracts tuberculosis, much to the displeasure of her mother-in-law. Nevertheless, to her husband, Namiko appears "slender and graceful," more ephemeral than *sakura* (cherry blossoms), which last a season. She is "the shy daisy dimly discovering itself in the dusk of a summer eve." Takeo, her husband, dreams of the beautiful, pale "face of the sick girl wrapped in a snow-white shawl," and envisions her as in the night, "as if a slender form in a white shawl were about to step out of the clear moon."[24]

But it was the myth of the tubercular as moral reprobate rather than erotic fixation that permeated Japanese culture and society, among both the unaffected and the afflicted. It was this misconception that *Hototogisu* also employs, although, in fairness to Tokutomi, he placed it in the mind of the antagonist—the mother-in-law:

> "Because of consumption—you want me to divorce Nami?"
>
> "Yes, exactly, though I am sorry for it. . . . I pity Nami and feel very sorry for her parents, but *isn't it wrong to fall ill?* Whatever they may think of us, it is far better not to bring the house of Kawashima to an end. You speak of injustice or inhumanity, but you can find many cases like this everywhere. It is right to divorce a wife when she is not contributing to the prestige of the house; it is right to do so when she fails to give birth to an heir; and it is right to do so when she contracts

---

22. Mitani, 77, 83.
23. Hardacre, 181.
24. M. Aoki, 118; Fukuda 1999, 180; Fukuda 1995, 136–37; R. Tokutomi, 207–8; Ito, 521; Y. Tanaka, 61; Karatani 1993, 100–101. In his *Origins of Modern Japanese Literature*, Karatani Kōjin discusses illness as metaphor at least as well as Susan Sontag does, if not better. It is, sadly, overlooked in most American scholarship on the subject (Karatani 1989, 331).

a dangerous disease. This is the rule, don't you know? There is no need to bring in questions of justice or humanity."[25]

Placing the blame at the feet of the victim was not only demeaning but also served to perpetuate the myth that recovery was possible through some force of will. The propensity to germinate the seeds of tuberculosis marked the victim as weak, either physically, morally, or both, unable to resist disease. In *Hototogisu*, Nami's husband urges his wife to amend her mental state in order to cure herself: "You will be cured if your will is strong enough. If not, it will be due to your lack of love for me. If you do love me, you will surely get well."[26]

This perception continued—and not merely within unafflicted society, but within the beliefs of the tubercular as well. Poet Ishikawa Takuboku, in his final days in the sanatorium, wrote a litany of tanka (lyric poems) about his experiences. Although only published posthumously, they reveal a man at once awash in self-pity and convinced that such a weakness condemned him to death by tuberculosis:

Oh how sad it is
That in my mind and in my heart no wish to heal exists
What sort of mind and heart is this?[27]

The self-conviction of the irresponsibility of the victim continued well into the Taishō period (1912–1926), when Kasai Zenzō wrote his semiautobiographical short stories about tubercular protagonists. Kasai, whose work was considered by a number of literary scholars to be the epitome of the semiautobiographical genre, often referenced his own beliefs about the disease that afflicted him in the comments of the protagonists of his short stories. In "Suikyōsha no dokuhaku," Kasai's hero comments to his nurse that she misunderstands the nature of his disease, which he maintains is the fault of his own will: "You've got my disease all wrong. . . . Considering the kind of life I've led, it would be odd if I had *failed* to contract the disease. I'm really not surprised at all. People who can vent their fantasies and passions do not suffer. Those who cannot and turn in on themselves—it's those who get TB."[28] Whether Kasai's narrator truly embodies the sentiments of all of his fellow victims, that the misconceptions about tuberculosis were as culturally rampant in Japan as in Europe ensured the country that its population, too, would be fed a series of misconceptions about the illness and those suffering from it.

Thus, like the nurse of Kasai's story, medical officials often felt the burden of their diagnoses. A simple statement of medical pathology could ruin lives. True,

25. R. Tokutomi, 156. He also uses the character of the mother-in-law to iterate the stigma that tuberculosis was genetic. Though Tokutomi presumably permits no negative stigma to survive his novel, the eroticization of Nami, and, thus, the romanticization of the disease, does a disservice to the victims (Tokutomi, R., 154).
26. Sontag, 44; R. Tokutomi, 143.
27. Goldstein and Shinoda, 215; Ishikawa, tanka 141, 181. Although I am using the edition translated by Goldstein and Shinoda, I find their translation of the poem to be a little terse. Thus, I have offered my own translation here, based upon the original tanka the editors courteously provided.
28. Hijiya-Kirschnereit, 220; Fowler, 287.

these lives were often shortened by the unacknowledged disease, but, in a battle against a foe with no known weakness, some believed that there was little to be gained by being direct. Throughout the world, various euphemisms came to signify tuberculosis without mention of the dreaded term: consumption, stomach ulcers, asthma, scrofula, phthisis, pneumonia, catarrh, cold, pleurisy, truly anything that referenced a condition less severe than tuberculosis. As Kafka lay in Kierling, the sanatorium in which he would die, he wrote that his physicians refused to make any mention of his disease beyond "swelling at the rear" and "infiltration," preferring instead to use "a shy, evasive, glass-eyed manner of speech."[29]

Within the last century, psychophysiologist T. Holmes has postulated that stress and mental health before diagnosis played a role in tuberculosis infection or deterioration. In his work, it seems that adrenocortical activity, catalyzed by stress-related adrenal response, is involved in susceptibility to tuberculosis infection and in relapse. As medical sociologist, David Mechanic counters, however, it may simply be that "highly disruptive life patterns" lead to opportunities for infection, as locale and habits may vary. Nevertheless, no study maintains that mental health after diagnosis is affected negatively by awareness of the disease. In fact, Holmes noted that, for many patients, "their attitudes and life experiences made it unusually difficult for them to decide what was expected of them or what they expected of themselves." If kept in the dark about their condition, their lack of awareness might just as easily affect their prognosis. Though Holmes' work emphasized prior stress, the frustration of a patient like Kafka could just as easily add further stress to an already-taxed body. "As a consequence" of the stress, Holmes explained, "their attempts at adjustment were characterized by unrealistic striving which was not only unrewarding but also productive of cumulative conflict, anxiety, and depression."[30]

Thus, in failing properly to identify and, to the extent they were able, to treat the disease, physicians allowed stress and depression to control the patients, and myths and confusion to control society and, in doing so, presumably worsened the epidemic. In modern Japanese literature, the first instance of this obfuscation occurs even before *Hototogisu* in "Zangiku," a short story by Hirotsu Ryūrō, a member of one of the most famous contemporary literary coteries. When Okō, a young housewife, begins coughing blood, the wife and her mother-in-law consult a physician:

> "Doctor, it's consumption, isn't it?"
>
> The doctor smiled easily and answered with a nonchalant air, "No, it isn't . . . pneumonia. I think it is a bronchial catarrh."
>
> When Mother heard it wasn't consumption, the furrows fell from her brow and she heaved a sigh of relief.
>
> "That's wonderful," she said. "I'm thankful for that. Since it isn't her lungs . . . But doctor, what about the blood she coughed up?"
>
> "Oh, the blood?"

29. Johnston 1995, 80–81; Murray, 379; Keyes, 125.
30. Mechanic, 274–75; Holmes, 252.

> "Yes, can she cough up blood even if it isn't her lungs?"
> "Of course."
> The doctor looked at my face. I suddenly felt ashamed.
> "That's from an ulcer in her bronchial tubes. I don't think she coughed up that blood from her lungs."
> "It isn't from her lungs? Thank you so much. Is there anything else that I should be careful of?"
> "It will heal completely very soon. Be sure that she rests and eats well."
> "Yes, I shall. Thank you so much."[31]

The doctor is no fool. Neither are the mother-in-law or Okō, but they all perpetuate the myth that Okō will recover to spare themselves the discomfort of the truth.

The desire to dissemble was not limited to fiction. Novelist Kasai Zenzō interrupted the narrative of one of his short stories to comment that recently he "was spared my usual asthma attack. I had even thought myself fully recovered." Even in presumably private journals, euphemisms were employed, as if to deceive the author himself. Kajii Motojirō, an author whose career began during the Taishō era, recorded reams of thoughts on his disease, but still employed euphemisms in his journal, as was the case in an entry from February 2, 1931 in which he noted that his "cold is very malignant . . . [and] waking is hard work, walking impossible." Meiji era novelist and poet Kunikida Doppo, in a missive to painter Kosugi Hōan, informed him that his "illness has at last taken on the appearance of a real disease. Dr. Kikuchi diagnosed it as laryngeal catarrh and Dr. Kimura as pneumonial catarrh. . . . My right lung shows only mild (symptoms), but my left lung seems to have a catarrh that has advanced beyond pneumonia." Kunikida concludes his letter with a postscript, "By the way, don't tell anyone I have pneumonial catarrh. I'd hate to be treated immediately like a consumptive."[32]

For those who refused to employ euphemisms and sought to confront the true diagnosis, the social costs could be severe. On May 21, 1938, Toi Mutsuo, at the age of twenty-one committed the mass murder of thirty of his neighbors before taking his own life. A recently diagnosed tubercular, Toi left an extensive collection of suicide notes explaining the logic behind his actions. Upon learning that he had contracted pulmonary tuberculosis, Toi wrote, a local woman, Nishimura Tome, made him "the laughingstock of the entire village. My reputation, my credibility, everything people respected in me disappeared. She dirtied my face." The stigmatization of Toi, as originally perpetrated by Nishimura, spread throughout his village. "The way everybody looks with suspicion and disgust at a person with consumption" deeply hurt the youth. So, too, did the severance of sexual relations with another villager, who upon discovering his illness "had a change of heart. . . . Even a woman with whom I had had such a deep relationship suffered a change

31. Keene 1984, 391; Johnston 1995, 128.
32. Fowler, 62; Kajii, 398; Johnston 1995, 134–35.

of heart when I told her I had become ill. . . . She laughed down her nose at me and spread any number of rumors." Unlike his former friends and neighbors, Toi saw himself as no different after contracting the disease. There had been no moral or social stain on his character, until Nishimura sullied it.[33] If the gospel of germs ruled the day, then having a dirty face, both figuratively and literally, was the ultimate sin. Attitudes towards and opinions about the disease proved as damaging to health and to the health of the nation as the effects of tuberculosis itself. After all, in each of Japan's largest cities, the percentage of tuberculosis-related deaths in 1900 proved a significant increase over that in 1899, with Tokyo, Osaka, Kyoto, Kobe, and Nagasaki exhibiting rates during both years at or over 15 percent of total mortality, and Yokohama producing the greatest percent increase with a jump of 6.1 percent from a mortality rate of 12.8 percent of total mortality in 1899 to 18.9 percent a year later. The problem was clear—the solution, less so.

33. Tsukuba, 8; Kiryu, 31; Johnston 1995, 109–14.

3

"The Enemy of Mankind"

The Struggle against Tuberculosis

Germ theory would prove necessary for understanding the etiology of tuberculosis, but, as with the case of Toi, would also serve to castigate its victims unnecessarily. Yet that was never the intention of Japan's pioneers in germ theory, at whose head stood Kitasato Shibasaburō. A colleague of Koch and an 1884 graduate of Tokyo Imperial University's medical school, Kitasato would become a key player in the story of Japan's tuberculosis epidemic, both scientific savior and political wrangler, whose antagonism with many of Japan's bureaucratic and political elite would affect the course of public health in Japan, to the extent that it seemed his perceived superciliousness and pride cost the nation political attention to the epidemic.

But to analyze the importance of Kitasato (and his perceived pride) in Japanese tuberculosis reduction as both scientist and politico, one need examine Japan's medical and scientific history from the Edo period (1603–1868) into the Meiji period (1868–1912), and beyond. Thus, that Toi faced stigma for his disease well into the Shōwa period was certainly no indication of the level of knowledge of pathology among Japanese physicians and scientists. Throughout the Edo period, medical knowledge in Japan, both native and from the Dutch, had progressed tremendously. The first medical school in Japan predated the Meiji period by a decade. Nevertheless, within a year of the Meiji Restoration, the new government had decided to base its medical education and practice on the German model of laboratory medicine, and sent its students abroad to study. In addition, it imported Prussia's military chief of staff and its staff physician to establish and teach at the medical school of the Imperial University (now the University of Tokyo).[1]

Though not a monopoly, the German influence on scientific practice, including medicine, continued to grow exponentially throughout the period. As historian James Bartholomew discovered, during the 1870s, over a quarter of Japan's scientists were sent to Germany. By the early twentieth century, almost 74 percent had trained there. More importantly, 90 percent of all medical scientists and researchers who studied abroad had done so in Germany.

To credit this entirely to the superiority of German medical knowledge would be a mistake. Relations between Japan and Germany had proved amiable, and the

1. Fujikawa, 60, 63; Kuriyama, 21; Porter, 159; Lenoir, 19.

educational system allowed students to study at multiple institutions. In addition, it helped that Nagayo Sensai, the physician who would later establish the government's Medical Affairs Bureau (the predecessor to Japan's Ministry of Health and Welfare), as well as the Japan Health Society preferred Germany to any other countries visited on the fact-finding Iwakura Mission, the political mission to study the workings of the Euro-American powers. The American "professors of medical schools and hospitals treated us like children," which angered Nagayo, a distinguished doctor in his own right. In Germany, however, Nagayo enjoyed himself, and spent his first night drinking. As he reported back to his government, "I was happy for the first time since leaving Japan."[2] Nagayo's preference would shape his intellectual and political successors in modern Japan, ensuring German influence on Japanese scientists for years to come, including on Kitasato, a scientist who would prove determined to wipe out tuberculosis.

Due to Nagayo's work, a number of Japanese physicians also enjoyed German tutelage and research. Chief among these scholars was Kitasato Shibasaburō, a proud and stubborn scientist. At the behest of the Meiji government, for whom Kitasato worked in Nagayo's Bureau of Public Health, Kitasato was sent to Germany, to work under the tutelage of Robert Koch. With the assistance of Mori Ōgai, Kitasato was able to remain in Koch's laboratory longer than the government officials had deemed necessary. He proved a good fit for Koch's lab. Having isolated the tubercle bacillus in 1882, Koch offered a workspace that was a perfect classroom for bacteriology. Under Koch's advisement, Kitasato successfully isolated the tetanus bacillus, a problem that had dogged bacteriologists. Yet, like Koch, he never fully turned away from the continued crisis of tuberculosis.[3]

Kitasato's success, however, was not seen by Japan's government as sufficient justification to keep him on in Koch's laboratory, despite Kitasato's and Koch's requests. Both Koch and Kitasato had been studying the properties of tuberculin, and Kitasato was to leave at the height of Koch's tuberculin therapy work.[4] Nagayo intervened, and, in the most politic way possible, pronounced that Kitasato "alone has long worked as assistant to its [tuberculin's] discoverer and in the process contributed greatly to this tremendous accomplishment." With Koch's support, Nagayo pointed out, Kitasato had "an advantage beyond the grasp of others. If despite this opportunity he must turn his back to the light and return emptily to Japan, it will be an academic embarrassment, a great misfortune to the Japanese people, and a loss of face to the Japanese state." Despite being a Home Ministry bureaucrat, Nagayo spoke as the vice president of the private Japan Health Society, and funding for Kitasato's continued study was provided by the Imperial Household, whose minister, Hijikata Hisamoto, was a member of Nagayo's society.[5] Although granted a

2. Bartholomew 1989, 71–72; Ikawa, 42; Jannetta, 158.
3. Shadanhōmin, 24; Bartholomew 1989, 73; Miyajima, 20.
4. Johnston 1995, 199; KKS: "Kitasato Memorial Museum," 3.
5. Johnston 1995, 200; Miyajima, 23–24.

reprieve, it would not be the last time that Kitasato and his supporters clashed with other members of Japan's government.

Koch was pleased to have his friend and assistant remain, as he had come to realize that "that small Japanese figure had indeed the power and talent" necessary for bacteriological work. Unfortunately, the work that had been occupying the time and energy of both Koch and Kitasato turned out to be a considerable failure. Although Kitasato's protégé and supporter Dr. Miyajima Mikinosuke claimed that "not only was tuberculin successfully employed for the treatment of tuberculosis, but it also afforded greater facility in clinical diagnosis," he was only half right. Although originally celebrated as a cure for tuberculosis, tuberculin proved ineffective, particularly against pulmonary tuberculosis. Koch's career never entirely recovered from the debacle of the fallout of the rapid rise and even faster fall of the "cure." Nonetheless, tuberculin did establish itself as a fairly effective diagnostic indicator of the presence of a disease that had so often gone undetected previously.[6]

Kitasato's allegiance to Koch had placed him in the line of fire in Japan even before his involvement in tuberculin research. When Ogata Masanori, building on the work of medical scientist Takagi Kanehiro, claimed to have isolated bacteria for beriberi, much to the jubilation of some colleagues in Japan, including one doctor who, in an editorial to the *Yomiuri*, urged the government to repeat his experiments and, upon confirming them, give Ogata "10,000 yen for his work. It is our duty to announce this in order to extend Ogata's achievements to the people, and demand that all the gentlemen of the government and the people recognize [this discovery]." Presciently, as it turned out, not every scientist welcomed Ogata's news with such ebullience. Koch, and his colleague, Friedrich Loeffler, both found his discovery specious, even before the realization that a vitamin deficiency causes beriberi. They entreated Kitasato to refute Takagi's findings in Japanese. Despite Kitasato's misgivings, he agreed, thus shaming Ogata, his *sempai* (elder classmate) and former boss at the Public Health Bureau, and angering many in the Japanese intellectual community. The President of Tokyo Imperial University condemned his hubris, and colleagues employed by the government libeled him, including the physician and novelist, Mori Ōgai.[7]

Kitasato's return to Japan, in 1892, once again brought him into conflict with Tokyo Imperial University and the government. As the most famous of Japan's bacteriologists, it was understood, at least by the Meiji government, that Kitasato would join the faculty of the university, and, ideally, head up a national laboratory for further research. Not surprisingly, Kitasato had no interest in this, bristling at the loss of control. As Miyajima reported it, his mentor had "fully prepared himself to devote his life to the advancement of bacteriology. But Japan had not yet been awakened to the importance of bacteriology. As is the fate of most pioneers in

6. Societe, 50; Miyajima, 20, 24; Aoki, 26; Porter, 441; Griffith, 560; Nakase, 7.
7. Bay, 117; Low, 28; Linton, 57; Kanogoki, 2; Bartholomew 1989, 81. Takagi is sometimes referred to as Takaki. Both appear to be acceptable.

political, social and other spheres, he had not been rightly treated by his people, and even his merit and ability were ignored." While this might be a bit of a stretch, many in Japan's government were not, perhaps, awakened to the benefit of allowing Kitasato the freedom to pursue his research independently. Itō Hirobumi, the prime minister, concurred with his education minister, and continued to seek the creation of a laboratory under the auspices of Tokyo University. Independently, as always, Kitasato sought to create his own laboratory, and obtained the moral and financial support of like-minded government officials, industrialists, and intellectuals—including Fukuzawa Yukichi, Nagayo Sensai, and entrepreneur Morimura Ichizaemon—to do so. When the funding proved insufficient for the size of institution Kitasato required, he took advantage of his connection to the Great Japan Hygiene Society and its member, Hasegawa Tai, Nagayo's successor as head of the Home Ministry Hygiene Bureau, and an amateur tuberculosis scholar. Hasegawa supported Kitasato's desire for independence, and saw no reason to grant another laboratory to Tokyo Imperial University when it already had a hygiene laboratory under Kitasato's former and estranged colleague Ogata. Moreover, he acknowledged that the Ministry of Education had a rocky history with Kitasato, and the forced association would do little to support the necessary work that Kitasato was conducting. On the other hand, allowing Kitasato independence would appear as if Japan had no interest in public health and bacteriology, and might undermine the legitimacy of the Ministry of Education.[8] Nevertheless, Kitasato's sponsors, who had launched a successful media campaign, convinced the Diet to fund an independent laboratory for the world-renowned bacteriologist—the Institute of Infectious Diseases.

For almost two decades, Kitasato was able to work independently, despite the absorption of the laboratory into the Ministry of Home Affairs, but enmity between the scientist and the Ministry of Education and Tokyo Imperial University grew. Prince Konoe Takumaro, a cousin of the emperor, regarded Kitasato's isolation of the plague bacillus as a "credit on Japanese medical science [that] makes our civilization shine to the heavens . . . Such achievements can only raise the level of our nation and bring it acclaim," and Kitasato's independence continued to appear nationally indispensable.[9] Yet, in 1914, then Prime Minister Ōkuma Shigenobu, a politician whose involvement with tuberculosis will be discussed in Chapter 4, was convinced that bacteriological work belonged in the university, and should not be performed in competition with it. By 1916, without Kitasato's consent, his entire institute was placed under the jurisdiction of Tokyo Imperial University.[10]

The rivalry between Kitasato and a number of the nation's politicians and their friends in the sciences had over two decades to gestate. In addition to Kitasato's run-in with Ogata over beriberi, the bacteriologist had long lamented his alma

8. Sunagawa, 61; Miyajima, 24–25; Ise, 21; Johnston 1994, 261; Bartholomew 1989, 101–2.
9. KMM: *Kitasato Shibasaburō no hito to gakusetsu*, 42; Bartholomew 1989, 141.
10. National Science Foundation, 43; Komatsu, 117.

mater's inability to foster open scientific research. The vociferousness with which Kitasato and, particularly, his allies denounced the university had done little to ameliorate the situation. Tokutomi Sohō, the journalist and pundit (and brother of the author of *Hototogisu*), pronounced that the university itself was "suffocating" and lamented the rampant "disputes between the authorities and learned circles opposed to feudalism"—which was to say, between the intellectuals and those in charge of their funding. As did doctor and Tokyo Imperial University professor Wakasugi Kisaburō, many of Kitasato's colleagues condemned the dean of the university's faculty, Aoyama Tanemichi, the prime minister's personal physician, who unsurprisingly was no friend of Kitasato's, had little to do with the transfer of Kitasato's laboratory to Tokyo Imperial University.[11]

Despite a staunch faction surrounding him, Kitasato was not known for his amicability or acquiescence. As with his battle with the Ministry of Education, Kitasato had always maintained a desire to research, not to teach. When a young Noguchi Hideyo joined Kitasato's laboratory as a librarian, much to the young man's dismay he was expected to be an autodidact, and one who conducted his own education on his own time, in accordance with the needs and expectations of the laboratory.[12]

For Kitasato, the emphasis on education was misplaced. As one of the leading proponents of public health policy in Japan, he sensed that academic bureaucracy would limit the extent of public health research, as it was concerned with producing graduates, not a healthy populace. In fact, one could point out that it behooved medical schools to maintain an unhealthy populace, else there would be far less need for the education they provided. "Scientific achievements," the bacteriologist maintained, "should be for practical use."[13]

But Kitasato's achievements were not limited to research. After resigning his newly acquired post at the Ministry of Education, Kitasato began again, founding another institute with the revenue acquired from years of successful research into vaccines, the immunological failure of tuberculin notwithstanding. Kitasato had kept busy, too, as the head of the Central Hygiene Commission, the president of the Japan Federation of Medical Societies, the first president of the Greater Japan Medical Association, the instigator of the founding of private (and generally expensive) sanatoria, and, as if to further spite Tokyo Imperial University, the first dean of Fukuzawa's Keio-Gijiku University Medical Faculty.[14]

Kitasato's research and political activities ensured that, no matter how many enemies he made, he was still invaluable to the nation. Kitasato was by far the best known of his nation's many scientists, to the extent that he was viewed throughout

11. Liu, 53; Imperial University, 66; Batholomew, 203, 152; Miyajima, 41.
12. Plesset, 54.
13. KKS: "Kitasato Memorial Museum," 5.
14. Bartholomew 1989, 153–54; Steslicke, 35–36; Iijima, 64; Miyajima, 43–44.

the international scientific community as an accomplished scientist, not simply a Japanese scientist or a scientist who required further qualifications.

And, while the international scientific community was certainly no less rife with divisions than its Japanese section, Kitasato had a considerable number of colleagues and friends worldwide. In fact, it seemed as if his involvement in the international scientific sphere was much more amiable than within Japan. His amiability globally serves to offset his anger with those at whose behest he served. Even his competition with Alexandre Yersin over their research on the plague bacillus in Hong Kong in 1894, an analogue of that of Koch and Pasteur, was far less divisive than presumed. Although Kitasato benefited from Dr. James A. Lowson's assistance and friendship, while Yersin toiled in far less favorable conditions, Kitasato, who had met Yersin in Hong Kong just once, presented him with a prestained pure culture of plague bacillus. While there remains a question whether there was some competitive conspiracy on Kitasato's part, there appears to be no documentary evidence for this. Indeed, it was Lowson, the superintendent of the Civil Hospital in Hong Kong, who, in a humorous note to Kitasato, replete with sketches of both Kitasato and Lowson in the header, expressed distaste for Yersin in passing. "My sanguine professor (*Mein Blutreich Professor*)," Lowson jokingly opened, "I salute you, and hope that you will be able to prepare a new shell filled with Pest Bacilli for the damned Chinaman. If you can at the same time kill a man called Yersin, for God's sake do so. He has led us a dance [*sic*] in a way but Takaki will tell you we have got the better of him." Lowson informed Kitasato that Aoyama (Kitasato's future presumed adversary) and the other scientists who had accompanied both Kitasato and Aoyama to Hong Kong had returned to Japan, and asked Kitasato to "look after him." He closed by extending regards to two colleagues, one of whom "the sisters used to call . . . Adonis (if you know what that means)." Aoyama, in fact, was responsible for instigating the conflict, as he published an article claiming that Kitasato's isolated bacillus was simply streptococcus, thus making Yersin's the only true isolated plague bacillus.[15] Aoyama's conclusions were specious, and it appears that Kitasato did, in fact, observe the same bacilli that Yersin did, but Kitasato never seemed to dwell on the inequality as others within the scientific community had.

Inequality was a theme with which Kitasato was familiar, both at home and abroad. His work on blood serum therapy certainly was overshadowed by that of his colleague, Behring, both in the published findings and in the recognition of the work by the Nobel Committee. But if Kitasato's followers are to be believed, the only inequality on which he dwelled was that inherent in his government's failure to combat tuberculosis effectively. Takano Rokurō, the hygienist who served as the first chief of the Ministry of Home Affairs' Prevention Bureau, and a disciple of Kitasato, noted that Kitasato had begun establishing multiple sanatoriums throughout Japan

15. Bibel and Chen, 636; Molyneux, 104; KM: Letter from James A. Lowson to Kitasato. Aug. 20, 1894; Shadanhōmin, 80; Bibel and Chen, 638.

for the tubercular.[16] Indeed, he did open one, although not, perhaps, multiple ones. With the founding of Tsukushigaoka Yojo-en in 1893, Kitasato had accomplished the opening, according to his disciples, of the first private tuberculosis sanatorium, a fact that merits surprisingly little mention in historical literature, and, perhaps more important, is incorrect. As Fukuda Mahito points out in his biography of Kitasato, and much to the chagrin of Kitasato's relatives and aficionados, the first sanatorium in Japan had been established four years prior, although it had soon closed.[17]

But it is true that what Kitasato might have lacked in actual buildings he made up for in his dedication to the cause of tuberculosis prevention. Even though tuberculin remained an ineffective vaccine, Kitasato continued to spearhead the effort to combat the disease. Yet most of Kitasato's political peers were more concerned about the bovine equivalent than the human one. Until the end of the Taishō period, legal ordinances about tuberculosis in Japanese cattle outnumbered those for humans by more than three times over. Furthermore, human tuberculosis care remained legally nonexistent until 1919, and moreover, from then until the start of the Shōwa era it was only addressed three times in legal ordinances, with one instance concerned solely with the disease in Taiwan.[18] The health care of the colonies notwithstanding, it was Kitasato as both bureaucrat and pundit who attempted to spearhead the campaign to focus as much or more on human public health as on bovine care in Japan.

Unfortunately, much of this work took place outside Japan's borders. Thus, in his 1904 presentation on Japanese bovine tuberculosis, "The Behavior of Native Japanese Cattle in Regard to Tuberculosis (Perlsucht)," at the International Conference on Arts and Sciences of the world's fair in St. Louis, Kitasato decided to use the platform to address the human cost of tuberculosis in his country. Despite the fact that "cow's milk is employed but little by us for the nourishment of children," both pulmonary and intestinal tuberculosis were ravaging the populace. By Kitasato's calculation, the entire country saw an increase in tuberculosis mortality from 7.3 percent of all deaths to 7.9 percent in the course of the turn of the century, from 1899 to 1900. It also translated to a total of 0.16 percent of Japan's entire population in 1900 succumbing to the disease in that year alone.[19]

As the twentieth century progressed, so, too, did tuberculosis' swath through Japan, a fact that Kitasato continued to point out at international conference after international conference. In a Washington, DC, conference in 1908, Kitasato shared information gleaned from the field of public health, as well as the insurance companies. Among the "three most prominent life insurance companies in Japan," it was obvious not only that "the death-rate from pulmonary tuberculosis has been steadily increasing annually" but also that the insurance policies for those afflicted

16. Bartholomew 1998, 249; Satofuka, 41, KM: Dec. 12, 1890; Chung, 87; Bartholomew 1989, 153.
17. KMM: *Kitasato to sono sekai*; KKS: "Kitasato Daigaku: Kitasato seimei kagaku kenkyūjo," 2; Fukuda 2008, 69–70.
18. NA: Japan Center for Asian Historical Records (JACAR)—(www.jacar.go.jp)—three human ordinances to thirteen cattle.
19. Kitasato 1977a, 336–39; Kitasato 1977b, 348–50.

were becoming harder to come by. Thus, according to these insurance companies, the pulmonary tuberculosis rate of late appeared to have diminished slightly. This, Kitasato was quick to point out, was due not to the successful prevention of tuberculosis in Japan but instead could be solely "traced to the fact that these [insurance] companies have adopted a strict method of examination for persons applying for insurance policies." Moreover, Kitasato noted, though the mortality rate continued to range "from 20 to 25 per cent of all deaths," the rates from insurance companies also failed to include those who died under the age of fifteen, the minimum age for this insurance. Consequently, while tuberculosis had become "the most prevalent disease in Japan, and as such it is to be greatly dreaded," and despite improved detection among the medical community, the rate continued to climb as prevention remained slack.

Indeed, Kitasato lamented, there was "so much to relate in connection with the prevention of tuberculosis in Japan." Kitasato had tried to educate physicians through journal articles in Japan, but to no avail. Neither medical professionals nor the public seemed to apply this knowledge to prevention. And why should they? Even twenty-plus years after Koch's work, misconceptions reigned supreme in both spheres. Ogata himself remained convinced in 1904 of the hereditary nature of tuberculosis, and stated as much in his articles, which erroneously countered Kitasato's.[20]

Yet even as the educational war continued, the responsibility for both education and prevention also remained unclear and disputed. In America, laws were already on the books for nearly a decade to curtail the spread of tuberculosis.[21] Kitasato, never a friend of large government, toyed with the idea of placing the future of prevention and care in the sphere of philanthropy, though he spearheaded what would become the Home Ministry's 1904 Pulmonary Tuberculosis Prevention Ordinance. This law mandated that "spittoons shall be placed in all buildings for public use, and makes certain provisions concerning sanitary requirements in such places as public bath-houses, hospitals, etc."[22]

For obvious reasons, the ordinance was quickly dismissed as the "spittoon law," and proper expectoration proved hard to legislate, and so was also dismissed. Sadly, the continuing disagreement between medical professionals as to the nature of contagion also meant that further legislation was doomed from the start. Kitasato continued to insist on the importance of tuberculin treatment, while Ogata's insistence on heredity as the catalyst of tuberculosis meant that his insistence on government involvement in prevention was not only misplaced but also offensive.[23]

Unfortunately, Kitasato's medical disagreements about the utility of tuberculin would turn out to be equally and inadvertently as damaging to his goal of sanitary

20. Kitasato 1908, 3–4, 12, 16; Johnston, 224, 227.
21. Abrams, 427.
22. Komatsu, 119; Kitasato 1908, 16.
23. Kitasato 1908, 17; Johnston, 227–28.

and public health in Japan as his political antagonism to so many of his nation's politicians. Had he proven less intransigent, would Japan's epidemic have been so long and so devastating? Perhaps not, but with so many conflicting opinions surrounding the disease, it was hardly surprising that the government found it easier to continue shirking the responsibility that some would claim was its duty. Whether that job was the responsibility of politicians remained moot as the disease continued to make inroads unhindered. In a coup of understatement, Kitasato declared to his international colleagues that "the combat against tuberculous infection in Japan is yet in its infancy." That Japan failed to declare war on tuberculosis, Kitasato explained, was due to Japan's medical professionals having "been hard pressed in fighting some acute contagious diseases of severe nature, which prevented us from attending to the chronic forms of infectious disease." In truth, many of Japan's physicians were at the cusp of medical research into various diseases, Kitasato being prime among them. But there were reasons that tuberculosis prevention was not pursued, and Kitasato was not necessarily responsible for them. As it turned out, whether he was then aware of it, his assurance to his colleagues was false, as he informed them that since "of late we have been enabled to fight against those (diseases) of a chronic nature; and the attention of the nation has been turned toward such diseases. Japan will henceforth endeavor to keep step with the advanced nations of Europe and America in combating this dreaded national, nay international disease, the enemy of mankind—tuberculosis."[24] Sadly, as we shall see, owing to politics and the vagaries of the moral enterprise, his conviction was misplaced.

Epidemiologist Aoki Kunio theorized that the epidemic was due to the increasing birthrate in Japan from 1885 to 1910, with increased opportunities for infection through "changing working environments and living conditions." Although the epidemic may have been somewhat curbed by improved factory conditions after the enactment (and eventual enforcement) of the Factory Law of 1909, which was meant to introduce labor standards, Aoki noted that tuberculosis spiked once more during the 1918–1919 Spanish influenza epidemic, in bodies already weakened by the flu, which was also common in textile factories.[25] Ito Araki, a presenter at the Sixth International Congress on Tuberculosis, believed that the problem stemmed not from a lack of knowledge of contagion but from "faulty nutrition," and the "lack of fresh air at night and on cold days." Adding to that, the population density of Japan itself, particularly in the slums, as well as the poverty within these slums, all but assured the proliferation of tuberculosis. Regardless of the causes, it was ubiquitous in the textile factories, and in the bodies of the factories' workers.[26]

24. Kitasato 1908, 17.
25. K. Aoki, 483; Prang, 313.
26. A. Ito, 573.

4

"Justifying the Liabilities Which Had Been Incurred"

Political Strife over Tuberculosis

If politics was a balancing act, Japan was lucky in possessing enough political acrobats. One such politician, Ōkuma Shigenobu—who will be discussed in more detail later—was particularly adept at appearing well poised. Schooled in the political ideology of utilitarianism, purportedly the greatest good for the greatest number, Ōkuma was inclined not only to balance the needs of the many against those of the few but also the work of one organization or group against that of another. Like Ōkuma, Japan's politicians were congratulating themselves on their victories in the wars of modernization and colonization, while looking forward to future successes. As we shall see, an as yet unconquerable foe, TB, was understandably not one that most politicians were eager to pursue. And, though that foe was formidable and though it proved hard to overlook, politicians could take comfort in the fact that its victims were still primarily limited to particular groups of the nation's subjects—namely, female factory workers. That tuberculosis remained on the periphery allowed Japan's politicians the possibility of writing off their potential inaction in combating the disease as a sacrifice necessary to ensure the greater good and as justified by the lack of viable remedies. Interrupting factory work, particularly at the textile mills, would have forced Japan's modernization to a halt. Certainly, to fail to acknowledge the self-interest of politicians would be foolish, but these men were also interested in strengthening their nation, and the policies they undertook were meant to do so, even at the cost of a number of citizens. We will evaluate the political decisions about the disease momentarily. First, however, we must examine the ideological background of those decisions.

In a nod to the prevalence of British liberal philosophy over French among much of Meiji Japan's political elite, John Stuart Mill's definition of utilitarianism governed a number of the rulers. Kiyoshi Karl Kawakami, an internationally recognized journalist (and sometime apologist), commented that "the utilitarian theory was the animating idea not only of the Progressive-Conservative Party but of a greater portion of the people during a certain period." Yet, Kawakami acknowledged that the concept of utilitarianism was not the "lofty and noble . . . idea set forth in Mill's discourse on Utility." Rather, as will become apparent, utility was measured in practical terms—essentially utilitarian utilitarianism.[1]

This was a truly Meiji ideology—one that promoted the growth of industry and national wealth. Hayashi Fusao, a one-time Marxist literary and cultural critic, maintained that utilitarianism undergirded the bureaucratic elite, many of whom had political interests, and vice versa.[2] That the nature of utilitarianism as an ideology had been changed in Japan under the elite was hardly surprising, although the philosophy also proved popular throughout society without the alterations promoted by the Meiji government. Nevertheless, no matter how many subjects enjoyed Mill or Spencer or Samuel Smiles, the greatest good for the greatest number was defined by the government, not the populace.[3]

Since the so-called "restoration," the aim of the newly formed Meiji government had been one of *fukoku kyōhei*, a rich country and a strong army. For this government, therefore, practically regardless of the political factions or parties involved, utilitarianism was little more than the requisites to that end, since, presumably, a rich country and a strong army constituted the greatest good of the modern nation-state. As historian Andrew E. Barshay postulated in his analysis of the public sphere and its relation to the intelligentsia post-Meiji, the government rationalized its promotion of *fukoku kyōhei* as a national good, the requisite of every modern citizen or subject, whether or not such citizens or subjects themselves were aware of it as such. Barshay noted that politicians utilized a number of specific formulas to guide their work, two of which specifically apply here. The first of these was the concept of *kazoku kokka*, or "family-state," wherein the relationship between subjects was familial, and be it imperial, oligarchic, or both, the role of the government was that of the paterfamilias. As father, the government was responsible for the good of the family as a whole, while his children remained too naive or immature to know how to care for themselves. And although Barshay does not imply this, the government as father sought to care for his children in perpetuity. At no time could the children mature enough to merit independence, again both literally and figuratively.

The second formula by which the government pursued *fukoku kyōhei* was *kanson minpi*—"exalt officialdom, slight the people." In the same vein, the Meiji leadership, in the role of father, held the reins of power tightly, and, despite the first article of the 1868 Charter Oath, that stating that governance would be shared with the public, had no real intention of sharing it with the subjects.[4] Thus, the Meiji leadership saw fit to decide how to define the common good.

So, too, did it decide the value of human life. For a nation built on military and economic wealth, a soldier was more valuable than a farmhand. If he was the head of the Japanese nation, Emperor Meiji declared in his Imperial Rescript for Military

1. Ohtsu and Imanari, 37; Kawakami, 137–38.
2. Najita and Harootunian, 262.
3. Maeda, 111.
4. Barshay, 3–5.

Men, then the military was his limbs.[5] Thus, as with other national commodities, the government could determine the cost necessary to ensure the best output, even when the cost was not inherently economic. People were currency, and currency bought that which served national interests.

In fact, the rise of utilitarianism in Japan was not of Millian origin. As Mill himself noted, the term "utilitarianism" was one adopted from John Galt. In Japan, moreover, utilitarianism had roots beyond Mill and Galt. Japanese notions of utilitarianism can be traced to the Confucian philosophy of men like Ogyū Sorai (1666–1728). This was the politically expedient form later popularized as utilitarianism within the Meiji elite. For Ogyū, such ideology was seen as a functional representation of a utopian world, a world based on what he deemed "the Way of the Sages" or "the Way of the Early Kings":

> The Way of the Early Kings is the way of bringing peace and contentment to the world. Though it takes manifold forms, they all much conform to this end of bringing peace and contentment to the world. . . . Thus the Way cannot be spoken of in terms of one man but only in terms of millions of men collectively.
>
> If we look at the world as it is, who can stand by himself and not associate with some collectivity? Scholars and samurai, peasants, artisans and merchants together assist and nourish each other. They cannot survive otherwise. . . .
>
> In general, according to the Way of the Early Kings and Confucius, everyone had his own function to perform and his own purpose to serve, and the essential thing was to nurture and fulfill that capability. However, later men with a more dogmatic view insisted on "humaneness" as a comprehensive virtue and they could not help but leap upon it as one all-encompassing principle.[6]

Thus, it was Ogyū's philosophy of political utility that served as a basis for understanding utilitarianism, and it was to this root that Mill, Spencer, and Smiles unknowingly were grafted in Japan.

With the combination of Ogyū's Confucian ideology, supplemented by the diction of Mill, the notion of utilitarianism could be extended by Fukuzawa Yukichi, the so-called Benjamin Franklin of Japan, and philosopher Nishi Amane to expand throughout society.[7] Thus, by their lights, those who were not sages or kings could participate in utilitarian action. However, to preach the choice of pursuing happiness for the maximum societal benefit proved difficult to reconcile with the notions of *kanson minpi* that ran rampant within the Meiji intellectual and political elite. Fukuzawa particularly was dismissive of the populace, even as he courted his categorization as a liberal. To see Fukuzawa's distaste for his country's populace, one need only read the anecdote in his autobiography in which he forcefully commands a peasant to mount his horse, ordering him to comprehend his equality, and then dismissing him as ignorant and fearful. For Fukuzawa, this was a sorry state—that

5. Shibusawa, K., 443; Keene, 367.
6. Jun, 130; Ogyū, 39; de Bary, 164.
7. Chamberlain, 366; Havens, 218.

the people remain so ignorant was wrong, yet the fact that they continued to toil in this way was worse. Accordingly, in his work, *An Encouragement of Learning* (1872), Fukuzawa proclaims that the country, whose health must be ensured, consisted not of the people but of the government alone: "The government is the living force [of this body] and the people are the outside stimulus." Whether a lamentation or a statement of fact, the continued and perhaps willful ignorance of the populace beyond being unfortunate, kept them from fulfilling a capacity for self-governance. As historian Julia Thomas pointed out, even Thomas Hobbes refused to bar the populace from the leviathan, while Fukuzawa had no such pretensions of inclusion.[8]

Fukuzawa was considered liberal, and, indeed, an adherent of utilitarianism, but more significantly, he was a pragmatist, not an idealist, and both his liberalism and his utilitarianism were based in practicalities. According to Keio University professor—and thus Fukuzawa devotee—Miyamori Asatarō, "Utilitarianism as a system of philosophy may be unintelligible to the masses, but Mr. Fukuzawa's adaptation of the leading principles of this system may be understood even by a man who has enjoyed few educational advantages. Of what does and what does not conduce to the welfare of society most people are very fair judges." To liberals and allied utilitarianists, society trumped humanity.[9]

A leading intellectual light, Fukuzawa spurned a political career, leaving his many political opinions in the realm of idealism, even as he preached pragmatism. Fortunately for him, however, there were a number of politicians who concurred with his positions. As renowned postwar political theorist Maruyama Masao commented in his analysis of Japan's ultranationalism, the notions of Millian utilitarianism were couched in the ideology of this ultranationalism, wherein state morality was internalized to the extent that it ruled out the individual freedom one might associate with Mill's conception. As he noted, Kōno Hironaka, leader of the Jiyuto, the Liberal political party, proclaimed that his ideological epiphany following his reading of Mill meant that his "entire way of thinking was revolutionalized [*sic*]." Where before he had adhered intellectually to Confucianism and other classical Sino-Japanese ideologies, upon reading *On Liberty*, "All these earlier thoughts of mine, *excepting those concerned with loyalty and filial piety*, were smashed to smithereens. At the same moment I knew that it was human freedom and human rights that I must henceforth cherish above all else." Where Maruyama cites evidence of the failure to distinguish between political power and morality, it is also clear that utilitarianism in Japan differed from that of Mill, who preached the greatest good for the greatest number.[10]

Yet, as Kōno unwittingly expressed, while the *genrō*, the elder statesmen of Japan, respected Fukuzawa's philosophical analyses (and, perhaps, those of John Stuart Mill), few had time for such justifications—what they did, they did for the

8. Najita, 92; Fukuzawa, 243–44; Thomas, 68.
9. Miyamori, 189.
10. Maruyama, 4–5; Scalapino, 170.

nation, without need of utilitarianism qua justification. Indeed, it really was not until the rise of political parties, and thus, electoral politics, well into the Taishō era, that justifications were necessary, as the group of likeminded individuals could no longer monopolize the government. Up until that point, there need be no check on legislation—every action could be pursued without the hindrance of legitimation, at least not to the populace.

Meiji politicians did, however, believe in legitimizing their actions to their Euro-American counterparts. Both the *genrō* and the next generation of Japan's leadership were eager to prove themselves and their nation as worthy to their international counterparts, yet some politicians, particularly those who rose to power (or continued to rise in power) after the decline of *genrō* influence, were more adept at courting the desired approval. For a man like Ōkuma Shigenobu, with one eye on his Euro-American peers, utilitarian justifications would prove a significant influence in his political ideology and his moral enterprise.

Ōkuma Shigenobu was a politician whose involvement in Japanese politics merited twice serving as prime minister (once for a few months in Meiji—specifically, 1898—and once during Taishō, from 1914 until 1916). A former samurai from the province of Hizen, Ōkuma was among the outside of the inner circle of Meiji period politics who quickly rose up to take his place among the new nobility of the nation.

Because his career included prominence in both the Meiji and Taishō periods, Ōkuma provides a very salient and important example of Japanese politics. His personality, or the perception of it, allowed many Japanese subjects, even those unable to vote, to view the politician as a kind patrician, regardless of the policies he enacted or refused to enact, including a number of public health initiatives on tuberculosis. Moreover, both his nature and his contacts in Japan and overseas often permitted foreign evangelists to consider him a friend, notwithstanding the fact that he often derided them. Even when out of political office, he remained "one of the most distinguished statesmen of our country," according to the 1904 Department of Education. For our purposes, Ōkuma also personifies the acknowledgment of governmental responsibility for the Japanese subjects, including those not yet born. He and his followers were concerned not only about the role of politics in the people's lives but about how those lives appeared to their counterparts worldwide. Utilitarian, politically long-lived, and concerned about the presentation of his nation and himself, Ōkuma was very the definition of a savvy politician and moral entrepreneur.

Ōkuma, though involved in Japanese governance since the start of the Meiji period, considered himself a bit of an outsider. The fact that he was from the former domain of Hizen, not Satsuma or Chōshū, the homes of the majority of the elder statesmen, allowed him to float within the Meiji government without being hindered by the associations deriving from his origins. His intelligence permitted him to undertake various political positions, including minister of finance, minister of foreign affairs, minister of agriculture and commerce, and, eventually, prime minister. His political longevity and, indeed, his political resurrection owed much to his ability to present himself in an amicable light to various factions (notwithstanding his 1889 attempted assassination by Kurushima Tsuneki, who decried Ōkuma's revisions of Japan's unequal treaties), both within and outside Japanese politics.[11] Since Ōkuma was considered a politician first and foremost, let us analyze the man's politics here as a means by which to understand his relationship with foreign evangelical groups and their work on tuberculosis later.

Ōkuma's grasp of Japanese economics was quite evident, as was his emphasis on the importance of education, particularly vis-à-vis the primacy of political economics. Organizing and reorganizing multiple political parties, he was not an intransigent man and showed a penchant for flexibility when it proved politically expedient. Yet it was both his legacy of and his opinions toward factory legislation (which was the closest Japan would get to national tuberculosis public health legislation until the Law for the Prevention of Tuberculosis of 1919, which itself did little to assist financially or enforce) that seem confusing.[12] To what extent did Ōkuma seek to protect both the rights and the lives of factory workers, including those most at risk of succumbing to tuberculosis? As historian Hyman Kublin notes, the very first national factory law intended to be submitted to the Diet the following year was debated by the Higher Council of Agriculture, Commerce, and Industry and Agriculture in 1897, and thus, under Ōkuma's prime ministership. This was to end what labor organizer and correspondent (in both America and Japan) Takano Fusatarō termed the "many years of perfect indifference to the welfare of laborers" by the Japanese government, which had finally "awakened to its proper duty and is showing a disposition to stretch helping hands to the downtrodden people by enacting a factory law purporting to remove great evils rampant under the factory system." Yet, much to Takano's discontent, the legislation stalled when Ōkuma resigned and his administration collapsed. The next factory legislation would not be presented to the Diet until 1909, where it was debated for the next two years, and not enacted for another five.[13] Despite this trailblazing, Ōkuma was hardly a staunch defender of labor rights.

Ōkuma was on record as promoting the paternalistic state, claiming Confucian ideological preference for those in charge (the bakufu in the case of the Edo period) maintaining the well-being of the populace: "From ancient times, our statesmen have espoused ideas of state socialism." He assured British Labour and Liberal politician Percy Alden that "in Japan the strong would always come to the rescue of the weak and oppressed." Thus, while not advocating the labor movement, the politician did acknowledge that "labor troubles, owing to our industrial changes,

11. Lebra, 19; Kataoka, iii; Ōkuma 1909, 1.
12. Monbushō, 19; Ramseyer and Rosenbluth, 44; Röhl, 588; Takahashi, 127.
13. Kublin, 125; Takano, 250; Dore, 438; Sato, 13. Labor historian Nimura Kazuo provides a complete website of much of Takano's work. For this, and for his own work on Japanese labor history, I am indebted to him (http://oohara.mt.tama.hosei.ac.jp/nk/index.html).

are likely to occur. Japan has been socialistic, and tends naturally in the direction of trade-unions. With the effort to better our coolies by education, their demands will increase. But I do not regard this as an evil."[14]

Yet, Ōkuma also publicly negated these positions. In 1897, as minister of agriculture and commerce, he announced that he was a staunch believer in laissez-faire and "have been opposed to intervention. Free competition is very essential to the development of business. It is necessary to promote a spirit of independence in businessmen." Either way, his paternalism was not the safety net that one might think. Japanese economic interests were intertwined with politics, and with respect to the zaibatsu family business combines, the two became symbiotic. Ōkuma himself had been affiliated with Mitsubishi, a Meiji shipping conglomerate, in order to counter the Satchō clique, the coterie of politicians who controlled much of Meiji politics since its inception, particularly the influence of head statesman Itō Hirobumi. Thus, as political economists Banno Junji and Ohno Kenichi conclude, Ōkuma entered politics believing in the economic principle of a balanced budget but soon became an advocate of government involvement in the Keynesian model of fiscal activism. Yet the content and timing of his statements seem off; fiscal activism, utilized during the Sino-Japanese and Russo-Japanese Wars, would not be fully adopted by the Meiji government until after the Russo-Japanese War, and then it would be promoted by Itō and the Seiyūkai, the Conservative political party.[15]

Where Ōkuma could be proclaimed as being "a statesman without solid group affiliation," as Banno and Ohno do, so, too, could he be seen as the epitome of the politician—a man who is not beholden to a party, ideology, or creed. Ōkuma was rather a man desiring to be accepted by specific individuals and also a generally canny public relations manager, the perfect moral entrepreneur. He could tell the people from whom he desired something—money, influence, power—what they wanted to hear, without necessarily having to stick to the party line. He felt no need to be entirely truthful (one political cartoon labeled him "big liar"), but it is by no means a foregone conclusion that he was aiming to deceive. It is interesting to note that he claimed, "Lying is the biggest sin."[16]

Janus-faced or not, Ōkuma proved particularly popular among the foreign community. A talented speaker, with the gift of congeniality and humor, he presented himself as a capable, if genuine, bureaucrat, despite his canniness in politics and public relations. Not just a politician, he was politic as well. So too was he disarmingly charming, striking his Euro-American counterparts abroad as a true patriot, regardless of his actual beliefs or intentions. To them, he was "one of the most earnest, sagacious, and truly patriotic statesmen that the present era has produced," a man "endowed with a bright, cheery disposition, possessed of most genial

14. Garon 1987, 11; Alden, 590; Humphreys, 897.
15. Marshall, 23; Nakagawa, 109; Kataoka, 261; Calman, 5; Banno and Ohno, 8; Ohno, 58, 88–89.
16. Banno and Ohno, 8; WUA: "*Waihan* Cabinet Formed." *Marumaru Chinbun*. No. 1170. July 1898; Kataoka, 381; Ōkuma 1964, 85.

manners, and . . . brilliant and entertaining to a degree in his ordinary conversation . . . (of) remarkable mental vigour and activity."[17]

Yet, despite his jovial and agreeable countenance, it seemed Ōkuma had no love of the foreign powers of Europe and America. When Indian historian and nationalist Taraknath Das wrote his 1917 book *The Isolation of Japan in World Politics*, after a study tour in Japan, and concluded that the Anglo-Japanese Alliance was doomed to failure, due to the unequal treatment of Japan at the hands of the Euro-American powers, Ōkuma applauded the book vociferously. This was not a new turn of events. When pressed by British ambassador Sir Gerard Augustus Lowther on his nation's foreign affairs at the turn of the twentieth century, Ōkuma showed himself to be both "tiresome" and "far from 'coulant' [easygoing]." Similarly negative was Ōkuma's opinion of the United States, which diplomatic historian Walter LaFeber claimed was notable for its "marked dislike and fear."[18]

Likewise, Ōkuma did not see Christianity as a religion or an ideology worth pursuing, either personally or nationally. Before the 1873 legalization of Christianity, as a Meiji government official, Ōkuma had assisted in the arrest of Japanese Christians in Urakami village, and had defended his actions and those of his government to foreign dignitaries. When he described the encounter, in 1902, some forty-five years later, he noted his zealousness but did not denounce his sentiments. His remarkable screed bears quoting at some length:

> I said: "I am one of those who arrested and examined Christians in Nagasaki. . . . We cannot grant your request for releasing the prisoners and withdrawing the prohibitions against Christianity. Foreign countries are not justified in interfering when we punish our people according to our laws. Hence we do not think it necessary to discuss the matter with you."
>
> Sir Harry Parkes, the English Minister, was very angry. He shook his fist and struck the table as he said: "This is insolence; this is going too far. Religion and truth are universal. Men are free to follow this religion or acknowledge that truth as they deem right. Among civilized nations, there is none that does not permit liberty of belief. To have laws punishing people who have done nothing wrong, to erect barriers for shutting out the truth, is a shame for even a barbarous country. You do not realize what you are doing. You are rejecting the friendship of other lands. You ought to consider the condition of Japan and think of its future."
>
> I answered: "You cannot hope to move us by such simple arguments as these. I know a little about religion and religious history. Christianity, indeed, contains some truth; but it must not be forgotten that its history is filled with evil. A historian has said that the history of Europe is the history of strife; and a religious writer says that the history of Europe is the history of Christianity. If these authors are correct, the history of Christianity is a history of strife. Christ has not given peace to the earth but a sword. After the birth of Christ came the age of the popes. What was it that gave rise to great tumults and continually plunged the people of Europe

17. Lanman, 177; Lebra, 85; Palmer, 177; Morris, 246.
18. Aydin, 118; Ruxton, 186–87; LaFeber, 107.

> into deep misery? From ancient times the rulers of different countries have often done cruel deeds; but what is it that has gone beyond kings in cruelty? How about the dungeons and the torments for punishing those who, as you say, simply held opinions differing from those of others? Of late, this evil has somewhat decreased in the West. This is because men's minds are expanding and they are not controlled by religion alone. In our country, conditions at present are different. From the first, Shinto has controlled men's minds. Buddhism also has had great power for over a thousand years. We are not lacking a religion. If at this time we should remove the edicts against Christianity and at the same time release its followers who have been arrested, Shintoists and Buddhists would rise up in anger and there would be a great disturbance. Of all disputes, none are more violent than those connected with religion. They suck out the blood, crunch the bones, and are never satiated. We cannot tell what sort of strife would arise in our land. Our statesmen must carefully consider this. In what happened at Nagasaki our Government did not make the first move. The people of different places came with their complaints and urged us to take action against the Christians. We were forced by reasons connected with the internal affairs of the country to take action and strictly suppress Christianity. We thank you for your benevolent thoughts; but the facts being as stated, what else can we do?"
>
> Parkes became more angry and said: "You are cowardly. If you wish to accomplish anything you must expect some loss. If you hesitate because of unwillingness to face difficulties, you can never attain success. Is not this an era of re-organisation? Why not destroy evil customs and come out into a broader world than you have known? Christianity is now accepted by all civilized countries. Though some evils may have appeared in its history, its fruits are seen in the civilization of this nineteenth century. Its excellence and truth are evident. Nothing is worse than to regard as an enemy what the whole world knows to be good; nothing is so foolish as to reject the truth. You ought to open your eyes. It is truly said that Oriental officials are so in the habit of looking only at what is directly before them that they never turn their gaze upwards. If you repeal the edits and pardon the prisoners, you will find that your fears were needless. If you do not take this action, I am sure that Japan is doomed."
>
> I answered with a laugh: "The day that we blindly follow the commands of foreigners will surely be the time of our nation's destruction. We are better acquainted than you with the state of affairs in our country. You think that what you desire can easily be done; but it is not so. Religious views that are the product of past centuries cannot be overcome in a single day. We cannot endure to add another to the many things that are disturbing our country. In making purchases, one should not pay more than a reasonable price. We do not like to pay too high a price, as we should by purchasing Christianity at the cost of many human lives."

Ōkuma also noted angering the French minister, who threatened to send the French navy to protect the Christians in Nagasaki. To this Ōkuma countered, "Your threat shows how good reason we have to fear Christianity; for as soon as trouble arises, there is instantly talk about gunboats." Though he had once toyed with the notion of utilizing Christianity to create a religious amalgamation of Confucianism, Buddhism, and Protestantism for national purposes, the idea was never pursued.[19]

Ever the pragmatist, however, Ōkuma's relationship with Christianity did not predetermine his personal relationships with Christians, particularly foreign Christians, including those who would assist his government in public health care. Much of his work with foreign evangelical organizations and his utilization of these groups with respect to medical missionary work, not the least of which was care of the tubercular, would prove the politician's commitment to both utilitarianism and moral entrepreneurship.

Moreover, what he did pursue with a dogged determination was the cultivation of a positive relationship with journalists and those who could best facilitate good press for both himself and his ideas. Domestically as well as internationally, Ōkuma engaged in public relations bids that both made use of the press and rewarded it for spreading the sentiments necessary to ensure his popularity. In addition to purchasing journals and newspapers, often as political outlets, and staffing them with protégés, Ōkuma presented himself as a friend of free press, as when he insisted on more favorable treatment of journalists and their trade as a precondition of his entry in Prime Minister Matsukata Masayoshi's 1896 cabinet.[20]

Ōkuma was particularly shrewd with the foreign press, and had established a close relationship with the somewhat caustic American journalist and autodidact Edward Howard House. This relationship would ensure that Ōkuma could court foreign investors to condone the moral liability and to foot the economic bill that Ōkuma would incur politically. House, who spent the first half of his life traveling and writing for such publications as the *Tribune*, the *London Times*, *Harper's Magazine*, the *Atlantic Monthly*, and the *New York Times*, originally came to Japan to report on the bakumatsu period, the fickle time leading up to the Meiji Restoration, and, having fallen in love with the inchoate nation, soon returned to begin work in education and journalism, meeting Ōkuma, who assisted in founding House's *Tokio Times*.[21] To many outside Japan, House seemed, as eulogized in the *Publisher's Weekly* periodical, "a sincere friend of Japan," but, in fact, his allegiance was to the Japan that Ōkuma provided him. The distinction might seem slight but actually speaks to nuances in the like-mindedness and the working relationship of the two men, whose relationship with evangelicals proves interesting, as will be seen.

For House, Ōkuma's patronage guaranteed an inside scoop of Japanese affairs—not merely social, but political and economic, as well. For Ōkuma, House offered his tenacity and determination in presenting both Ōkuma's ideas and person in the best light in the English language press, both at home and abroad.[22] For the handful of literati who followed the careers of both men, the intentions were obvious, as

19. Cary 1909b, 310–11; Ozaki, 46–47.
20. De Lange, 120; Huffman 1997, 115; Ozaki, 49; Hirayama, 231; Kasza, 15; Reischauer, 124.
21. "EDWARD HOWARD HOUSE," 1902; Huffman 1987, 234.
22. "Obituary Notes," 96.

each praised the progress of the Japanese nation, and as House lauded Ōkuma as the perfect statesman of this progressive nation. It was not particularly libelous for contemporary Keio politics professor W. W. McLaren to claim that "we do not look for an unbiased account of events in the writings of E. H. House, nor in those of Nitobé [Inazo, the Japanese Christian author of such works as *Bushidō*], Okuma [Shigenobu] and [Frank] Brinkley [the editor of *Japan's Weekly Mail*]." House himself had declared in his periodical that the paper was the "vehicle of expression for the views of a single person . . . the direct manifestation of his thought and feeling." It seems that both House and Ōkuma were perfectly content to promote the other, either in occupation or in print, and in each other, the changeable statesman and the oft-cantankerous pundit found a kindred spirit, though not necessarily a friend. Ōkuma failed to attend House's 1901 funeral, sending his personal secretary in his stead.[23]

As with Ōkuma, House's personality could be off-putting. His friendships could end as quickly as they began, but even those who found him gratingly caustic admitted that his talents were considerable and his determination impressive. As his colleague and competitor Brinkley recalled, "The great effect which Mr. House's brilliancy and dogged persistency" wrought was that he succeeded in his charges, although his undertaking often cost him considerably. Tokutomi Sohō, another journalist, noted that House had no mind for subtlety, and his methods were like "murdering *tōfu* with a kitchen knife." Yet House's travels brought him into contact with a number of international and influential figures, many of whom remained charmed by the "good fellow, handsome, well-bred, winning in manners," who appeared when House made the effort to be sufficiently charming. He had met and befriended Georges Clemenceau in 1860, and insinuated himself into the bohemian community that met in the vault at Pfaff's pub in New York, which counted among its clientele, besides both Clemenceau and House, Emerson, Greeley, Poe, Whitman, and Twain.[24]

Nevertheless, it seems that, until he met Ōkuma and settled in Japan, House's charm was lavished primarily on the literati. House embraced his role as Ōkuma's bulldog abroad with the same gusto he had shown in publishing. Thus, both employments actually dovetailed nicely. As he wrote to Ōkuma in 1888, his goal was "to keep the facts of Japan's condition before the public of America . . . [and] to create such a state of feeling as will make it essential for the Government at Washington to take notice of the affairs of Japan, and to proffer aid and encouragement to your nation." This would surely benefit evangelists in Japan, as House pushed for equal relations between Japan and the Euro-American powers in discussions with Clemenceau, then a member of France's Chamber of Deputies, and with his opposition. He did the same to Premier Leon Gambetta, E. J. Reed—then a member of England's Parliament and former lord of the Treasury under Gladstone's third

23. Hornbeck, 775; McLaren, 323; Huffman 1987, 235–36.
24. Huffman 1987, 243; Browne, 154; Baldensperger, 18.

premiership—and to both Charles Dickens and Ulysses S. Grant, of whom House wrote, "He belongs to us. . . . He represents the best of what is common to us all."[25]

Ōkuma, backed by the evidence of his champion, House, remained staunchly perched between his compatriots in Japan's government and the elite of the so-called Western powers. In so doing, he placed himself in a position to play each against the other, primarily to his benefit, the true moral entrepreneur.

Yet it seemed that House, *Japan Punch*'s "naughty Yankee boy," was just as concerned with promoting his beliefs as he was with voicing Ōkuma's. The tumult over an 1887 Peace Preservation Law, which prohibited all secret meetings and associations (in addition to confiscating all pamphlets believed to disturb the public peace, seen by many of Japan's foreign evangelists, William Elliot Griffis foremost, as an attack on missionary activity), inspired House's vitriol against evangelists, particularly the actions of Griffis, his former friend and colleague.[26] Missionary activity was "false and injurious," and evangelists' "angry quarrels, in which they often invite publicity . . . their frequent fondness for gain . . . their sharp dealings with the poorer class of tradesmen and laborers, which are notorious wherever they dwell; these and other unpleasant features of their life in Japan are by no means calculated to endear them to the populace." His polemical novel, *Yone Santo*, attacked the evangelical institution in Japan, and pronounced that, try as one character might, he could find no "missionaries whom I could hold in honor, whose characters I could unqualifiedly respect, whose methods of dealing with the Japanese seemed to me worthy of approval," and not a one "in whom the loftier spirit of devotion, unselfishness, and willing sacrifice might be found." The reaction was pronounced, and, as House predicted, "the missionaries will do all they can to tear down my work. How they do buzz and sting!"[27] House was, in the words of Tokutomi Sohō, newspaper raconteur, "a good hater," and refused to hide his animosity, as when he admitted to believing that Japan's foreign evangelists were "lazy people who received money from their homeland, yet did nothing but live by selfish pretence."[28]

While both House and Ōkuma grew to despise Harry Smith Parkes, the British Minister to Japan for almost twenty years, due to the Urakami incident mentioned above and the continuing issue of the unequal treaties, their regard for and relationship with evangelists proved more divisive.[29] Certainly, Ōkuma had been at the forefront of prosecuting (and, indeed, persecuting) Christians early in the Meiji period, but he seemed to have more of an issue, as House had, with the Christians themselves than with the creed or ideology. It was to his credit, therefore, that Ōkuma, regardless of his personal beliefs, proved less myopic than House, and thus still succeeded in convincing Americans, Christians, and especially American Christians of

25. Huffman 2003, 206; WUA, Sept. 3–4, 1881; Huffman 1987, 248; Huffman 2003, 203, 145.
26. Uyehara, 104.
27. Yakhontoff, 308; Huffman 2003, 208–9, 211; House, 145.
28. Huffman 1987, 245.
29. OM: Ōkuma kasōhan, From House to Ōkuma, Meiji 12; Vittinghoff, 332; Burkman, 148; Huffman 1987, 250.

his appreciation of them and their assorted missions, particularly their involvement in Japanese public health, including the fight against tuberculosis.[30]

Should most Americans and, particularly, American evangelists have researched Ōkuma's opinions and statements a bit more, they might have seen, as only a small handful did, that the statesman had the uncanny ability to tell his audience what it wanted to hear. Three years after stating that Christianity had no influence in Japan in 1909, he happily pronounced that the religion, though boasting few adherents, "has poured into every realm of Japanese life."

More significant, Ōkuma included himself among those under the influence of Christianity, even as he pronounced the lack of influence throughout the country. In 1909, when Christian politician and journalist Shimada Saburō, in a text edited by Ōkuma and included in his treatise on modernization, noted not merely the superb influence of "the missionaries and educators, whom the United States sent to Japan . . . [who] were all men of piety, moderation, and good sense," but also emphasized the education of Ōkuma at the hands of one such man, Guido Verbeck. Verbeck and his compatriots, thus, with "their sincerity and kindness produced on the minds of our countrymen a profound impression, such as tended to completely remove the suspicions hitherto entertained towards the Christian religion."[31]

The evangelists savvy enough to do so realized that, like many of his other stances, Ōkuma's attitude towards Christianity in general, and evangelical activity specifically, was utilitarian. But, at times, the fact that Ōkuma never became a Christian seemed paradoxically to undergird the conviction of the evangelists both in the verity of the Christian faith and in Ōkuma's acknowledgement of this truth. That Ōkuma agreed to speak to and work with foreign, Protestant evangelical groups in Japan was indicative of "the power of Christianity" and its "recognition" in Japan. The reception Ōkuma held in honor of YMCA leader Dr. John R. Mott and his colleagues proved that the statesman, though "not in any sense a Christian," truly believed in "the power of Christianity and in the influence of Christians to maintain peace and righteousness in the spirit of brotherly love." Never mind that, had he truly believed in the truth of the word, would not he, too, have converted?[32]

Regardless, Ōkuma was far more welcoming to foreign evangelists than to Japanese Christians. At first this might seem arbitrary, but it was actually quite calculated. Certainly, he had Japanese Christian colleagues, including Shimada, but few domestic Christians were capable of the utility Ōkuma believed their foreign counterparts possessed. In exchange for lip service and nominal private assistance from the pockets of Ōkuma and his monied colleagues, including entrepreneur (and textile mill owner) Shibusawa Eiichi, these men and women undertook work that both fulfilled their need and desire to assist and addressed a public service lacuna in providing for the nation's tubercular that Japan's government had no need or

30. Y. Abe, 122.
31. Robinson, 241; Shimada, 91.
32. "Signs of the Times," 401.

desire to fulfill itself. This lacuna, moreover, became a significant niche for foreign evangelical organizations to supplement proselytizing. By ensuring that foreign evangelists' social work was presented well in their home countries, Ōkuma knew that their domestic supporters would continue to fund their work in Japan. Indeed, it was hardly difficult to declare that William Booth, the founder of the Salvation Army, "would ever be remembered in Japan," and it meant that the Army would continue to pursue the social work on which it prided itself.[33] The significance of this calculation with regard to public health work by Ōkuma will be examined in later chapters; suffice to say, the man was adept in playing individuals as pawns.

The question of whether Ōkuma believed in his statements to foreign evangelical organizations can, of course, be debated, but, in fact, it really did not matter if, as he claimed, "the origin of modern civilization is to be found in the teachings of the sage of Judea, by whom alone the necessary moral dynamic is supplied." Nor did it matter if the Young Men's Christian Association believed that Ōkuma, as "one of the leading statesmen . . . gives his endorsement to the Association," so long as these individuals continued to pursue social work in Japan, even if this work was meant to promote a foreign religion, albeit one that may have supplied "the necessary moral dynamic."[34]

In addition to his vocal approval of these organizations, Ōkuma often indicated a desire to extend his support monetarily and organizationally, although such support never seemed fully to come to fruition. In 1905 both Ōkuma and Shibusawa Eiichi claimed to have been convinced by British evangelist Hannah Riddell's earnest desire to assist those in Japan with Hansen's disease (leprosy). Ōkuma, particularly, declared himself to be stirred by the assistance of foreign aid in caring for Japan's unwell, to which he insisted that Riddell's work must be added. And, in fact, he did provide aid to Riddell's hospitals, donating cherry and maple trees to line the grounds. True, Ōkuma was known for his green thumb, but the arboreal donation was hardly in line with what Riddell had been given to expect. She had been clear about her need for funds, writing to Ōkuma that she desired "the Endowment Fund" for her hospital, and questioned if Ōkuma thought that money would be forthcoming, thus presumably making an indirect request for funds from the statesman as well. Ōkuma did not appear to have donated the funds she wanted. Ten years later, when Ōkuma was once more in office, Riddell sent him a request, thanking him for his earlier assistance but noting that the "great step in the right direction" still demanded Ōkuma "give a little consideration to the important question of how to relieve Japan from the terrible loss which she continuously and increasingly sustains, financially and morally, by the many lepers within her Empire." There is no evidence that Ōkuma responded in kind or as desired, paralleling his lack of response to TB, although Riddell was able to continue her work.[35]

33. SANA: "Japan." *The Salvation Army Year Book*, 1916, 46.
34. Speer, 117; Woodman, 93.
35. OM: Letter from H. Riddell to Ōkuma, Oct. 15, 1915; Tobimatsu, chs. 14–16.

While Riddell never took Ōkuma to task for his potential evasion, other foreigners in Japan were more direct. American teacher and journalist, F. W. Eastlake, by no means otherwise rancorous with respect to Japan, accused Ōkuma of contrarianism, noting that he had "received the enclosed reply (to an enquiry placed to Ōkuma on behalf of the government), which is *quite contrary* to what was written in your Excellency's favour."[36] German translator Baron Alexander von Siebold, too, informed Ōkuma that his missteps had not gone unnoticed. The *London Times*, according to Baron von Siebold, noted that a governmental pamphlet on Japan's financial policy, written by Ōkuma, was equal parts apologist and obfuscatory, "with the evident object of vindicating the policy of the present Government, and of endeavouring to prove that the results obtained quite justify the liabilities which have been incurred."[37] Few were as forward as muckraker Andrew Melville Pooley, who accused Ōkuma of personifying educator Sawayanagi's pronouncement that the Japanese had "no moral courage to help those who are down, or to support those who are oppressed, though they have the physical courage to kick the weak and the defenceless." For Pooley, not only was Ōkuma a notorious vacillator and obscurantist, so, too, had his obfuscation prevented Japan's government from pursuing social work, including that for victims of the tuberculosis epidemic.[38]

But if Ōkuma's characterization as a vacillator, or, more positively, an *Ō-buroshiki* (large carryall) containing promises to various interest groups emboldened by his "Hizen [Province] penchant for vagueness," meant that he lacked the moral courage to help the unfortunate, he nevertheless knew who could aid them, and he ensured their continued assistance within his nation.[39] Regardless of his true feelings about Christianity, Ōkuma was an unabashed devotee of medical missions. Even his bulldog, House, approved of medical missionaries, writing in *Yone Santo* that such men and women were "honest and well disposed, and the least disputatious of mortal men," and whose work "enlarged their understanding and endowed them with broader human sympathies" that their fellow evangelists failed to possess.

Whether Ōkuma found the evangelical peers of medical missionaries as distasteful as House did, he certainly made the effort to encourage, and to allow his name to be attached to, the Salvation Army's hospital and tuberculosis sanatorium and to St. Luke's Hospital, as will be seen in later chapters. Moreover, in the case of St. Luke's, Ōkuma went so far as to submit a joint memorial to the Carnegie Association asking it to fund the Japanese hospital, promising that it would "exert in a most practical way far-reaching influence for International Peace." More influential than the possibility of achieving world peace, however, was the "very obvious gap" St. Luke's was filling as it provided a "thoroughly modern hospital under foreign

36. OM: Letter from Eastlake to Ōkuma, Jan. 8, 1892.
37. OM: Letter from Siebold to Ōkuma. Aug. 4, 1881, including *London Times* article "Japanese Finance," from June 27, 1881.
38. Sawayanagi, 167; Pooley, 344.
39. Lebra, 147–48.

management where the nursing, diet, heating, sanitary arrangements, and control of the patients are best suited for the care of foreigners and where they may at once secure the services of the best specialist in the city if necessary," since "the heating, sanitary arrangements and general regime in a Japanese hospital are not satisfactory for the care of a foreigner." Although, presumably, Japanese nationals needed less sanitation and heat, Ōkuma and his cosigners noted that, since "none of these hospitals (currently in Tokyo, both private and governmental) . . . are conducted as are general hospitals in America where a patient may call in consultation any reputable physician, or specialist, as the case may demand," St. Luke's also required "50 charity beds for the city and a large free dispensary giving treatment to 100 or more charity cases a day." Since only 150 beds were planned for the hospital, the memorial was requesting that one-third of the inpatient facilities be provided free of charge. Moreover, as there were few truly impoverished foreigners in Japan at that time, let alone in Tokyo, it is hardly surprising that these beds would be occupied by Japanese subjects. With funding coming from outside Japan's government, the hospital could afford, as planned, at least three foreign doctors and six Japanese physicians, selected entirely from graduates of the Imperial University of Tokyo. It would also be able to afford, in expectation of proper funding, consultations with professors at the University and with "the Imperial Government Laboratory, under the direction of Professor Kitazato [*sic*]," undoubtedly Japan's most renowned medical scientist at the time. And, again, despite the original point that the hospital was necessary for Japan's foreign residents, the composers of the memorial concluded that "a hospital built in Tokyo in the interest of international peace, largely through the generosity of Americans" was truly desired by the Japanese (for whom the hospital had been deemed unnecessary some seven pages earlier). St. Luke's was a Japanese utilitarian venture, and one that, through the hard work of Ōkuma, could serve as a public relations boon. Through his dedication to utilitarianism, Ōkuma had successfully courted evangelical organizations to commit funds and personnel to combat national health issues, including tuberculosis, that the savvy politician had seemed to ignore.[40]

Certainly, St. Luke's International Hospital might have been desired by the Japanese, and it certainly did assist foreign nationals in Japan, but it did not prove extremely necessary for their care, despite assurances to the contrary, since presumably they could afford care anywhere. Ōkuma was not unaware of this fact; moreover, he knew it was his fellow countrymen and women who would benefit from the creation of effective charity hospitals to fill the lapses in the social welfare system of the Japanese state.

40. House 10, 146; "General Missionary Intelligence," 952; "Notes, News and Gleanings," 94; "The Church and The World: Missions," 424; "An International Hospital for Tokyo: Memorial to the Trustees of the Carnegie Endowment," 77–84.

The actions (and inaction) of Japan's government were predicated on utility. As philosopher and educator John Dewey observed during his post–World War I visit to Japan, the nation's industrial transition was hasty:

> In 1918 alone the number of factories in Tokyo doubled in spite of extraordinary increases in prior years. The last five years have practically transformed Japan from an agrarian into an industrial state. For there is today actual shortage of farm labor in that country, although the wages of farm hands have more than doubled. The urban factories have been absorbing labor at such a rate that for the time being at least the old plea for territorial expansion to take up the growth of population does not hold. In consequence of this expedited development Japan has been plunged into the labor problem—and plunged with exceedingly little preparation.
>
> The remote and speculative observer is given to supposing that a new country which is undergoing the industrial revolution at this late date will surely learn from the experience of the other countries that passed through it earlier. Why wait for all the evils of child labor, woman's labor, long hours, unsanitary factories, congested housing, slums, and so forth to show themselves, when experience has demonstrated how surely they follow upon a laissez-faire policy, and also how legislation and administration may at least alleviate their worst evils? Especially would it seem as if a paternalistic government like that of Japan would do something, if only because of the general influence exercised by her model, Germany. But practically no foresight was manifested. Certain factory laws on the Western pattern were indeed passed, but their execution was postponed for a term of years—up to twelve—on the plea of giving capital a chance to adjust itself. As a matter of fact, greed for immediate profits irrespective of ultimate results has taken possession of industrial Japan. . . .
>
> It was a cynical Japanese—there aren't many—who told me that Japan's factory legislation was solely for the benefit of the Westerner. Being tired of telling curious visiting foreigners that Japan had no labor laws, they put some on the statute-book and suspended their execution for the most part. . . . The effect of this absence of regulation in conjunction with the rapid development of industry and trade during the past five years has been what every Westerner would have foretold. The labor crisis has arrived and it is unmitigated, acute.[41]

In the fight against tuberculosis, as part of the labor crisis, outsourcing the solution to foreign medical missionaries permitted government officials to save government funds while addressing the epidemic, as Ōkuma and his cronies were no doubt aware. Morality, meanwhile, was the self-proclaimed purview of Japan's foreign evangelical groups, and it was with this in mind that so many evangelists hoped to ameliorate the conditions in which the emperor's subjects lived. Many, however, first found a land that was more willing to welcome them if they addressed other needs first.

41. Dewey, 161–64.

5

"The Nazareth of the Orient"

The Particular Work of the Evangelists

For many Western evangelists, Meiji Japan seemed, if not a promised land, certainly a promising land. In it they sensed both a need and a yearning for salvation among an intelligent populace they believed was desperate to ameliorate its ignorance. And, for most evangelists, the desire to assist in that salvation was neither naive nor imperious but was motivated by a deep faith in the rectitude of their beliefs and a true devotion to their mission. Often highly educated, these men and women volunteered for the difficult life of the evangelist, many turning down a myriad of other opportunities, including evangelical work closer to home. One such person was William Merrell Vories, whose work we shall consider in a later chapter. Vories trained as an architect yet still planned to pioneer evangelism in "some Nazareth of the Orient where no missionary enterprise had ever been established, or would ever be established otherwise."[1]

Nevertheless, as Vories evidenced, the desire to serve did not preclude the desire to merit acclaim. For evangelists, working for the common good also included working for one's own benefit, regardless of whether personal preference was defined by an aesthetic or ascetic life. So, too, did it include the good of the nation, although what evangelists considered that to be did not necessarily correspond to the considerations of the government, as defined by many of the government's employees, as I shall discuss later. What the common good did seemingly preclude was often the specific goals of other, though not of all other, missions.[2] The desire to serve, therefore, did not prevent a sense of competition with other missions, particularly those affiliated with other Christian sects.

Complicating the competition was the fact that its currency was denominated in the souls of Japanese converts. This soteriological value was the basis for moral entrepreneurship with the evangelists. This was obviously a slippery measure. Besides the difficulties of haggling over actors, not objects, evangelists in Japan and back home had no standard by which to measure success. What constituted

1. Vories 1936, 7.
2. Ransome, 108. This, however, was natural, as many felt that those who subscribed to a "false" religion or "false" interpretation of the same religion were much further beyond educating in the "correct" religion or interpretations than those wholly ignorant of, in this case, Christ's gospel. Thus, while not wishing other missionaries ill, there existed a tendency in Japan to focus evangelical work solely on the Japanese populace.

victory? Conversion generally indicated an individual saved, but converts were difficult to define and even more difficult to procure. Victory also meant an increase in donations and income for the mission, but the monetary economy and the human economy were not necessarily symbiotic, as we shall see. What many evangelical organizations discovered was that in Japan there was a fine balance between attracting converts domestically and acquiring funds abroad. This would become even more important in medical missionary work, as among the victims of tuberculosis. Yet, as conversion rates rose, or were perceived to rise, evangelical supporters in the States often assumed that domestic income would supersede their donations. This, however, was rarely the case. In part, this was the nature of the work: most converts lacked the funds of the wealthy philanthropists abroad. More important, however, was the fact that all evangelical organizations promoted supplemental programs, from English lessons to the sporting events that distinguished the "muscular Christianity" of the YMCA, and many counted mere participants as professing Christians.[3] This was somewhat disingenuous. The majority of the Japanese subjects who attended the extrareligious offerings of the evangelical organizations did not consider themselves Christian, nor did they intend to become Christians.[4]

Nevertheless, as no coercion was involved, those who attended extrareligious events were identifying themselves as supporters of the organization, though not necessarily ideologically or economically. And, in a country with a history of hostility toward Christianity, evangelists marked this support as a significant triumph. In many ways, this became analogous to the relationship between many evangelical organizations and the Japanese state.[5] Rather than professing belief in Christ, such supporters maintained a belief in the efficacy of Christianity. Just as Ōkuma was staunchly not a follower of Christ, he was a believer in the effectiveness and utility of evangelists in Japan. Still, at best, such a believer was, in the words of Motoda Sakunoshin, the first Japanese Anglican Bishop, "the Pseudo-Christian," who might "believe in ethical Christianity but know(s) nothing of spiritual Christianity."[6] Despite Motoda's disappointment, "Pseudo-Christians" would become the most important Japanese figures in the maintenance of the evangelical movement in Japan, particularly in work with the tubercular.

The very existence of "Pseudo-Christians" among the public enabled a number of Japanese government officials to reconsider their hostility to the cultural

3. I. Abe, 119.
4. That sentiment can be deemed somewhat moot, as many people who convert to a religion begin to study it without intending to convert. Nevertheless, the majority of the Japanese subjects discussed above continued to attend organizational events and programs without showing an interest in converting to Christianity. For most, it seems, the activities and services offered filled the void that evangelists hoped Christianity would.
5. It is important to note the difference between evangelical organizations and churches in Japan, particularly with regard to the relationship to the Japanese polity. Most evangelical organizations had foreign connections that many churches lacked, either in terms of foreign leadership or counterparts. Thus, the relationship between the government and the YMCA or the Salvation Army is not mirrored by that of the government and, say, Uchimura Kanzō's mukyōkai.
6. "Attitude of the Japanese People towards Christianity," 146.

imperialism they feared manifested by the evangelical presence. Among the offerings of the evangelists were linguistic training, physical fitness, moral education, and, eventually, medical work, all of which contributed to a populace that assisted the nation in its quest to modernize along the lines of the Euro-American colonial powers. To lose a few individuals to a foreign religion that placed its god above the nation was not desirable, of course, but neither was it unacceptable. So long as the foreign Christians did not attack the government itself, there was little harm in allowing them a handful of converts.[7] What proved particularly appealing was the fact that the potential betterment of the populace, whether spiritual or physical, was funded by the evangelists and their supporters, and not by government coffers. Moreover, at little to no cost to the government, apart from its tacit acknowledgment of Christianity, were the beneficial international relations it could nevertheless claim to have fostered by utilizing the work of the evangelists.

Both organizational perquisites of moral enterprise, endorsing the state good and the evangelical good, promoting modernization and providing independent funding, were further enhanced by the introduction of medical missionary work. Certainly, evangelical organizations had long offered spiritual therapy for the infirm, but the existence of evangelist-funded dispensaries had failed to interest government officials early in the Meiji period. This was due less to the nature of the work than the timing and intended recipients of the evangelical enterprises, the utility of this work to its beneficiaries. It was not so much that the work itself was different or better than previous attempts, but it was seen as more useful than previous attempts. After all, in order to make the work palatable to a still-unwelcoming land, missionaries needed to be seen as utilitarian. Indeed, Dr. James Curtis Hepburn, one of the first Protestant medical missionaries to Japan, garnered political renown not from his busy dispensary or his later appointment as head of a Christian medical school, but for his popularization of a romanization system for the Japanese language. This early indifference was hardly surprising. After all, many evangelical organizations themselves thought that there was far less of a need for such extrareligious work in Japan than in the rest of Asia. Hepburn's own Presbyterian Church soon abandoned his medical position, preferring to employ evangelists who specialized in teaching and moral suasion.[8] Nevertheless, while many foreign evangelical organizations saw Japan as a nation desperately in need of spiritual guidance, they felt that it had become equal to their motherlands in terms of medical practice. The Japanese government, however, knew differently, aware that while knowledge was great, deficits

7. Indeed, the occasions of such were rare among foreign evangelists, who avoided Japanese politics. To have addressed political issues publicly was not a necessity in saving Japanese subjects, and, depending on the legislation of the time, could have seriously affected their work, to the point of imprisonment or extradition. Unlike foreign evangelists, Japanese Christians were rarely as taciturn, although, again, many were both savvy enough and compartmentalized enough to avoid addressing issues that would have proved too incendiary for the government to ignore.
8. Griffis 1913, 125; Whitney, 347; and Bradt et al., 423–25; Gordon, 172.

in distribution and lack of equity were still greater, as the tuberculosis epidemic could testify to.

Japanese scientists excelled at medical research, and the Meiji government had urged many researchers to pursue their investigations abroad, at the finest laboratories in Germany and America. In addition, toward its goal of *fukoku kyōhei* (rich country, strong army), the government had employed many of its top physicians in military medicine. Thus, while many physicians were occupied in research or military medicine, most of the populace lacked even the most basic level of medical care. Indeed, thirty years after the Meiji Restoration, only 136 public hospitals existed to serve almost forty-five million subjects.[9] There were, of course, private hospitals, but as one bedridden doctor, Kondō Tsunejirō, remarked,

> As for the [private] hospital, it is exactly like a brothel that is greedy for profit. The sick who should be pitied are viewed as shady characters. They will not be set free until they have emptied their pockets. The assets of the average man, earned over ten years, would be completely exhausted when his wife enters the hospital for a single stay. . . . The attitude of the hospital director is like that of the madame of the establishment, while the staff doctors and clerks are like accountants and bouncers, respectively, and the nurses are like prostitutes who have just started in the business.[10]

Their opposition to brothels notwithstanding, the state of Japanese public health provided a niche in which to work for those evangelical organizations willing to dedicate the necessary resources but a bargaining chip, namely moral entrepreneurship, with which to relate to the Japanese government.

Such was the appeal of this niche and bargaining chip that organizations did attempt to accumulate the resources needed to perform such work. While obtaining staff and funds abroad was an arduous task for any evangelical group, those offering a medical missionary branch also faced far greater difficulties acquiring buildings and equipment domestically. Foreigners were not allowed to enter into land contracts in Japan until 1899, which made early attempts to establish missionary centers, let alone hospitals, difficult without a willing Japanese intermediary. Even with the issues of legality cleared, many landlords or sellers remained unwilling to engage foreigners. Neither were medical appurtenances readily available, least of all to unknown interlopers in the community.[11] When the wife of Protestant Episcopal bishop John McKim prepared the small house that was to be the first home of St. Luke's Hospital in Tsukiji, Tokyo, before medical missionary Rudolf Teusler's arrival in 1902, she lamented, "How dismal the little hospital seemed when we went in—it was so small, so barren, so forlorn. We did our best to cheer up the rooms with flowers, and a few homelike arrangements, but could not help wondering how the

9. Anesaki, 58; Ikegami, 125; Longford, 17.
10. Irako, 19; Burns, 173.
11. "Proceedings," 111; Gordon, 87.

place might impress the Doctor fresh from the wonderfully equipped hospitals at home."[12]

Despite these impediments, evangelical organizations hoped to maintain a standard far above their means (or the means which they were allowed). As Dr. John Cross, stationed in China, argued at the Central Presbyterian Church meeting on April 30, 1900 in New York:

> No medical missionary should be without a hospital, with a good supply of surgical instruments. It seems to me cruel and unchristian to send a man who has a medical degree to any place, and say to him, practically, "You must exercise your science, remove your tumors, set your broken limbs, cure the fevers as best you can with the title at the end of your name, or little else."[13]

The disconnect between the desires of the evangelical organization headquarters and the reality of the situation in which evangelists in the field found themselves continued, often until the prospects became so prohibitively expensive as to require immediate action. In part, organization headquarters needed the medical missionaries' work to continue—not merely for its proselytizing potential, but also because their institutions were frequently the only ones in which foreigners, including evangelists, felt comfortable seeking treatment and convalescing. It was to Teusler's credit, therefore, that he was able to build a working hospital from the small house he was given, as his became one of the most famous medical missionary enterprises in Japan, if not in East Asia. (We shall meet Dr. Teusler again in a later chapter.)

It was also a testament to the power of the "Pseudo-Christians" who recognized the great service evangelists were performing with regard to public health. As awareness of the hospitals grew, so too did the assistance provided by the wealthier Japanese subjects. This was often given as much out of a charitable impulse as out of a self-serving one. Such a sentiment ruled the minds of a few government officials as well. Unlike a donation to a church, such gifts could be seen as assisting all subjects, regardless of religious conviction. They could also be seen as promoting cross-cultural relationships. Thus, a small handful of Japanese politicians chose to donate (and donate vociferously) to evangelical organizations as "private" citizens. Doing so allowed them the freedom to garner the rewards of encouraging international relations and assisting the national welfare without the potential imbroglio that could arise from trying to push for charitable funding politically. Moreover, in donating as individuals, these men could dissimulate as though they were merely philanthropists, not seeking political gain from their donations. They could present themselves as officials who felt so strongly about Japan's welfare that they were unwilling to chance sacrificing it by politicizing it, a clear instance of moral entrepreneurship. Take Ōkuma, for example, whose donation of trees to Riddell's mission among the victims of Hansen's disease could be seen as supporting missionary work privately.

12. Robbins, et al., 29.
13. "HEATHEN CRUELTY."

Nevertheless, evangelically promoted public health remained enough of a controversial prospect that many were reluctant to provide monetary gifts without also limiting its prospective beneficiaries to those politically acknowledged to be in the national interest, specifically the Japanese military forces. With the stipulation that the donations fund evangelical assistance to Japan's fighting men, more top Japanese officials were willing to be identified by evangelical organizations as "Pseudo-Christians." Again, to do so was also seen as promoting international relations, and it was not as suspect or as politically controversial as donating to an evangelical dispensary in some working class slum. It was with this intent that the imperial household, intended to be viewed as transcending politics, donated a few times to such organizations, as for instance when it presented the YMCA with a gift of 10,000 yen on April 19, 1921, for its work with Japanese soldiers (and their Soviet prisoners of war) on an extended, and governmentally unpopular, deployment in Siberia following World War I and the Bolshevik Revolution.[14]

Let us not forget that, above all, this was the epitome of moral entrepreneurship. By supporting foreign work, which might otherwise appear suspect, the imperial house was promoting its moral suasion and appeal, just as the foreign evangelists, by working on an unpopular expedition, were. Both the imperial family and the YMCA could then proclaim itself to be sacrificing money or work for Japan's greater good, here represented by the deployed soldiers.

The success of work with the military, however, meant that evangelical organizations, gratified by the growing acknowledgment of influential Japanese officials of the organizations' utility to the armed forces of Japan, often abandoned plans to initiate or to continue public health promotion outside Japan's army bases. From the first recognition of such work during the Sino-Japanese War of 1894–1895, many evangelical organizations placed their hopes for acceptance in their assistance to Japan's war effort, in terms of charitable donations, and winning souls. They were assisted by their pronouncements of ideological support for Japan's wars. In his polemic *What Shall I Think of Japan?*, George Gleason, YMCA secretary in Japan, wrote not only for foreign Christians but also for domestic officials when he proclaimed that the "outbreak of hostilities [in 1894] does not show that Japan had any other desire than self-protection," and that "Japan's demands were the customary rewards of successful conflicts with China, as the dealings of the European nations with the Celestial Empire clearly prove." Where their Japanese Christian compatriots were often the loudest voices denouncing Japan's modern wars as imperialist (particularly those after the Sino-Japanese War)—as did Uchimura Kanzō, whom we will discuss below—foreign evangelists were quick to voice their support, both to demonstrate their allegiance to their new home and to promote sympathies abroad for purposes of fund-raising. Indeed, Gleason's epigraph provides his own

14. This was not even one-sixtieth of the cost of the services provided, to add a bit of perspective.
KFA: Letter from S. Saito to A. C. Bookwalter. May 12, 1921.
KFA: "Imperial Grant to The Y.M.C.A." The Japan Times and Mail. Wednesday, Apr. 20, 1921. p. 8.

thoughts on the subject: "The people of Japan are too often disliked, or as they say 'misunderstood.' Neither they nor their neighbors fully comprehend the reason. Dare we Americans delay a sympathetic attempt to interpret her struggles and help Japan find her place among the family of nations?"[15]

That the organizations' leadership in Japan was insistent in its support of the nation in the Japanese press was hardly surprising, particularly given the tumultuous history of evangelical-Japanese relations. Nor was it odd to promote the Japanese in Western periodicals as a people similar to their Western counterparts, especially for fund-raising purposes, as few wanted to assist a truly alien nation, no matter how desperately ignorant of salvation it was thought to be, either spiritually or medically. What was interesting was the need evangelical organizations' leadership (particularly those strongly affiliated with larger international umbrella organizations like the YMCA) felt to present Japan as a nation interested only in self-defense. To continue work within a nation perceived to be bellicose was to risk curtailment by their headquarters, either because such work was seen as wholly anti-Christian and hopeless or because it was deemed too dangerous. This was to prove even more pressing during the Russo-Japanese War of 1904–1905 (a conflict we will discuss at length below), as Japan was fighting a Christian empire, albeit a Russian Orthodox one. Evangelists were assisted by then prime minister Katsura Tarō, who assured Christians worldwide that Japan's fight was not based in antagonism to Russia as a Christian nation, merely to it as an aggressor. His assurances were manifested further by his earlier establishment of the Anglo-Japanese Alliance in 1902, which evangelists could identify as proof that Japan was not the anti-Christian nation its opponents, most stridently Russia, claimed it to be. As evangelist Daniel Crosby Greene remonstrated, "The so-called abyss which separates the Japanese from the peoples of the West is far less wide and deep than is often supposed. The common ground of humanity on which we all stand is broad and firm. It is not difficult to reach and when reached affords a solid basis upon which to build the structure of a warm and sympathetic social intercourse."

Indeed, Japan's experience in the war proved notable not merely for its victory but for its own, far more decisive humanitarian work.[16] Japan's entrance onto the charitable stage during the Russo-Japanese War was, in many ways, astonishing. Already less than half a century since the Meiji Restoration, Japan's branch of the International Red Cross was the largest in the world, with over nine hundred thousand members. This impressive figure is both somewhat misleading and also indicative of the national conception of humanitarian work. First, membership in the organization was seen by the government as obligatory for those ineligible for compulsory military conscription. Though such a mandate was difficult to enforce, the

15. Y.M.C.A. shi, 22; Kowner, 22; Gleason, 52; K. Lee, 158; Gleason, frontispiece.

16. Though many of the evangelical organizations purport to be nondenominational, they remained staunchly Protestant. Thus, such organizations had little contact with the Russian Orthodox Church, which did have its own missionaries in Japan. Parker, 64; Greene 1904, 11; Checkland, 64; Yokote, 177.

fact that nominal leadership posts were held by imperial family members, including the imperial couple, meant that many subjects subscribed on the basis of perceived imperial sanction alone. Each war won or national tragedy overcome also swelled the ranks. Moreover, the Japanese Red Cross Society (JRCS) remained at the behest of the government, and worked under the auspices of the War Department. One can clearly see the level of national responsibility vested in the JRCS in the statement of Dr. Ariga Nagao, international law professor and (as ordered by the war ministry) drafter of the JRCS' wartime regulations:

> In Japan the Emperor is the personal leader of the nation in arms, and the soldiers are his soldiers, not in theory only, but by the fact of historical tradition. Hence the nation, which loves and respects the Emperor literally as children do their fathers, naturally loves the soldiers whom the Emperor cherishes so much, and does everything in its power to help them in order to please the Emperor by so doing. We owe to the Emperor the independence and prosperity of the empire, which he maintains by means of his soldiers, and the best means of paying back this immeasurable debt is to give aid to his soldiers while risking their lives on the field of battle.

The fact that the JRCS became financially solvent under the presidency of the nation's most successful finance minister, Matsukata Masayoshi, moreover, indicates how tightly the organization was tied to the government.[17] That a government would mandate philanthropy or that a war office would control humanitarian efforts did not strike Japan's leaders as unusual. Nor did it seem misguided that the philanthropy would be aimed toward the war effort and not necessarily toward those struggling in other "wars," including that against epidemic disease on the home front—namely, tuberculosis. The JRCS became a huge boon to Japan's image worldwide during the Russo-Japanese War, and, as such, attracted and required government involvement and control.

One of the most important aspects of government efforts to control the JRCS was the symbolism behind the organization. Although the Ottoman Empire introduced the use of a red crescent as an emblem for the work of the International Red Cross, seeking to assuage Muslims that the work performed by the organization was neither limited to nor dependent upon Christians, the Japanese government, as organizers of the national Red Cross society, did not feel the need to alter the symbol of the red cross on a white background. Instead, it sought to separate the image, and thus, the mission, from Christianity. The red cross (and the Red Cross), therefore, became a national symbol in 1887, representing national values, strength, and jurisdiction.[18] While a boon to Japan's national image, both at home and abroad, such a tactic confused the nation's evangelists. Was it a denial of Christian values?

17. Checkland, 8–9; McCaul, 30–31; Hutchinson, 208; Seaman, 144; Kawamata, 419.
18. In many ways, this is an organizational analogue to Andersonian constructs of national consciousness (Anderson, 37). While the methods used for such a task are beyond the purview of the current work, for an excellent analysis of this phenomenon, see N. Margaret Kosuge, particularly "The 'Non-religious' Red Cross Emblem and Japan." Benthall, 160; Kosuge, 77–79.

Or was it a claim that Christian values mirrored and were mirrored by Japanese values, despite the denial of the religion's authority?

In the face of this uncertainty, Japan's evangelists renewed their efforts to present themselves as being of service to the nation. Regardless of Japan's own humanitarianism, their role was to enhance the good within Japan itself, to instill Christian morality within the nation without undermining Japan's own authority. Rather than work on campaigns that might embarrass the host nation, such as open attacks on prostitution or combating shamefully high industrial disease casualties, including those of tuberculosis, many foreign evangelists took the opportunity of the war to demonstrate their support of Japan, and thus embrace moral entrepreneurship. Sidney L. Gulick, of the American Board of Commissioners for Foreign Missions, reiterated the modern evangelist (and Protestant) goal in his 1905 analysis of the Russo-Japanese War by differentiating it from that of the Portuguese Jesuit missionaries to Japan of the sixteenth century. In his treatise *The White Peril in the Far East*, Gulick proclaimed that "it is safe to say that no form of Christianity which seeks to subordinate the state to the Church will ever find permanent lodgment in Japan. She builded [*sic*] better than she knew in excluding from her land an organized religion with political aspirations."

So, too, did evangelists utilize Japanese humanitarian efforts to emphasize the putatively Christian morals that they hoped undergirded the nation. After all, by 1912 the Japanese government had sponsored Christianity as one of the eponymous "three religions" of the "Three Religions Conference" (the other two being Buddhism and Shinto).[19] Similarly, they pointed to the JRCS' activities as evidence of a merciful nature. As Gulick proclaimed, "the Red Cross Society truly stands for a national movement and the national spirit," but this spirit was one that evangelists believed had not existed previously. What changed, then, was the acquisition of an appreciation of the "regard for others as individuals with rights and feelings such as we ourselves possess." This appreciation—which fed national values that, regardless of whether they were recognized as Christian by Japan's government—was, evangelists like Gulick believed, sparked by the permeation of Christianity within the nation.

This was not only what evangelists claimed but what they knew that their headquarters and domestic contributors desired. While a number of their Western peers feared a proverbial "clash of civilizations," which they felt was evidenced by the Russo-Japanese War, many evangelists saw the war as an opportunity to redefine the split thought inherent between the occident and the orient. In their view, Japan, with seemingly new values instilled by Christianity, was no longer threateningly "oriental," having transcended "her gross superstitions, her ancient polytheism, her unethical religions, and her empty ceremonials."[20]

---

19. Ion 1999, 84.
20. S. Gulick 1905, 14, 105–8, 122.

As suggested above, the Russo-Japanese War of 1904–1905 provided Japan with the opportunity to prove how successful it had been at Westernizing and Japan's foreign evangelists with the chance to prove their utility and their merit to Japan. As a heightening of the evangelical embrace of moral entrepreneurship, which we discussed previously, and as the occasion for the growth of medical work among evangelists (the nature of which will be discussed later), the war proved a significant moment in Japanese history. Its importance thus extended beyond the momentous achievement of the nation's military-industrial complex. Yet, like the achievements of the nation itself, Japan's evangelists required time and energy thereafter to reshape their relationship both with the nation's government, and with each other.

To begin with, in order to convey both how much Japan had changed and its potential for future change, evangelists needed to portray the nation in the best light possible. After all, in order for the moral enterprise to work, both sides needed to view the other as a near equal, slightly less civilized than itself, to justify the work performed by the other on behalf of the nation. The one had to see the other as requiring the charity of the former. The work of the JRCS did, indeed, make this considerably easier. But such a portrayal also required that evangelists utilize the war to paint a clear polarity between the Japanese and the Russians. Never mind that, in order for the Japanese Red Cross to be as effective as possible, the Japanese government repeatedly emphasized that Japan's opponents were not the Russian people but their government; for the evangelists, Russia and not merely its government had to become Gulick's eponymous "white peril in East Asia." Similarly, the fight against a domestic scourge had to take a backseat while worlds collided.

To paint such an image meant not only assuaging potential racial fears of Japan but also stoking the flames of bigotry against the Russian Orthodox Church, which practiced under the auspices of the czar's government. In the former task (though not the latter), evangelists were assisted by Japanese officials. On May 27, 1904, in an interview with the English-language periodical *Japan Mail*, Prime Minister Katsura proclaimed that while the war's object was for "the security of the empire and the permanent peace of the East, I say also and with equal emphasis, that the war is not a war for the supremacy of race over race or of religion over religion. With differences of race or religion it has nothing to do; and it is carried on in the interests of justice, humanity, and the commerce and civilisation of the world." It is interesting to note, however, that Katsura precedes his assurances with a comparison to the Greco-Persian Wars of the fifth century BCE, insofar as "the position of Japan is closely analogous to that of ancient Greece in her contest with Persia; a contest for the security of Greece and the permanent peace of Europe. Japan is Greece and Russia is Persia."

Ōkuma furthered Katsura's metaphor by pronouncing that "Oriental as Japan is in her geographical situation, she, none the less, identifies herself with the progress of the world, and cheerfully adjusts her interests to those of humanity and peace. The conduct of her soldiers during the war must also have shown their moral constitution to be akin to that of their European brothers, for they added the chivalrous refinement of the Athenian to the invincible fortitude of the Spartan." Ōkuma, known for his gregariousness, often at the cost of forethought, could perhaps have been questioned on his use of the term "adjusts," implying that Japan's earliest impulses may not have been as humanitarian as presented. He counters this soon after, however, by claiming that "the rigorous discipline of *Bushidō* had taught the Japanese soldier not only to be brave in battle, but also to be considerate to his enemy."[21] In any case, the racial notions of clashing civilizations that had become so prominent in the minds of intellectuals and politicians around the turn of the twentieth century loom even larger in the philosophies of Japan's ideologues, precisely because legitimization of global power required them. As far as antipathy to Russian Orthodoxy, however, the evangelists were on their own.

Like Katsura, Japanese officials were unwilling to denounce the Russian Orthodox Church, particularly in the Western press. Indeed, then bishop Nikolai, Japan's first Russian Orthodox missionary, later canonized by the Russian Orthodox Church for his work in Japan, felt secure enough to stay in Tokyo throughout the war, and urged his congregation to pray for Japan's victory. Nevertheless, in order to remain relevant to their headquarters and donors, Protestant evangelists needed to separate Russian Orthodoxy from Christianity and deny it any positive involvement in Japan. There was no way that men like Nikolai could be credited with the same permeation of Christian values for which they honored themselves. Certainly, in terms of numbers, there was no contest between the influence of Russian Orthodoxy and that of the various sects of Protestantism, who haphazardly banded together for their survival. Similarly, unlike many of its Protestant counterparts, the Russian Orthodox Church lacked a clear missionary protocol and a grassroots base from which to draw funds.[22] But the Orthodox Church's true offense in the eyes of men like Gulick was its association with the czar's rule. Because it remained under the thumb of an autocrat, it could not truly be Christian. To evidence as much, Gulick reported one specific incidence in which a group of fifteen Russian prisoners of war wrote an open letter to Emperor Meiji via the Japanese press requesting that, once the war ended, they might be able to become Japanese citizens. While such an event may not be seen as an overt attack on the Russian Orthodox Church, Gulick provided a small detail on which his indictment turned. The prisoners, he mentioned parenthetically, were Jews.

To be sure, Russian Jews had little to look forward to at home. While Jews were no longer forced to serve as cantonists, conscripted into the czar's army for some twenty-five years, Russia's antisemitism was infamous worldwide. The "success" of the Kishinev pogrom of 1903 provided the momentum for some 650 more pogroms throughout Russia's Pale of Settlement for the next three years. Faced with continuing violence at home and on the frontlines, why would Jews return to a homeland

21. Imbrie, 208–9; S. Gulick 1905, 163; Imbrie 207; Ōkuma 1909, 52–53.
22. Pospielovsky, 169; Wilson, et al., 2; Stolberg, 287.

that made its distaste for them so clear? Indeed, it also prompted Jewish American banker and businessman Jacob Schiff to assist in bankrolling the Japanese war effort. The history of Russian antipathy toward the Jews allowed Gulick the evidence to suppose that the Orthodox Church in Russia lacked the very basic Christian values that all sects of Christianity were to uphold. While Sergei Witte, Russia's chairman of the Committee of Ministers and, later, prime minister, claimed in his memoirs that it was the Church and its teachings which kept Russians from complete savagery and "distinguishes the Russian people from beasts," Gulick denied this distinction, deeming the Church "the disturber who claimed to carry to the heathen the religion of the Christ. . . . The white peril . . . cloaks its crimes with the very religion which condemns them."[23] It was in Japan, then, Gulick believed, that these prisoners saw the authentic essence of Christianity, for it was in this nation that, despite lacking the conversion rates to suggest it, true Christianity was gaining power.[24]

Yet Christianity was simultaneously also losing power. Many of Japan's earliest converts, young former samurai and members of the intelligentsia, Kenneth Pyle's "new generation," had dabbled in Christianity in their youth, like the so-called "Kumamoto Band," only to commit apostasy upon reaching maturity. Each ideological threat had to be counteracted or coopted to assure the success of the moral enterprise: disaffection among former Christians, rationalism, Darwinism, and so on.

For many, the reason for this rejection lay in a realization of the very goal they had wished to achieve by conversion in the first place. At the beginning of the Meiji era, Christianity became a way for young men to individuate themselves after losing their social cachet with the self-destruction of the samurai class. While most of these students went to mission schools and missionaries for purposes of English language acquisition and a general understanding of Western ideologies, many saw within Christianity a validation of the individual, both in the abstract and in the literal. As young men wrestling to find their place within a particularly protean society, Christianity seemed to offer not only that identity, and that place, but also a chance for these boys to thumb their noses at their elders, as many youths are wont to do.[25] Yet some of the most outspoken of these youths grew up to be some of the most outspoken apostates. It seemed that too many still saw Christianity as a means to an end, and that end was not their own salvation. Certainly, some students did mature within the faith, and a few, like Ebina Danjō, became very famous throughout Japan for their works and their views. Nevertheless, faced with prolific apostates like Tokutomi Sohō and equally prolific heretics like Uchimura Kanzō, evangelists in Japan suffered pointed critiques. Such critiques could call into question the entire

23. S. Gulick, 1905, 103; Lambroza, 287; Falk, 651; Best, 315; Witte, 191; S. Gulick, 1905, 153.
24. Indeed, it was in Japan that Christianity was proving enticing to Jews. For Gulick, this was a double coup, despite the fact that Eastern European Jews had far lower conversion rates than their Western European counterparts. In any case, it remains moot, as I have been unable to uncover these prisoners' postwar fate.
25. Pyle, 5; Lee, 71; Harris, 36; Gordon, 55; Scheiner, 54–60.

moral enterprise, on both sides, the Japanese and the Christian, even before questioning the efficacy of the medical mission.

For Tokutomi Sohō, conversion had been an act born out of peer pressure and of admiration for his teacher, Captain L. L. Janes (about whom, more below), but his apostasy emerged from much self-reflection. The teachings of Christianity were not at odds with his beliefs, but he could not "feel the intimacy with Christ that is the backbone of Christianity." The religion was empty, and his relationship with it, as he was quick to note in a memoir, "had no meaning." As Tokutomi Sohō renounced his previous allegiance to and affiliation with Christianity, Uchimura Kanzō had already dismissed ties to foreign evangelical organizations.[26] In the evangelical organizations both in Japan and of the world, Uchimura saw cultural imperialism and greed, neither of which had any basis in Christianity. For Uchimura, the word of Christ was pure, but it was the interference of man that adulterated Christianity. In this view, regardless of the righteous motives of their members, these missionary groups answered not to the almighty God but to the almighty dollar. In relying on these groups for their salvation, Japan's Christians were belittling both themselves and their faith. Both halves of this base equation fed the other, producing a sordid symbiosis, as Uchimura illustrated in his memoir, *How I Became a Christian*, in his description of a missionary meeting in New England (which he disparagingly deemed a "show"):

> The worst lot in these shows falls to some specimens of converted heathens who happen to be there. They are sure to be made good use of, as circus-men make use of tamed rhinoceroses. They are fetched up for shows; and such wonderful shows! Till but recently bowing before wood and stones, but now owning the same God as that of these white people! "O just tell us how you were converted," they clamour; "but in fifteen minutes and no more, as we are going to hear from the great Reverend Doctor So-and-so about the ways and means and *rationale* of the mission." And those rhinoceroses who like to be seen and petted gladly obey the behest of these people, and in the most awkward manner, tell them how they ceased to be animals and began to live like men. But there are other rhinoceroses who do not like to be used. They do not like to be robbed of their internal peace by being made shows to the people, all of whom cannot comprehend through what tortuous and painful processes they were made to give up the rhinoceros-life. They like to be left alone, and walk silently in God's green field away from the sight of man. But the circus-men do not usually like such rhinoceroses.

Uchimura's scathing evaluation would continue even more aggressively:

26. Pyle, 119; Fisher 1923, 154; Tokutomi S., 64 (trans. John Pierson); Davidann, 81. Tokutomi Sohō remains a fascinating, if misunderstood, man to this day. Often compared to his younger brother, Tokutomi Roka, the elder Tokutomi comes across as a shrewd, if somewhat immoral, apostate, who not only abandoned Christianity but also his liberalism. Such a conclusion is probably quite unwarranted, and is unfair to both brothers.

> Now I, a regenerate rhinoceros, advise the mission circus-men to be more considerate in this matter. On one hand, they spoil the tamed rhinoceroses, and also induce the untamed ones to simulate the tamed, for that they find the easiest possible way of getting things good for their rhinoceros-flesh. On the other hand, I believe you give false conceptions of what the Christian mission really is to the people whom you like to get interested in your work in that way. I do not read in the Bible that Paul or Barnabus [*sic*] brought a Titus or a Timothy to Jerusalem for the purpose of making him sing Gentile songs, and tell the brethren there in his queer half-incomprehensible way "ho he cast his idols into fire and clung unto the Gospel." I read how the great Apostle defended the cause of Gentiles with all his vehemence, and told God's people that they were no better than the godless Gentiles, that both were condemned in sins, and came short of the glory of God; —from all which I conclude that to Paul and Paully-minded people, Gentilism was nothing to make merry about, or even to be "pitied," but it was a thing to be sympathized with, to be taken as their own state, and hence to be treated with all reverence and Christian graces. I do not value those contributions raised by making a Hindoo youth in his native attire sing Toplady in his own Paoli, any more than I do money raised by showing tamed ourangoutangs [*sic*]. O do not call that a Mission-work that appeals to people's Pharisaic pride, and showing them that they are better than heathens, urges "the Christians at home" to "pity them." The best of missionaries are always upholders of the cause and dignity of the people to whom they are sent, and they are as sensitive as the patriotic natives themselves to expose the idolatories [*sic*] and other degradations before the so-called Christian public.[27]

Uchimura's was the more stinging critique, and the one not lost on the evangelists themselves. Captain L. L. Janes, who taught the Kumamoto Band, that group of young, former samurai, to which Tokutomi Sohō had (reluctantly) belonged, had come to provide English, scientific, and historical education at the Kumamoto Yōgakkō in 1871, at the behest of the former *daimyō* of the region. However, the American Civil War veteran was also a missionary, and felt it his duty, when permitted, if not openly to proselytize, at least to introduce Christian concepts to his students. As he wrote to his colleague, Jerome D. Davis, at Kyoto's Dōshisha, in 1876, "My work at the school has been accompanied, from the time when it was possible to speak of Christianity, by constant and direct religious instruction of my pupils; in fact, the whole work has been inspired from the first with one aim, on my part, of making it, under God, subserve the founding and upbuilding of the Kingdom of Christ." A soldier, Janes became a warrior for Christ, and many of his young, former samurai students appreciated the martial consideration he paid to them. His pedagogy echoed his rather Weberian belief that the Christian ethic undergirded Western culture, and that, in providing a background in this ethic, he was not only assisting soteriologically but culturally as well.

For his work with the Kumamoto Band, Janes is considered one of the most successful evangelists of nineteenth-century Japan. But he is also one of the most

27. Uchimura, 136–38.

controversial. After the backlash caused by the Kumamoto Band's mass conversion to Christianity, Janes left Japan, only to return to divorce proceedings and allegations of adultery.[28] His return, fifteen years later, saw a changed man. While Janes had always been wary of the evangelical establishment, his treatment at their hands following the scandal sealed his opinion. The need to pander to donors at home, Janes believed, fostered an environment abroad wherein the evangelists would "occupy political, military, social and religious relations toward the people of three fourths of the human race, that would disgrace heathens not only, but devils." Like Uchimura, Janes had no love for organized religion; his Christianity would be quite his own, one which did not dabble in the moral enterprise medical missions seemed to require.[29]

For evangelists tied to umbrella organizations or specific Protestant sects, these men were more dangerous to their cause than either nonbelievers or apostates. For unorthodox Christians like Uchimura and Janes, the existing channels of organized religion were too easily corruptible, too stained by the desires of intermediaries. "The odium of Christianity is in its churches," Uchimura polemicized. "Christianity minus churches is the Way, the Truth, and the Life." Yet Uchimura, like Janes, was a pious Christian. To be attacked by your presumed peers was damning, but many of Japan's evangelists dismissed Uchimura as a heretic. Janes, as both a Westerner and a successful missionary was harder to ignore, but his potentially scandalous past proved a godsend for that purpose. Nevertheless, not all Christians who refused to ascribe to an organized sect were as easy to denounce.[30]

As Uchimura was renouncing organized Christianity, a young orphan named Kagawa Toyohiko began his English lessons at a missionary school. Within the year, he was baptized, and soon thereafter, determined to enter the seminary. He was to become Japan's most famous Christian export; philanthropist, minister, social worker, and author within the small, frail (and tubercular) body of a devout believer. Though ordained as a Presbyterian, Kagawa never truly subscribed to any Protestant sect, preferring what he deemed "a religion of life."[31] Nevertheless, Kagawa was not perceived as the same sort of threat as Uchimura. In part, this was due to the nature of his work. Kagawa was neither the ideologue nor the leader that Uchimura was. Although lauded by Professor Kenneth J. Saunders of Berkeley's Pacific School of Religion as "a Gorki in literature, a Saint Francis in piety, a Tolstoi in loving sympathy with the poor," Kagawa was unable to equal the legacy that Uchimura left to both Japan and Christianity.[32] Kagawa's religion of life required no church, whereas

28. Gordon 53–54; Davis 1894, 74–75; Scheiner 2002, 85; Scheiner 1966, 183; Cary 1909a, 256.
29. Notehelfer, 237.
30. Ohara, 121; Ishida, 8; Park, 47.
31. Kagawa 1998, 38.
32. Saunders 1931, 308. The employment of Tolstoy in Saunders' metaphor was hardly unique, either to him or to Kagawa. Many of those Christians in Japan who worked outside organized Christian sects earned such comparisons, more often positive (as above) than negative, although the sentiment remained similar. Indeed, as Sho Konishi pointed out, Tolstoy's rise in Japan (both as a novelist and as a Christian) occurred as the Russian Orthodox Church had decided upon his excommunication. Thus, Tolstoy makes a fascinating counterpoint

Uchimura's religion created his "No-Church" (*mukyōkai*). While both men conceived of a religion beyond the bounds of organized sects, only Uchimura was able to devise a perpetuating religious endowment to future generations of Christians. Unlike Kagawa, Uchimura bequeathed manifold treatises on his interpretations of and belief in Christianity to an audience of followers, philosophers, and curious seekers on both sides of the Pacific. Although perhaps most famous for his autobiographical work, Uchimura's essays on the Bible, Christ, and the role of Christianity were both prolific and influential. Kagawa, with his semiautobiographical novels, poetry, and his (by contrast) scant lectures (also primarily autobiographical) could not compete with the ideological output of a man who presented sixty lectures on Paul's Letter to the Romans alone.[33] This is, of course, about Christianity, not the Christian enterprise. The former was challenged by the two men, thus motivating further the moral enterprise. As Uchimura and Kagawa railed against the evangelist enterprise as it appeared in Japan, the enterprise needed to redouble its efforts to counteract the slights against it.

It is in Kagawa's discussion of Western Christians, however, that he truly differentiated himself from Uchimura. Kagawa, while not pandering to his Euro-American counterparts, never produced diatribes of the same level of intensity as Uchimura. "The peoples of the Occident have lived under the aegis of the Christian faith for nineteen hundred years," Kagawa reported. "Consequently they utterly fail to comprehend their deep indebtedness to Christ."[34] Thus, Kagawa sought to remind Christians of their religion, while simultaneously introducing the faith to others, and in this he never shunned the assistance of foreign evangelists. Indeed, he welcomed both the monetary and ideological help these men and women offered. As a self-proclaimed man of action, he saw such assistance as necessary for his mission. His "A Million Souls for Christ" campaign (later renamed the Kingdom of God Movement) only became feasible with the assistance of John R. Mott (YMCA general secretary, president, and Nobel laureate) as well as the support of many Protestant missionaries in Canada and the United States.[35] His awareness of his dependence shaped his publications. Thus, while never attacking the Protestant evangelists on whose funding he depended, he lamented in his diary after receiving their support:

> I differ from the established church in the course I am taking. The church today chatters on noisily about minor sins, overlooking entirely the major sin of capitalism. In this regard I do not wish to accompany the church down the easy path it is taking. Thus I do not think I'll adopt the simple methods of the gospel evangelists.

to Uchimura, Kagawa, Tokutomi Roka, and a handful of other Japanese Christians (Konishi, 235).

33. Howes, 86.
34. Kagawa 1934, 110.
35. Kagawa 1935, 167; Ryder, 127; Wright, 173.

> . . . We need an inner evangelism. And this will be an evangelism directed inevitably against capitalism.[36]

In many ways, Kagawa now seems a paradox, a Christian who worked outside organized sects while simultaneously depending on them. In this way, too, he remains a contradiction, the Christian socialist who could afford to denounce the capitalism that philanthropically funded him. Not surprisingly, the sects he rejected could hardly afford such contradictions and paradoxes. And, in avoiding such controversy, so, too, did members of the organized sects and evangelical groups relegate themselves to a far less prominent existence.

But the lack of recognition did not deter many evangelists, either foreign or Japanese. And many of Japan's politicians appreciated their work, celebrating it as the epitome of the moral enterprise—not merely because Japan's government could reap the rewards of social work performed in the name of God, but also because their work seemed far less antagonistic than that of men like Uchimura and Kagawa, and even Janes. This appreciation allowed evangelism to continue throughout most of the early twentieth century, even during periods of backlash against perceived "Westernization," evidencing the success of the moral enterprise strategy. Indeed, the rise of evangelical organizations in Japan coincided with the first recrudescence of popular sentiment against the government's push during the first two decades of the Meiji period for modernization and industrialization following the example of France, Prussia, Britain, and the United States. The lack of government opprobrium despite the political climate permitted a small minority of Christians to subsist throughout Japan.

What evangelists did see as having the potential to be far more harmful to their cause was the "incoming tide of rationalism," believed to be as much a concomitant of Westernization as was Christianity. To the undiscerning, to be "rational," and thus to be a modern man of science, medicine, and reason, threatened the evangelical organizations' ability to maintain their appeal as modern institutions and their extrareligious work, particularly within the classroom or the hospital.[37] In other words, as J. Merle Davis, the general secretary of the YMCA in Nagasaki, later lamented:

> Materialism, the religion of educated Japan, is the greatest obstacle to the spiritual growth of our work. The upper classes and students in general pride themselves on being scientific, and to them Science and Religion travel opposite roads. While with . . . superficial spirits the name "Science" is a mere catch-word used to support a position of indifference and ignorance regarding religious faith, still with multitudes of the finest men of the country the supposed irreconcilability of Religion with the claims of Science, forms an honest basis for the doubt or contempt with

36. Bikle, 172. (From Kagawa Toyohiko, Shinpen Zakki, in Mutō Tomio, ed., Kagawa Toyohiko Zenshū. Vol. 24. Tokyo, Kirisuto Shimbunsha, 1963–1964, p. 6.) This presented a different challenge, then, to the moral enterprise.

37. Taylor, 21; Frank, 177; Greene 1901, 93; Schwantes, 153.

> which they consider the claims of Religious faith. The sad statement of a student in one of my Bible classes, "Science only increases our spiritual agony," expressed a frame of mind that is typical of great numbers of thinking men and which challenges the Christian worker in Japan to his utmost efforts in attempting to solve this fundamental problem.[38]

Japanese intellectuals were certainly not unaware of this conflict inherent in the works of their teachers from America and Europe. In the writings of Thomas Paine, particularly *The Age of Reason*, these men saw opportunity for modernization without a concomitant acceptance of Christianity. In the teachings of Edward S. Morse, Tokyo University's first professor of zoology (and the son of a preacher), they learned of Darwin's ideas of evolution even before his work had been translated into Japanese.[39] At this nexus of science and reason, the heart of the Enlightenment, was a modernity that did not require an otherworldly power. This was a modernity that was easier to control, for it was under this banner of reason and enlightenment that Japan's oligarchs claimed to have established their nation. Still, as long as this modernity ruled, it was also in the oligarchs' best interest to allow for a Christian presence, particularly after the first age of Meiji leadership gave way to the new generation, both through faculty and mortality. And, interestingly, this was even as the tide of public sentiment turned against infatuation with the West. The two facts, however, were not as paradoxical as they may seem.

As historians Kenneth Pyle and Irwin Scheiner illustrated, many of Japan's new generation of leaders in the nineteenth century had dabbled in Christianity. As this trend continued into the next century, however, men like Fukai Eigo, a rising economic statesman, dismissed their own immature dalliances with the religion. Notwithstanding this, for such men rigorously to denounce or to attack their past was dangerous, as it could call into question their entire intellectual and political legitimacy. Thus, by merely writing it off as the folly of youth, Fukai and Tokutomi not only enabled themselves to maintain face but connected themselves to the lineage of Japan's leaders, who had averred as much previously.[40]

These dismissals of Christianity were often explained as a maturation of rationalism. Nonetheless, these were not necessarily a promotion of Darwinian ideals. In fact, a number of Japan's foreign missionaries proposed a far more generous view toward Darwin than their compatriots had done abroad. Though an admittedly extreme example, the Reverend John Thomas Gulick, a YMCA missionary and uncle of Sidney Gulick, was well known outside his more parochial sphere for his work in evolutionary biology, even vying with Darwin and Wallace for a complete

38. KFA: Annual Report, J. Merle Davis. Oct. 2, 1911, p. 4.
39. Schwantes, 124–25; E. Morse, 318, 316. In his polemic The Christian Stake in Science, chemist Robert E. D. Clark cautioned his readers not to equate science and reason, but acknowledged that "the two are nevertheless closely associated in the minds of most people" (Clark, 116). The Japanese were no different.
40. Pyle, 29; Scheiner, 4; Smethurst, 128.

theory of evolution. Still, some of Gulick's evangelical peers in Japan were willing to dismiss Darwin.

For Japan's leaders, too, Darwinism was awkward. The problem for Meiji's elite was how Darwinism was interpreted. Despite their earliest introduction by the biologist Morse, Darwinist theories proved far more popular in social, not biological, doctrine. Social Darwinism became the order of the day, and one that was often wielded in an uncomfortable way for Meiji's oligarchs. In social Darwinism, young ideologues found a "scientific" paradigm for their beliefs in natural rights, the unstoppable power of nature, or the march of progress without regard to national origin, none of which rested comfortably on the nation's leaders, who promoted Japan as singular and paramount. Thankfully for them, Katō Hiroyuki, president of Tokyo University, and a former proponent of natural human rights some eight years prior, pronounced his new belief in social Darwinism, though not in the same sense as the young ideologues had maintained. For Katō,

> survival of the fittest is easily proven by the historical evidence of societies from ancient times to the present and, perforce, wipes out any specious proof of the existence of natural rights to liberty, independence, and equality. . . . The proponents of wild fancies, not being able to know this indisputable and clear principle of truth, have eagerly advocated natural rights. These people do not know that such rights as we do have are those which have been taken by force from others.

By the 1880s, Katō's treatises gained widespread acceptance in Japan's government—not only in the realm of international politics, but also, perhaps, in a Malthusian analysis of disease as a necessary scourge, justifying the prioritizing of modernization above health care. Certainly, in Katō's work, the Meiji oligarchs saw a bridge between the rationalism that was still in vogue, the preeminence of the imperial family, and the goal of national power that would come to depend increasingly upon a doctrine of imperialism. It was hardly surprising, therefore, that Katō's treatise immediately preceding the Sino-Japanese War was entitled *The Struggle for the Rights of the Strongest.*[41]

41. Sakura, 341; Shimao, 100; J. Tucker, 174; Amundson, 122–23, Unoura, 215–16. While Shimao's article provides a worthwhile overview of Darwinist theory in Japan, he does make a few errors. One worthy of the reader's attention is his claim that Aoikawa Nobuchika's tract Hokkyōdan of 1874 utilized Darwinian theory to denounce Christianity. Yet Aoikawa's polemic appeared three years before Morse's lectures introduced Darwin as a conceptual whole to the Japanese public. It is implausible that Aoikawa, if he had read Darwin, ostensibly in the original, would use a still-unknown biologist to justify anything.

Unoura's brief article offers one of the most comprehensive views of Katō's thought, a subject deserving of far more attention than can be paid in the current work. Particularly interesting is how Katō allowed himself to be caught by his own interpretation of Darwin, as was the case when Toyama Masakazu, a sociology professor from the same institution over which Katō presided, questioned the possibility of the end of imperial rule, should someone fitter than Meiji emerge. Katō, unable to respond, shifted his theory to maintain the power of the imperial family. Thus, Katō was more concerned with the maintenance of Japan's leadership than he was with theoretical Übermenschen. This, again, was not surprising, since his pension and livelihood were controlled by the leadership.

As Katō was lauding the Darwinism that promoted Japanese leadership, Gulick maintained the balance between political power and religious freedom that his evangelical compatriots had come to understand very well. As both biologist and evangelist, Gulick supported Darwinism, even in the social sense that a proponent like Katō could hardly find distasteful. Yet Gulick tempered social Darwinism, distinguishing between the struggle for survival of animals and a society of humans. Animals, Gulick determined, were nonrational, while humans were rational. As such, animals might be ruled solely by Darwin's evolutionary biology, but humans required an explanation for their struggle. Like Katō, Gulick allowed for the social Darwinian aspects of survival that pleased Japan's government, but unlike Katō, Gulick sensed that humans needed something else, something both to justify devotion to the nation and something to nourish the individual. Religion, particularly Protestantism, Gulick believed, would serve that purpose. As noted by the editors of *Bibliotheca Sacra*, the oldest theological journal in the United States, Gulick's own findings provided "a far-reaching argument both for Darwinism and for Theism, for they rule chance out of the problem, and reveal a law whose source is invisible but all-powerful, and which can be no other than the eternal, omnipotent fountain of all orderly movement."[42] In the original letter from 1861 that was later reprinted in the journal, Gulick declared,

> Man is rational & he finds himself part of a universe that is capable of being interpreted & used by reason. The arts & sciences, through which his power is constantly advancing, are proofs that he is justified in the assumption that every part of the universe is constructed on principles that will yield an ever expanding meaning to his search for unity, law, & order. The progress of science rests on man's faith that he cannot be wrong in applying this assumption to new realms; and the rationality of the assumption is justified by the result. But rationality includes not only the adjusting of means, but the weighing & choosing of ends;—not only intelligence, but morality;—not only knowledge, but love guiding in the use of knowledge. Man finds himself part of a social system in which regard for the good of all is the guiding principle that brings order out of confusion. The history of social evolution shows that in proportion as man gains faith in this principle, & applies it intelligently to wider groups of society, & to each & all of the relations of social organizations, in that proportion has he advanced in happiness & dignity. We also find that a very large share of this advancement has been due to Christianity. Though other systems of teaching have dimly apprehended the ideal, they have none of them been able to inspire men with new motives that are able to hold the brutal tendencies of the race strongly in check. In populous regions there seems to have been a slow biological evolution through which altruistic instincts have gained increasing force; but no power outside of Christianity seems able to take man as he is, in any & every land, & set him on a new course. The cause of this wonderful power in Christianity, seems to lie in its ability to assure men of the fatherhood of God, as well as of the brotherhood of man. Indeed judging from

42. J. Gulick 1896, 69.

> my own experience & from what I have observed in China & Japan it seems as if a strong hold on the latter idea, such as will awaken the enthusiasm of humanity, is attained only by those who are filled with the former idea.[43]

Similarly, Gulick noted later, "The fact that although I had always worked in scientific lines and was one of the earliest believers in evolution" only served to emphasize the importance of Christianity, because "I still retained my faith in Christ and considered Christian evangelism the one work most worth while." This fact, perhaps more than Christ's teaching, "had a strong influence on the young Japanese men with whom I was brought in close contact through the school in which I was a teacher."[44]

Besides, without religion, there was neither impetus nor strength to make the sacrifices necessary in the struggle of the survival of the fittest. Thus, Gulick maintained that when a man "sacrifices himself to the good of his family, or nation, or race, he knows that he is making sacrifice. He cannot, like the beast and bird, sacrifice himself without any thought of the consequences." Sacrifice was not to be avoided, Gulick noted, but was to be supplemented: "The law of nature seems to provide for the success of the race, without regard to the fate of the individual. But religion offers the highest blessedness to the individual while devoting himself to the service of the race, through love of God." Kato Naoshi, however, a Japanese writer for the YMCA publication *Kaitakusha*, saw neither a need to supplement sacrifice nor to juxtapose individual and nation, particularly with regard to the role of Christianity: "Christianity will bring to fruition the spirit of the nation. . . . The spirit of the nation cannot be realized until the spirit of the individual is in harmony."

Like Gulick, many Japanese Christians, too, saw no reason to view evolution as antithetical to Christianity. Kozaki Hiromichi, one of the Kumamoto band and a student of Gulick, who would become a leader in the upper echelons of Tokyo's YMCA, dedicated a considerable amount of time to explaining the symbiosis he saw as inherent to both Christianity and to evolution. As man progresses through history, Kozaki maintained, so, too, does he come to better understand the divine.[45]

Discussions of both the fate and role of the individual became of utmost concern to the methodology of evangelists in Japan, particularly with regard to the moral enterprise. It was Christianity, such men maintained, that not only affirmed but introduced the Western concept of the individual in Japan. Individuals were to be valued as part of creation—not solely as a part of a gestalt, but as an end in and of themselves. Part of the moral enterprise in Japan at the behest of the evangelists was having converts and "Pseudo-Christians" cherish the individual at every level. By valuing the individual, each Japanese subject became worthy of salvation—either of the nation or the church, or, ideally, both. As missionary author Ernest Wilson

43. JTG Papers, Bancroft Library: Letter to George H. Romanes, Mar. 7, 1861; later sent to Thomas Gulick, Jan. 5, 1892; sent by Thomas to G. F. Wright for publication in Biblitheca Sacra, Jan. 1896, pp. 1–2 of original letter.
44. JTG Papers, Bancroft Library: Outline of my life by John T. Gulick (18 May 1906), p. 50.
45. Amundson, 128; Davidann, 106; Miyahira, 118; Dohi, 30–31.

Clement contended, "In 1853, the individual was swallowed up in the family, the clan, the nation; by 1903 the word 'personal' had been introduced into the language by Christian teaching, and individual worth, rights, and responsibilities were acknowledged in the codes, the courts, and the Constitution, the latter itself a fruit of Christian civilization."[46] In many missionary fields of endeavor, such work would have been seen as too meager, too simplistic to qualify as evangelism.

But Japan, pioneering evangelists of the late nineteenth century quickly realized, was not like other such domains. For some twenty years after the Meiji Restoration, foreign Christians acknowledged the continued unique nature of much of their work. In an 1871 letter to his elder brother and fellow evangelist, Orramel Hinckley Gulick, John Thomas Gulick advised him that the "surest way to reach the people & make your work tell will be to start a newspaper. The people are so eager to learn foreign news & foreign science that a paper well managed would pay for itself & in time would have a very great influence. I believe Yokohama or Yedo would be the place for gathering news, rather than Hiogo. If you are to stick to the ordinary lines of missionary work China is the place."[47] This letter is from June 22, 1871, not long after the Meiji Restoration, and thus, the restoration of a foreign evangelical presence in Japan (although two years before the repeal of the ban on Christianity). What is notable is not merely that Gulick believed that Japan was not ready for "ordinary lines of missionary work"—that is, direct preaching—but that he also promoted the newspaper as a potential proselytizing vehicle (presumably somewhere beneath all the "foreign news & foreign science") that would not require outside support. While missionary boards were always eager for self-supporting evangelism, Gulick seemed to acknowledge that such a newspaper, without its overt Christian teachings, would not garner the same kind of philanthropic support from Christians back home that "ordinary lines" of evangelism would elsewhere, that the moral enterprise would be more difficult when not couched in soteriology but in practical terms, including scientific information.

Many evangelists utilized their fluency in English to proselytize outside ordinary lines. Such men and women were far more sought after for their cultural currency than for traditional preaching. In a nation where everyone was ostensibly equal, the promise of a meritocracy led many Japanese subjects to pursue English literacy, even with a dose of Christianity. Eliza Talcott, a missionary and cofounder of Kobe College, suggested, in 1873, the same year that the ban on Christianity in Japan was lifted, that English teachers take advantage of the situation and "use the 'Peep of Day' for a Reader." *The Peep of Day*, written by British evangelical author Favell Lee Mortimer in 1836 with the subtitle *A Series of the Earliest Religious Instruction the Infant Mind Is Capable of Receiving*, became a "standard textbook" of English in Japan within three years. Julia A. Gulick, John's sister and Talcott's assistant and coevangelist, found the work extremely helpful: "The children are

46. University of Chicago Alumni Council, 68; Clement, 145.
47. JTG Papers, Bancroft Library.

learning the Old Testament stories while studying the corrected English language," and they continued to do so for another two years. It was telling that Talcott saw Kobe College not as a school but as a pretense for Bible study. During her tenure, the school had no commencement ceremonies.[48] Thus, despite the lifting of the ban on Christianity in 1873, evangelism continued to take place within the confines of some trade: teaching, reporting, medical work. This was, of course, the epitome of the moral enterprise—appearing to serve the nation selflessly while seeking acceptance and promotion of one's own agenda.

By the late 1880s, however, for some evangelists, their work had become seen as commonplace and ubiquitous within Japan enough to merit a division of labor between employment and proselytization. The promoter of extraordinary lines of missionary work, John Thomas Gulick wrote to his brother Halsey that the Japanese Christians in Kyoto wanted Julia, his sister, "to train the nurses to be Bible Readers & evangelists while acting as nurses. There are of course opportunities for such work but of course it would be easy to overdo that line, as in the case of a dentist who always preaches to those whose teeth he is filling."[49] But such a division was not to compartmentalize the evangelist's Christianity. In all work, such men and women understood, one's values and morals could and should be imparted, but there was no longer any need for subterfuge. As Gulick suggested to the home mission in the late 1890s, "The necessity for a miss'y [missionary] to devote himself to mere teaching is largely past, unless he sees in that work a wide opportunity to influence his pupils for X'y [Christianity] as well as others whom he may reach through them. It is our thought that the miss'y should be always an evangelist in whatever lines of work he may be engaged, & that he should seek those places in which he can best accomplish his work." It was, of course, a fine line between being the sermonizing dentist and being the missionary who imbued his work with the spirit of evangelism.[50]

It was this delicate distinction that medical missionaries had to respect. Arriving later than many of their counterparts in English language education, they were not as limited in their evangelism, but remained sensitive to the division between science and religion that so many philosophers had distinguished after the Enlightenment in Europe, and certainly after the growing acceptance of the veracity of Darwinism. Although certainly not medically naive, these men and women also perceived illness as a spiritual problem, and medicine as concomitant to a spiritual salve. Neither could spiritual health and physical health be separated, nor could spiritual obligations and medical responsibility be divided, and the medical missionary knew that better than anyone. "The aim of the medical missionary is twofold," noted Canon Charles Henry Robinson of Ripon Cathedral, the editorial secretary of the Society for the Propagation of the Gospel in Foreign Parts:

48. Ishii, 83.
49. JTG: Letter to Halsey Gulick, Dec. 8, 1887.
50. JTG: Suggestions to the Mission, n.d. (but likely 1896–1898).

> (1) To alleviate suffering and to train those who in non-Christian lands are ignorant of the art of medicine in order that they may be enabled to alleviate the sufferings of their fellow-countrymen. (2) To co-operate with the Christian evangelist by interpreting the Divine compassion and breaking down the prejudices of those who would not otherwise be willing to listen to the gospel message. Some of those who have advocated the extension of medical missions have laid exclusive emphasis upon the latter objects, but have failed to grasp the importance of the former. The charge given by Christ Himself to His first missionaries was to preach the gospel and to heal the sick, but there is nothing in the context to suggest that in places where the preaching of the gospel was welcomed they might consider themselves absolved from the obligation to heal those who were sick. It may with confidence be asserted that apart altogether from any consideration of the fact that medical missions have proved a powerful evangelistic agency, it is the duty of the whole Christian Church to establish missions which have as their object the alleviation of bodily suffering, and that it is the duty of the individual missionary who possesses a knowledge of medicine that is not shared by any of those amongst whom he works to use his knowledge with the object of alleviating human suffering, and to continue his labours with this object in view until such time as the medical practitioners of the country are in a position to carry on the work which he has inaugurated.[51]

The Right Reverend William B. Stevens, Episcopal bishop of Pennsylvania, voiced similar thoughts, in his Epiphany missionary service on "Medical Missions; their Origin, Scope, and Influence, Especially in Connection with China, Japan, and Mexico," as reported in the *New York Times*. Caring for the infirm and ill was "a Divine command. . . . In nearly every land where early hospitals were founded they came in with Christianity, and Christian charity supported them." The bishop was quick to point out, incorrectly, that China and Japan, though populous, "have no medical science." Instead, "they have quacks and magicians. They know nothing of anatomy or physiology. They do not know of the circulation of the blood; they know nothing of the lungs, the eye, the ear, or the brain. All their medical works contain doctrines long since exploded by science. The medical profession there is a very low one. The first missionaries to those countries saw the necessity of introducing medical service."[52]

The first missionaries (and, indeed, those who followed) also saw the benefit to the mission of the divine command. In practical terms, those who required medical care had both the time and the desire for guidance, be it spiritual or otherwise. In convalescence, Dr. Sarah Craig Buckley wrote in 1887, "the people are very willing to hear the truth, and we certainly have them where their minds are most plastic to mould. In hours of sickness the Japanese, like ourselves, think most seriously. I often think we have the most promising Christian work in Japan."[53] She was not mistaken;

51. Robinson, 28.
52. "HEALING THE HEATHEN SICK."
53. Buckley, 67.

hers was an audience that, if not necessarily wholly receptive to her ideological message, was certainly open to her medical assistance. As William Elliot Griffis, missionary and educator, reported almost two decades later, medical missions, particularly, had proved fairly successful:

> This gate of opportunity, at first view seemingly small, opens on a boundless field. As we traverse it, we see another gate of opportunity, that of charitable work, and here in Japan we note one of the great moral revolutions of the world wrought within fifty, perhaps we might say in thirty, years. The Japanese are as a nation getting to have what they did not have before,—ideas, and a conscience concerning their duty to the blind, the insane, the starving poor, the orphans, the outcast, and criminals. When first in Tokyo, I remember reading, with, I confess, an irreverent and comical feeling, the notice boards, especially the one that hung right under the anti-Christian edict and sandwiched in between the old text and the new proclamation. It read: "Human beings must carefully practice the principles of the five social relations. Charity must be shown to widowers, widows, orphans, the childless, and sick." Why widowers should be first pitied was not clear, and why the starving and hungry were not thought of seemed strange. In pagan Japan hospitals, orphanages, schools for the insane, blind, and dumb, systematic or voluntary famine relief, reform of the criminal, tender relief of the sick paupers, were practically unknown. The Japanese were benevolent, but only in a narrow way. They answered the question, "And who is my neighbor?" in the spirit of Confucius, not of Jesus. Now, thanks to the statistics of Dr. J. H. Pettee, we see that the Christians of Japan have thirty-one orphanages, four homes for discharged prisoners, three blind asylums, three leper hospitals, two homes for the aged, five schools for the Ainos, four free kindergartens, ten industrial schools, ten other schools for the poor, ten boarding-houses for students, and fourteen hospitals. That is to say, a fraction, one two hundred and fiftieth part of the population of the empire, support about one-fourth of the organized benevolence of the land, and that fraction of people consists of the Christians.[54]

As medical missionaries, more so even than as spiritual or political educators, guides, and preachers, foreign evangelists became the neighbors most acceptable to the population they sought to assist. The success of the moral enterprise was rooted in this acceptability for soteriology, as we will see shortly in the case of the YMCA.

54. KFA: Griffis 1904, 269–70.

6

"Now Is the Day for Japan"

The YMCA

Of the nearly one thousand foreign evangelists proselytizing in Japan at the time of the coronation of the Taishō emperor in 1912, arguably the most successfully moral entrepreneurial groups (though not in terms of combatting TB) and certainly the most recognized were those associated with the Young Men's Christian Association.[1] Working in the country in one (sometimes protean) manner or another since the 1880s, the workers of the YMCA had, from the start, relied more on labor than on preaching to make their mark.[2] Cognizant that their exoticism would not carry them as far as their utility, the men and women affiliated with the YMCA left privileged lives in the expanding United States for labor on the frontlines of Protestantism's battle to gain acceptance in Japan, and thus to save souls. As we shall see, however, for the YMCA, saving lives was another matter altogether.

The task ahead of the organization seemed simple enough—to educate the Japanese populace, primarily using the gospel. Therefore, though the official arrival of the American evangelists under the auspices of the YMCA was not until 1889, the concepts upon which the YMCA was based, both religiously and organizationally, had been introduced by foreign teachers at the start of the Meiji period, and had been adopted by a few of their more eager Japanese students. Consequently, because the domestic branches of the Japanese YMCA predated those established by foreign evangelists by almost ten years, the men who founded Japan's first YMCA divisions were students of foreign Protestant teachers, the vast majority of whom were affiliated with the organization in the United States. At the behest of the fledgling autochthonous student groups, American missionaries from a variety of Protestant sects sought to incorporate these separate groups under the auspices of the international YMCA organization.[3]

As noted previously, Japan's position, the American evangelists believed, was unique. Unlike the great empires of India and China (and so many other countries in Asia), Japan had managed to escape colonial or semicolonial status. Within twenty years of the Meiji Restoration, the modernization along Western lines that

1. Eddy, 74.
2. Davidann, 40; Y.M.C.A. shi, 4.
3. KFA: Galen M. Fisher. *Japanese Young Men in War and Peace*, pp. 10–11.

Japan's leadership had undertaken was already creating a Japan that seemed to have disassociated itself from China and Korea. This fact was, of course, not lost on the Japanese themselves, regardless of their religion. Such influential men as Fukuzawa Yukichi and Taguchi Ukichi had been identifying the dichotomy between Japan and the rest of Asia for years.[4] But theirs was more than untempered pride at Japan's new stature in the world; they also acknowledged confusion in placing Japan neither in Asia nor fully in the West. This ambivalence, however, was far less pronounced among the foreign Protestant evangelists, particularly those of the YMCA. For these men, Japan's disassociation from Asia was something to be lauded. As Charles Kellogg Ober, then co-national secretary of the YMCA intercollegiate work, wrote in 1889, over 30 years since the Meiji Restoration, in the YMCA publication the *Watchman*,

> Now is the day for Japan! . . . Here is a land that eagerly seeks all the treasures of the West and is ready for religion. . . . Not only is it a crisis in Japan, it is a crisis in Missions. Success here means very much for all Asia—failure here is an alternative we dare not contemplate. As the Christian world knows, Japan is just now the center of the fight. Here the enemy is weak—let us pour in our forces. A day here now is worth a year in China or India.[5]

Yet it would be foolish to believe that, despite any slight confusion as to their position on the part of Japanese intellectuals, the leaders of the YMCA missions and those of Japan's elite saw Japan similarly. After all, Japan was still held by unequal treaties that predated the Meiji Restoration, and no promise of Westernization or Christianization would alter that. The relationship, therefore, between the Japanese and foreign evangelists was one of an obvious power imbalance. Because the foreign missionaries of the YMCA were wont to show disdain for the Japanese, they could not help but condescend. The Japanese seemed to the missionaries to be charges, men and women who showed progress, but required guidance. The "enemy" Ober identified was weak in Japan, but the Japanese themselves, he imagined, were incapable of addressing the "crisis" he identified on their own. Nor were they able to do so long after the unequal treaties were nullified. As Dr. John Lincoln Dearing, a Baptist missionary to Japan and the editor of the annual volume *The Christian Movement in the Japanese Empire*, noted in 1914:

> No nation in the East is so well prepared for a great religious awakening as is Japan. There is a widespread and generally correct estimate of the value and character of Christianity. There is no special prejudice existing against Christianity which cannot be removed with far less difficulty than in any other Eastern land. . . . The present is an unusual opportunity for Christian propagation and progress. Famine

4. S. Tanaka, 37–38; Pyle, 90; Gluck 2005, 1227.
5. Schwartz, 688; Davidann, 39.

> and disaster and social problems are all adding their emphasis to the call of the hour for the nation to turn to God for help.[6]

If Christianity could be propagated in Japan more easily than elsewhere, it was not merely, as Dearing noted, due to the ideological predisposition of the populous. The presence of tragedy and uncertainty, as was the case of an epidemic, were believed to be an asset to the spread of the religion, an asset that the foreign YMCA officials were not only well aware of but well willing to utilize. To do so was not callousness but pragmatism, and even faith. How could this opportunity not be attributed to divine action? Moreover, such occasions provided evangelists, particularly those associated with the YMCA, opportunities to assist the general population, regardless of the spiritual beliefs of those whom they supported. In this way, the YMCA's ministrations spread, both religiously and philanthropically. During the same period to which Dearing referred, John Merle Davis, former YMCA secretary of Nagasaki and then secretary of Tokyo, reported to the home office that, though "the quarter [of the year] has been a period of heavy national calamity," comprising

> in January the greatest volcanic eruption of modern Japan in the far South, [*sic*] (which) was more than matched by appalling famine conditions, which still continue in the far North. The response of the nation to these disasters has been generous, but the provincial officials have not been able to properly disburse the large sums placed in their hands for famine relief. It is distressing to learn that hundreds of people are starving to death in the snow-bound villages of the North, because of the red-tape and inefficiency which stands between them and the funds actually given to save life. The fact that the funds for famine relief being handled by Christian agencies are splendidly administered, has already been widely commented upon, some Japanese newspapers even urging that all relief funds be placed in the hands of Christians for disbursement.

That Davis' branch of the association donated funds and food, including thirteen hundred bags of rice, merited distinction, both by his report, and by those of the newspapers he cited.[7] Caring for the entire population, regardless of evangelical potential, actually also provided a niche that most earlier evangelists, particularly those without a larger organizational community within the country, never realized they could thus occupy.

The first evangelists had tried to maintain themselves solely through preaching—before engaging in the moral enterprise—or, at least, by insinuating their ministry into the moral enterprise, using the aspects of cultural exchange provided

---

6. Franklin, 163; Eddy, 75–76.
7. Condliffe, 66; KFA: "Report for Quarter." J. M. Davis, Tokyo. Apr. 6, 1914. The eruption both men refer to was that of Sakurajima, a volcanic island in Kagoshima Bay (Kinkowan). Though the eruptions of mid-January were some of the most violent in modern Japanese history, actually shifting the location of the island, and though the eruptions were also accompanied by earthquakes and were not far from the major metropolitan center of Kagoshima-shi, the loss of life was minimal. For more on this geologic event, see the works of Professors Kotō Bunjiro and Ōmori Fusakichi (Ōmori, 31–33).

to them by the Japanese government. By the time of the rise of the YMCA, however, the evangelists who associated themselves with the organization had come to realize the precarious position such single-minded pursuit imposed. This was hardly surprising, of course. Whereas previously, foreign evangelists were only answerable to the Japanese government, the association of the YMCA with evangelism meant that these missionaries were to work under the auspices of two organizations as moral entrepreneurs—the Japanese government and the American YMCA board. Thus, while the YMCA could provide funds and, in some rare cases, a modicum of legitimacy,[8] it restrained the work that such men and women could undertake.

The men of the YMCA were essentially employees, and, while dedicated, they had to reconcile the assumed necessity of Japan's spiritual awakening with their own limited economic resources. This was not done out of selfishness but out of an awareness of the futility of stretching oneself and one's resources too thin. Japan needed pragmatists, not martyrs, and it was through pragmatism, the essence of the moral enterprise, that these men believed the Japanese would best be persuaded.

While obtaining converts was a major component of all evangelical enterprises, the YMCA, particularly those branches with a strong foreign presence, also concentrated on establishing amicable relations with and support of influential Japanese nationals, including politicians, bureaucrats, businessmen, and even imperial household members. Whether such men were saved was not always as important as whether they provided a show of goodwill and support for the organization and its members. As such, it was hardly surprising that, in noting the success of the 1907 World's Student Christian Federation Conference in Tokyo, Davis lauded not the influence of the conference on Japan's Christian population but its effect on the Japan's heads of state, business, and culture: "The leaders of Japanese National life, prominent statesmen, politicians, editors and professional men and the great student community of the country were deeply impressed by the conference."[9] The impact that the YMCA had was fostered strongly by the Japanese YMCA's foreign members. Skilled in public relations, men like Davis believed that positive native perceptions of the YMCA served the organization better than essentially preaching to the converted. As long as the organization did not antagonize influential and intellectual Japanese subjects, the YMCA could maintain itself long enough to do good for the nation, and, ultimately, for itself and its converts.

The guiding light of these efforts was moral enterprise as in the war effort, in peacetime and within limits for the sake of the poor. Their pursuit of the moral enterprise required the YMCA to address some problems and to neglect others, all the while cultivating the support of notables and fulfilling the policies and wishes of their headquarters. Indeed, nothing illustrated this strategy better than the YMCA's concentration on army work. In a nation that was dedicating so many resources to

8. However, when the YMCA began its work in Japan, most missionaries were regarded similarly, regardless of whether they possessed the credentials such a connection could provide.
9. KFA: Report of J. M. Davis, Nagasaki, Apr. 1–June 30, 1907.

strengthening itself militarily, an offering of martial assistance led many Japanese elite to view the organization in a new light. By the Russo-Japanese War, the YMCA, like the Japanese Red Cross, sought to assist the injured—primarily Japanese, but also Russian—to the approval and surprise of the Japanese government. General Terauchi Masatake, the minister of war, admitted to the Tokyo branch of the YMCA after three months of observing the work that the association had undertaken, that he recognized the power of the assistance offered. "I wish to express my deep appreciation of the splendid work being done by your Association in behalf of our soldiers at the front," he stated.

> At first I had slight interest in the matter, thinking that, like many other propositions presented to us, it would pass over with little result. When your work was first launched I had some feelings of anxiety concerning it, but I may say now that all apprehension has been turned into admiration, and I express both the opinion of men at the front and in Tokyo, when I say that this work has proved successful beyond our expectations.

Such words were, as Galen M. Fisher happily noted, "the most striking endorsement of Christianity ever given by a Japanese army official. It is obvious that such words from a quarter so near the throne will do much to place all Christians and Christian institutions even higher than present in general esteem."[10]

Esteem like the general's was earned through great effort in difficult circumstances by the young men of the Japanese YMCA. Indeed, at the outbreak of the war, as Terauchi later admitted, the campaign that the association sought to undertake was beset by "the problems connected with so vast an undertaking but also had to overcome the difficulty of securing from the War Department permission to go to the front." Where other evangelists had failed, however, the YMCA succeeded, a triumph of moral entrepreneurship, eventually persuading the Ministry of War to allow it access in August to begin work at Antung, the base of General Kuroki's troops stationed by the Yalu River.[11] From that foothold, the association managed to open another post in the port of Yingkou (at the mouth of the Liao River) that November, at Fenghuang Cheng in Zhangjiajie by February, and beyond thereafter.[12]

While evangelists continued to assist troops domestically, only the men of the YMCA undertook a significant effort abroad, working side by side with Japan's combatants in the best capacity they could. As news of their mission spread to Japan and to America, the YMCA became a paragon of evangelical work. Mrs. F. S. Curtis, a reverend's wife and missionary to Kyoto, wrote excitedly to her home church of the success of "the Y. M. C. A. workers [who] are there with big tents for meetings,

10. "Association News & Notes," 248; KFA: Galen M. Fisher. *Japanese Young Men in War and Peace*, pp. 9–10.
11. KFA: "With Japanese Soldiers at the Front: The Minister of War Grants Special Permission to the Y.M.C.A. to Follow the Army." *Japanese Association Army Work News Service*. No. 1. Dec. 12, 1904.
12. *Cassell's History*, 217; KFA: "The Y.M.C.A. Army Department." *Japan Weekly Mail* (from *Asahi Shimbun* article by Ikeda Suyeo), p. 145.

and all the paraphernalia for helping and benefiting the soldiers."[13] The benefit to the soldiers, according to YMCA heads Fisher, Hibbard, and Gleason, included the following:

1,547,483 sheets of paper used.	26,168 books loaned.
757,159 envelopes.	18,500 used laundry at
1,053,381 postcards.	Fengwangcheng.
101,229 portions of Bible distributed.	764 visits to hospitals.
312,033 religious tracts.	1,752 gramaphone [sic] concerts,
3,385 Testaments.	lantern lectures, and
877,485 men received letter supplies.	other entertainments.
87,940 men received supplies like	1,566,379 men entered the buttons, thread, soap, etc. different branches.
152,213 men used barber's outfit.	At least three-fourths of the entire army was reached by the Association.[14]

Certainly, this was no small feat, and was one that required a significant amount of coordination. But at what cost? It seemed a wise investment to many Americans, a small donation meant that three quarters of the Japanese army were introduced to Christianity. Yet the work often ended there. In a war where victory proved pyrrhic, how could the success of support be measured accurately?

Yet for both the YMCA board in America and for the Japanese government, the war work performed by the YMCA was considered a success. For the Americans, the foreign evangelists in Japan presented the Japanese as "plucky," full of "spirit and sagacity." They noted at the start of the Russo-Japanese War,

> The missionaries of Japan, China and Korea, with rare exceptions, regard Japan as a champion of righteousness, as an ally, unconscious as yet, in the Christianization of the East, as a Galahad deserving the sympathy and calling for the increasing cooperation of the Christian West, in order that she may become a conscious and more potent agent for the emancipation of her neighbors.[15]

Moreover, after its tremendous victory in the Sino-Japanese War a decade earlier, the Japanese Army had rapidly become the heart of the nation. Thus, as General Stewart L. Woodford, former US envoy extraordinary and minister

13. "Local News," 7; Loomis, 123 (also KFA: Rev. H. Loomis. "Christian Work among Japanese Soldiers." *Missionary Review of the World*. Feb. 1905, pp. 119–25.)
14. Odell, 604.
15. KFA: Galen M. Fisher. *Japanese Young Men in War and Peace*, pp. 3–4.
Fisher's use of the Japan-Galahad metaphor is poignant on two counts. First, Galahad is a distinctly Western archetype, a model of chivalric knighthood in medieval Europe, a beacon at the end of the Dark Ages. Second, Galahad, as both the perfect knight (kind, chaste, and righteous) and (depending on the treatment) the only hero of the quest for the Holy Grail is a true representation of Christianity, if not of Christ himself.

plenipotentiary to Spain before the outbreak of hostilities and the declaration of the Spanish-American War in April 1898, YMCA work at the front was "the chance of a generation for Christianity in Japan: for if you capture the Japanese army for Christ, you capture the Japanese people."

The awareness of the political importance of army work reverberated beyond the political sphere, and was recognized by those at the forefront of this mission. As one pioneer of Protestant evangelism in Japan, the Reverend Doctor John H. DeForest, noted to YMCA student secretary in Tokyo C. V. Hibbard at their send-off meeting for association members embarking on war work, "This meeting is probably more important with respect to the establishment of Christianity in Japan than any other meeting that it will be given to any of is [*sic*] to attend." Hibbard concurred, and noted further that "in view of the high place which the army holds in Japanese life and the systematic opposition to Christian propaganda in the army which, to quote Dr. DeForest again, 'has been pushed to the verge of violation of treaty rights,' and which has been consistently manifested in the suspicion which our recent efforts to establish Army Work has encountered, in view of these facts, I believe that Dr. DeForest scarcely overestimates the importance of the Army Work." National secretary of the Japanese YMCA Galen M. Fisher reiterated Hibbard and Woodford's sentiments by pointing out to his colleagues on the American board that "the soldier is the man of the hour in Japan, and the association, as the only Christian agency permitted to work in Manchuria, feels that it represents as never before the whole Church."[16]

To the organization's leaders back home, the YMCA was not only at the forefront of evangelism in the most promising of Asian nations, it was, in truth, the only organization with the resources, the drive, and the desire to evangelize. This resonated in the United States with both the leadership and with those Christians willing to dedicate themselves to this most promising of missions. To join the YMCA was thought to be the most soteriologically successful of Christians, and the organization played upon such sentiments of superiority in its advertisements for volunteers, as the following shows:

> This is no call to ninnies and milksops. The Y. M. C. A. needs real men, preferably men who have had some broad and grueling experience of life; men of education, yes; but, above that, men capable of understanding, sympathy, and an infinite deal of hard, exacting work. Men who can turn a Ford inside out; men who can play the piano and lead five hundred others in singing; men who are trained in athletics; men six feet high and three feet wide and eighteen inches thick; men who understand what Christianity really means; men with humor and leadership who have been earning a hundred dollars a week and are willing to live on ten dollars a week. In other words, MEN.[17]

16. KFA: Galen M. Fisher. "The Mother of the Japanese Army." KFA: C. V. Hibbard. "Foreign Secretaries Reports, 1904–05," 235.
17. Odell, 604. That the advertisement reads like an army recruitment ad is no mistake. The YMCA did see itself as an elite force at the vanguard of the salvation of civilization.

Here, therefore, we see the emphasis on muscular Christianity as a promotional point, not for the Japanese but for the Americans the organization hoped to recruit to engage in the moral enterprise in Japan. And for good reason, since the Japanese government, too, deemed the YMCA's war work successful. Certainly, the politicians had no need to provide the promise of salvation, but they did require a military willing to fight for the nation. Such a daunting effort required high levels of morale. If, in their promises and their entertainments, the evangelists and volunteers of the YMCA could ensure that morale be maintained, then the presence of such workers was a small, often nonexistent, price to pay for a well-oiled war machine. Major General Kamio Mitsuomi, chief of staff at Dalny (Dalian), admitted that though "everything was completely provided for [by the government and military] for the prosecution of the war, yet I must frankly acknowledge that there was no provision made for the field recreation of the Japanese soldiers; it was entirely outside the Japanese army system." It was within this lacuna that the YMCA made its presence both known and vital, and in doing so avoided having to address health inequities at home. By employing the "MEN" of the advertisement above, the YMCA was able to promote itself as engaging in the war effort seemingly so successfully that both the evangelists and their charges became recipients of moral entrepreneurship, as below:

> In all eleven places where work was definitely organized, the Young Men's Christian Association provided suitable buildings, divided into meeting and music halls, library, reading-room, tea-room, barber shop, letter-writing room, etc. To these rooms soldiers were given free access day and night. The men who had charge of the Association received the innumerable soldiers with untiring zeal and kindness. They gave soldiers healthy recreation and everything else they needed, which made them almost forget that they were in the field of war.[18]

The work, admittedly, often separated the YMCA's workers from their wholly evangelical roots. Secretary Hibbard noted a conversation between himself and a soldier in which the soldier approached him and asked, "Where does this '*gun-tairokwai*' [soldiers comforting outfit] come from?" Hibbard reported that he explained the organization and added that he hoped that "this thing will be a practical example of the spirit of Christianity," the nature of which he explained to the recruit. "Do you make many converts," asked the soldier. "No," Hibbard admitted, "we don't have opportunity for the sufficient teaching here but we hope that some of you fellows will have enough interest to follow it up later." "Naruhodo [I see]," the soldier exclaimed. "Well, most of us haven't enough religion to hurt us."[19] The men and women of the YMCA had to compromise their values, a position to which they were rapidly becoming accustomed.

18. KFA: "What Japan's Army Thinks of Christian Methods."
19. KFA: Bishop Harris. "Association Secretaries in Manchurian Hospitals: Timely Service to Badly Wounded Men, Hair Cut a Luxury." *Japanese Association Army Work News Service*. No. 6. Apr. 15, 1905.

It was from this vantage point that Hibbard happily reported on the coverage of the YMCA's inclusion in the celebrations of the imperial birthday in the field:

> We were invited to take part in the celebration of the emperor's birthday. When the phonograph began its grind the crowd started from everywhere. A Japanese *gendarme* ran a rope around our big tent and by a vigilant patrol we managed to keep the entrance open. Free saké (Japanese wine) in small portions had been distributed to the soldiers, and the proverbial saké thirst sent them straight across the parade ground for a cup of celebration tea at the Y. M. C. A. tent. The commandant came in while I was stooping over the fire, slapped me on the back right cordially and said it was good work. Nine-tenths of the commissioned officers visited our tent, and it was impossible to estimate the number of soldiers. Many thanked us heartily. It was something to be the representative of the only religion that has followed the men here.[20]

The inclusion of alcohol, much to the delight of the soldiers, was certainly not in keeping with the YMCA's policy on providing only wholesome refreshments to keep their charges from immoral forms of recreation.[21] Nevertheless, while the cost of the sake somewhat undermined the mission, the value of a cup of sake proved immeasurable, bringing the organization the recognition of the imperial household, as well as a 10,000 yen donation from the Meiji emperor and empress. As minister of war, General Terauchi wrote following the war's end, on behalf of the government, the YMCA "at large expense of money and labor, and by a great variety of means . . . filled the leisure of our officers and soldiers, far from home, with wholesome recreation. The completeness of the equipment and the success of the enterprise were universally tested and recognized by our troops in the field. I am fully assured that the recipients of all this generous service are filled with deep and inexpressible gratitude."[22]

The gratitude so many felt toward the YMCA did not always translate into souls saved. But, for the government, it did save the relationship with the American public. In their work, the men and women of the YMCA presented Japan as following the West, and by allowing these men to work on the frontlines, the Japanese government ensured for its constituents that American Christians would view them as worthy of assistance.

On both sides of the Pacific, the role of the YMCA was boosted by its activities in support of the Russo-Japanese War. While the war had, according to Associate National Secretary V. W. Helm, "interfered to a certain extent with certain regular lines of work and certain previously planned policies," so, too, did it present the organization with a number of

20. KFA: Galen M. Fisher. "The Mother of the Japanese Army."
21. Davidann, 113.
22. KFA: "What Japan's Army Thinks of Christian Methods."

> opportunities which for the future will much more than make up for whatever may have been apparently lost. Through the war and opportunities in one connection with it the Association has been brought more vividly and more commendably to the attention of the Japanese public, Christian and non-Christian, and particularly to men in highest authority in government, than would have been possible in several years of ordinary growth and progress.[23]

One of the most auspicious of opportunities for the association was actually one of the most troublesome for the Japanese. As mentioned, the war was pyrrhic, with casualties upwards of 130,000 dead and wounded. Not surprisingly, the Japanese government had little desire to share this information at home or abroad, but still needed to provide hospital care for those whose deaths were not instantaneous and those who survived, but were scarred and maimed.[24] It was to these hospitals and convalescent homes that the YMCA next turned. Yet despite having a number of men trained or training as physicians among its ranks, the YMCA never attempted to aid or to interfere with the medical regimen delivered in these facilities. Rather, as before, it was decided that the association should instead concentrate on the moral and recreational rehabilitation of these unfortunate men. It was not, as general secretary at Kyoto G. S. Phelps iterated, a physical but a psychological and mental healing that the YMCA provided, a potential twisting of the medical mission. Thus, he reported, "the social side of the work is one of our greatest opportunities."[25] And, thus, as casualties began to steadily increase, the men and women of the YMCA dove into this aspect of one of their greatest of opportunities.

Not surprisingly, the work in the hospitals, which often included such luxuries as "magazines, games, writing materials, a phonograph, barber outfit, and some homely decorations," was quite popular among the invalids and the infirm. Supplying basic needs not provided for by the overworked hospital staff, the association men and women rapidly became among the most popular in the institution. C. V. Hibbard recounted to Bishop Harris his encounter with one injured soldier desperate for the most basic of hygienic necessities then lacking in the facility:

> Late in the afternoon one man spoke to me as I was crossing the yard and asked me to please wash his face. A glance and I had no thought to refuse. Both hands torn by a field gun, were neatly dressed and hung from slings from his neck. His hair, which had not been cut since Christmas, was all down over his face and ears. His face, which he said he had not been able to wash for five days before he was wounded, naturally had not been washed in the fifteen days since and was unspeakable. I cut his hair, shaved him, washed head and face and as much of his body as possible without undressing him and found a more than unusually fine face under the grime. He said frankly that he could not speak his gratitude and wouldn't try.[26]

23. KFA: V. W. Helm. "1903–04 Foreign Secretaries Reports," pp. 216–17.
24. "JAPANESE WAR CASUALTIES," C3.
25. KFA: G. S. Phelps. "1903–04 Foreign Secretaries Reports," p. 237.
26. KFA: Bishop Harris. "Association Secretaries in Manchurian Hospitals."

Similarly, the wounded, often in physical and mental pain, as well as increasingly bored, frequently welcomed the visits as a respite from both the anguish and the ennui. The most successful technique to combat both, association workers discovered, was employing music, an approach that Secretary C. V. Hibbard recommended utilizing, proclaiming, "When I ran out of material there was the phonograph to fall back on." The hometown paper of Troy, New York, the *Troy Times*, offered its readers a glimpse into this aspect of YMCA work, noting the association's work in the hospitals and adding that "the most popular thing the Secretaries do is to give gramophone concerts and entertainments at the hospital, as the poor fellows are glad of any break in the monotony."

Monotony could also be broken by the sheer sight of a foreigner or a woman, or both. Again, the association could provide this "interesting curiosity . . . to the average Japanese soldier, who is from the country." The attention paid to such a soldier, especially if he was far from home, alleviated some of the loneliness and the tedium of hospital residence.[27] So, too, did the gift of literature. Certainly, the association volunteers had little to offer casualties by way of halfpenny "dreadfuls" or dime novels, but the New Testament, both in English and in translation, provided a form of escapism to those seeking a fantastical story, and an answer to some of those seeking an explanation to counter existential crisis and impending death. Miss Elizabeth P. Milliken, a teacher at a female mission school in Tokyo and, later, the superintendent of the Women's Missionary Society, wrote to the YMCA mission board about her experiences distributing literature to hospitalized soldiers:

> Last Sunday afternoon Miss Mizuto and I took a supply of Testaments and tracts and went to one of the hospital wards, where men are badly crippled and cannot get out to the meetings. They are so ill that they are in little rooms, only three beds in a room. They said they rarely had visitors, and expressed much pleasure at our coming, and especially over the books. A number of them said they had heard of the Bible, and had long wanted to see it. One man said he had read "Hototogisu" (Mr. Tokutomi's famous Novel) and always remembered the girl who found "Kofuku" (happiness) in the Bible. He was going to search the Testament through and see if there was "Kofuku" in it for him.
>
> As we went down the hall, and the men found that flowers, singing and books were coming, they made ready for us by straightening out their bed clothes and pulling themselves up on their elbows to listen. Their politeness always finds some way of expressing itself. A few of them, who were able to walk on crutches, hopped out of bed and followed us rom [*sic*] room to room.
>
> We had not quite finished the round when the hour came for visitors to withdraw. We were hastily sending flowers into the yet unvisited rooms, and writing down the names of a few men with special requests, when I heard a plaintive voice saying, "Ask them please not to go away without giving me a Testament." I followed

27. KFA: "Japanese War Department and the Y.M.C.A.: Army Officers Pleased with the Organization." *Japanese Association Army Work News Service*. No. 2.
KFA: "Y. M. C. A. in Japanese Hospitals." *Troy Times*. Troy, NY. Dec. 27, 1904.

up the voice and found a man wasted to a shadow, and quite too ill to raise his head, but he stretched out to me a tract "The story of the Crucifixion." This was given to me in Hiroshima," he said, "I have read it over and over. They say there is more about the same story in the Bible."

I gave him a Testament, and asked his name, promising to see him the next time. "Dont [*sic*] forget" H said eagerly, "Next time." I was glad indeed that I had the Testament to give him then, for I almost doubted whether there would be a "Next time." . . .

Last Wednesday four men, from a ward which we had never yet visited, sent us their cards asking that we come and talk with them.[28]

Such experiences were common in the association's visits to military hospitals across the country. While not female, Reverend H. Loomis' work with the YMCA was met by hospitalized soldiers in a similar manner:

We visited the main hospital in Tokyo last September, where formerly I had found that only a few of the soldiers were favorable to Christianity. It was, therefore, important at first to overcome prejudice, so that we might convince them that we were their friends, and that Christianity was adapted to meet their greatest need.

The introduction of music secured for us a hearty welcome. The joy manifested in their faces was sufficient evidence that we had touched a sympathetic chord. Scriptures and tracts were offered to all, and none were refused. Then we decided to learn whether the men really desired the books, as we had no wish to impose upon them or to waste our ammunition. The question therefore asked in each ward as to how many wished a portion of the bible and a tract. Almost every hand was raised, and quite an eager desire was evident on many faces. We discovered that those whose hands were not lifted had failed to do so only because of inability on account of wounds. We visited twelve wards and supplied four hundred men.

The appreciation of the infirm was such that the approbation continued for the organization, even to the extent that the evangelists became ambassadors of America's goodwill toward the Japanese, something the YMCA capitalized on in the correspondences to the mission board:

The next day we went to one of the larger hospitals, where there were some three thousand sick and wounded. The head surgeon was very cordial and evidently pleased to see us. Directions were at once given to have all the officers assembled to meet us, and as they came in one by one it was a most impressive sight. At the sound of music their dark and stern faces lighted up with satisfaction and joy. Soon a little nurse came tottering in, bringing on her back an officer much larger than she, but unable to walk. He had caught the sounds of the music, and was anxious to see and hear. After some songs and instrumental music, a colonel, who was suffering from a severe wound, stepped forward and said:

"In behalf of my comrades, I wish to thank you for your visit and the great pleasure you have given us. We appreciate very much the kindness and sympathy

28. Sasakuba, 90; KFA: "Work among the Sick and Wounded."

> of the American people, and we wish to make this known. Such kindness is beyond our power to repay. My great desire is to recover as soon as possible, that I may return to the front and do all that is in my power to bring this war to a successful issue."
>
> We went from ward to ward among the men, and as the strains of music reached their ears those who were able to move rushed forward with eager faces and listened with intense interest to all that was said. After the music, the purpose of our visit was explained, and Scriptures were promised to all who desired them. This was evidently a welcome announcement, and was followed, in some cases, by the Japanese cheer or a clapping of the hands.[29]

Of course, these visits were not merely about fostering a passion for music or for solving boredom, and to the delight of the missionaries, some of the hospitalized soldiers proved receptive to their teaching. Beyond the care and attention these men and women paid to the infirm, the message they preached also resonated with a few of their charges. These veterans had seen death, both on the field and in the hospital, and some seemed to understand that, just as there were no atheists in foxholes, neither were there on deathbeds.[30] Thus, for some infirm and wounded soldiers, the gospel, as it was intended, was a comfort, and assured them that their suffering was not in vain. In that way, too, it comforted the missionaries, assuring them that their work was not without reward. As Miss R. J. Watson commented, the war work seemed a culmination of much of the YMCA's work in Japan up to this point. In the aftermath of the Russo-Japanese War, in the hospitals, "we have a fine opportunity to sow broadcast [*sic*] the seeds of Christianity,—then trust God to water and care for it, until it grows to perfect fruit."[31]

Such acceptance, rare though it may have been, may have surprised both the soldiers and the missionaries who served them. Certainly, both were looking for something to fill the lacunae each possessed. Miss A. E. Garvin, a teacher at the girls' missionary school in Osaka, was pleased to report that "the hospital work has been full of surprises from the start," the biggest of which "is the appetite which the men themselves evince for tracts and Christian books. . . . Since they have faced death, the great question is occupying a prominent place in their minds. . . . What impressed me is that these men want something that they think Christian missionaries can give them."

The missionaries' surprise turned to pleasure as they saw the effect that their visits had on the veterans and the medical staff. Garvin marveled, "In reply to a

29. KFA: Rev. H. Loomis. "Christian Work among Japanese Soldiers." *The Missionary Review of the World*. Feb., 1905. p. 120.
30. And, to the evangelists, the Japanese might well have been atheists of a sort. Within the Christian belief system, the amalgam of Buddhist and Shinto beliefs to which many Japanese professed was merely another way of denying the existence of God. Still, while many evangelists knew that proselytizing to atheists was futile—since atheism was based solely on a negation of everything in which the evangelist believed—to preach to so-called heathens was not, for such people, they imagined, lacked an insight into the truth, and, in their ignorance, worshipped incorrectly. This, however, is a discussion for another work.
31. KFA: "Work among the Sick and Wounded," p. 9.

modest request last spring the physician replied that the whole place, and all the other hospitals yet to be built, were at my disposal for Christian work. The under doctors and nurses were ordered to let me pass, and to give me assistance that I required."[32] The freedom of movement and the freedom to preach had, in fact, increased, particularly in the hospitals. Despite the best and continued efforts of anti-Christian factions within the country—often those among the elite who committed apostasy earlier—the war work was proving successful in turning the tide of sentiment in favor of the work done, if not of the religion itself.

Acquiescence further turned towards acknowledgement, and, thus, it was of little surprise that doctors soon saw the mental health benefits that the association's teachings could promote. While physicians employed by the Japanese military proved to be some of the most sophisticated in the country, if not the world, many saw that the physical assistance they could offer was rarely complete when there was no amelioration of psychological trauma. If nothing else, the association could offer something for this. Whether it was an afternoon's entertainment, a comforting visit, or the opportunity to occupy the mind with something other than death and fear, the YMCA's war work provided patients with both the patience and the will to heal. A man identified by Rev. Henry Loomis as the chief surgeon of the Imperial Japanese Army, Dr. K. Hayakawa, wrote to the association as "the Head Surgeon of the Kaijo Military Hospital in Manchuria," to report his gratitude:

> At the battle of Mukden I was at the Liau Yang Hospital and treated an enormous number of wounded men. Towards these men we were bound to discharge our duty as physicians by the most careful medical treatment; but I have always had the opinion that this is not enough. With the care for the bodies I have cherished the desire to add religious teachings.
>
> In consequence of these views I have tried to have the patients read religious and especially Christian books. As there was no provision for the spiritual comfort of the men at Liau Yang I had to read these books to the patients with the aid of my assistants.
>
> Imperfect as such a means of comfort was we were pleased to see that some of the patients died in perfect peace, confiding themselves entirely to God and to Christ; and still more of them returned to the ranks perfectly cured; for their belief in divine help, in addition to medical treatment, encouraged their hearts and hastened their recovery.
>
> In order to perpetuate such teachings, and also as a souvenir of war I proposed to publish a book entitled, "The Heart's Comforter" and to distribute about five hundred copies to each Division.[33]

32. Barrows, 447; KFA: "Work among the Sick and Wounded," pp. 10–11.
33. KFA: Rev. H. Loomis. "Among the Sick and Wounded." The publication of the book planned by Dr. Hayakawa seems to have never been pursued, either by him or by the association. Moreover, it appears that Dr. Hayakawa was Hayakawa Kiyoshi, a man now infamous as a colleague of Dr. Ishii Shiro (of the notorious Unit 731 during World War II), and quite possibly complicit in, though never charged with, biological warfare war crimes. (Powell, John W. "Japan's Biological Weapons: 1930–1945." *Bulletin of the Atomic Scientists*, vol. 37, no. 8, Oct., 1981, pp. 43–51.)

Mrs. James McCauley, a member of both the female counterpart of the YMCA and the Woman's Christian Temperance Union, was delighted to discover that their work reverberated outside the hospital walls, as "mothers and father thank us so kindly for coming to see 'Their boys.'"[34] Yet this did not mean that parents approved of their children converting, nor did it indicate that many soldiers chose to do so. It was nice, both for parents and for their sons, that not everyone in the country disdained their children, either for failing to complete their national duty or for their complicity in a war that proved unpopular postvictory.[35]

It was also nice for soldiers to interact with people who sought only to assist them. In truth, such assistance may not have been required, but the association missionaries were nothing if not attentive and committed. Nor did they discriminate within the hospital; officers and enlisted men were given equal time. Indeed, for the illiterate veterans, too, these men and women brought pictures, photographs, and illustrated works. Loduska Wirick, the missionary deemed the "Angel of the Hospital" and the "Florence Nightingale of the Orient," was particularly dedicated to assisting the men who had served their country yet still had not benefited from its educational reforms, and she reveled in her work:

> I am very glad indeed to have the pictures. I took the albums to the hospital and I wish you could have seen the men gather around-wardens and all-looking at them.
>
> In some wards (there are 60 in some) every man would put up his hand and ask if he might have one. When I told them I could give them but one in a room they looked disappointed; and as many as could get up would go to the one who had the book and eagerly wait his turn to get it. So many are confined to their beds I am sure these pictures will help them to more cheerfully pass the long painful hours they must suffer before they recover from their wounds.

The Angel of the Hospital continued her work long after the injured veterans had recovered and returned home, keeping in contact with many, who fondly remembered her, not necessarily as the woman who brought them to Christ, but the woman who cared for and about them. Indeed, one such soldier had encouraged his family, much to Wirick's dismay, to worship at her portrait in their home shrine.[36]

For the missionaries and, more significant, for their charges, there were hours to pass in the hospitals, and, without any other stimuli, this time was spent in the mind. For many, these were hours spent contemplating one's own mortality, a truly frightening prospect, made more so by the proximity to death in the military existence of these young soldiers. As Mrs. Gibert Bowles reported to Loomis, "The men literally devour anything given them to read. . . . They are inclined to seek for life eternal."[37] Bowles assumed this meant that such men had received a calling from God, but, more often, it was equal parts ennui and fear. Wirick was somewhat

34. *The Christian Movement* 1905, p. 35; KFA: Rev. H. Loomis. "Work in the Hospitals." *War Time in Japan*, p. 15.
35. Stolberg, "Review: *The Russo-Japanese War*," p. 444.
36. KFA: Rev. H. Loomis. "Pictures and Picture Albums." *War Time in Japan*; McLean, 218–19.
37. KFA: Rev. H. Loomis. "Work in the Hospitals." *War Time in Japan*, 17.

more circumspect, admitting that, while "during all these months, (now nearly two years) since the war began, all Christian literature and the Gospels have been gladly received by the soldiers and carefully read," it was similarly true that "while they [the infirm] are shut up in the hospital they are glad for anything to occupy their minds, but reading is the principal thing."[38]

Nevertheless, both the fear and the ennui were hardly hindrances to the growth of faith. Indeed, some soldiers claimed that their experiences, bored and afraid in the hospital, were the spark needed to enlighten them. One soldier wrote to the Tokyo missionary who visited him in the hospital that the missionary's gift of the New Testament "was indeed the beginning of my faith. I was wearied by long confinement on a sick bed and I began to read the books earnestly."[39] Perhaps the most famous anecdote among the association and their supporters in America was that of Takasaburo Yoshimasu. As Loomis reported,

> Takasaburo Yoshimasu is 26 years of age and was called to go to the war in the month of August 1904. He left a wife, and a little daughter,—born after his departure, which he has never seen.
>
> On the night of November 28th he was among the troops engaged in the assault upon Port Arthur, and was struck by a ball which deprived him of both of his eyes.
>
> After he was thus wounded he was very much depressed in spirit; and he felt that life to him in such a condition would be of no value. He had never heard of Christ; and had no source of comfort for this life, or hope in the life to come.
>
> Rather than be a burden to his family, and endure the some [*sic*] wretched condition of mind and heart he determined to take his own life; and thus put an end to has [*sic*] misery. But in his sightless condition he was unable to carry out his purpose; and was sent to the Toyoma hospital in Tokyo.
>
> There he was found by Miss Wirick, who told him of Christ, and how He would give him peace of mind, joy in his heart, keep him from sin, and give him eternal life in heaven.
>
> In the words of Miss Wirick, . . . "Life was now a different thing to him. He was completely happy; and he began to make plans for the future." . . .
>
> Miss Wirick has procured a small instrument for making the raised letters, and with it he has written to her a letter, the translation of which is as follows.
>
> "Teacher of Christ; I am very thankful to have recently learned of God's great love to the world; for, when I was first wounded, there could be nothing greater than my suffering, and my life was filled with anguish all the time.

38. KFA: *War Time in Japan No. 3*, 13. This YMCA work was also extended to Russian prisoners of war, despite the vast majority of these men being Christians (although the wrong sect). However, it is interesting to note that the response from these men was also included in Loomis' reports. What amazing work the association was doing when "even [a] Russian POW wrote thanks: 'We have here only a few Russian books, read and re-read for a long time. Imagine then our lively joy when we received your papers, which besides the pleasure of reading them gives us plenty of material for work, for many among the prisoners are studying the English language.' From L. de Bagretzoff (Lieut. Of the Cossaks). Shizuoka, 2/26/05." The mere utility of the work of the YMCA was seen as a success, despite its failure to instigate mass conversions (KFA: Loomis, *War Time in Japan*, 22–23).

39. KFA: Rev. H. Loomis. "Soldiers Letters." *War Time in Japan*, 19.

> After coming to the hospital, and hearing the singing of hymns and the teaching of Christ's love, I knew my sins were great in His sight, and I repented and prayed that He would take them away and give me His love and peace. I was happy then, and my heart was filled with joy continually. All sorrow and anguish disappeared, and I now have happiness and peace that those who have eyes cannot know, and I rejoice to know that there is a living God for the blind, and thank you for helping me know the way of salvation."
>
> Miss Wirick adds "Daily we find him reading his Bible, with many other soldiers gathered around him; watching his face as it lights up with gladness as his fingers touch each new word, and listening to the truth as he reads it to them. As he sits up and tells them about what he reads, the Spirit shines out through his wounded, scarred face until it is beautiful with joy and peace. He is the happiest man in his building, and a comfort and help to every man in the wards. Hundred [*sic*] are asking for this Gospel that has saved him, and it is for us to supply them."[40]

Although no one in the association presumed that Yoshimasu's blindness was able to be cured by his dedication to God, they were aware of the assumed power of faith on one's ability to heal. Whether this could be attributed to divine intervention or some psychosomatic nature of belief was seen as irrelevant. What was known was that faith offered a desire and a drive to improve one's lot in life, even in the most dire and depressing of circumstances. Neither was this awareness limited to the missionaries practicing in Japan. Like Yoshimasu, other veterans had experienced the psychological healing brought by conversion. Such anecdotes were eagerly bandied about in the association and its home offices as illustrations of both the enormity and the practicality of God's divine power. Loomis dedicated considerable time and effort to recording examples of such works:

> A missionary wrote: "Only yesterday a fine young soldier who had lost his right leg was here. His misfortune seemed so great to him that he was wondering whether it would not be better for himself, his family, and society if he were to put an end to his life, when a Bible was given to him. It brought him new views of duty to his fellow men and to God. He is now a happy Christian, and hopes to be baptized on the first Sunday of the New Year." . . .
>
> A non-commissioned officer says, "The knowledge of God as our Father and Christ as our Savior from sin, which came into my sad heart while I was in the hospital ward, was brighter than sun light slanting across a dungeon."

Similarly, Japanese physicians had long recognized this effect, and some had commented as much to the men and women of the association, who, in turn, discussed it with men like Loomis. The latter proudly reported it back home, as in the following passage:

> One of the Head Surgeons, who was in charge of a hospital at the front, and who is not a Christian, makes the following statement, "All observations have tended

40. KFA: Rev. H. Loomis. *Among Japanese Soldiers*, 1–3.

> to show me the great need for soldiers to have a deep rooted faith in religion; and, so far as has been possible, I have given them religious books, especially Christian books to read, so that they might find much needed comfort. For this reason, I, and my under officers used to read to the men whenever time permitted.
>
> We have noticed the powerful effect of the Christian faith, and what a great factor this faith has been toward rapid recovery on the part of the less seriously wounded when they can believe in the presence of a prayer hearing God,—besides and beyond the works of the doctors and nurses."[41]

If spirituality was medicinal—and therefore virtuous—why, then, did the YMCA not attempt also to employ physicians to assist the injured and infirm, both in the military hospitals and in sanatoriums, as they so eagerly did missionaries in the former? Again, the question came down to utility. Although it may have proved equally as effective to save souls by saving lives (for what could convince someone of the power of the divine more than a chance for continued life), it actually served to distance faith from the equation. To be as persuasive as possible, science, although neither unknown to nor antithetical to the evangelists, could not be as large a part of the equation as trust in God. To ensure that the two were not seen as competitors in any true sense, particularly since many evangelists feared that the Japanese had, in only just being truly exposed to salvation, an inability to grasp that science and religion need not be a dichotomy, it was thought best to rely solely on faith. And, in doing so, the evangelists of the YMCA fostered the power of spirituality. In many respects, it proved successful, particularly among soldiers who felt they had been saved from certain death and among those who felt that they still required salvation from that eventuality. In such cases, men like Kano Eko, a converted Buddhist priest who fought on the frontlines, became illustrations of the strength of Christianity's power as both salve and savior. As Loomis reported to both the YMCA and the American Bible Society, Kano wrote to him from the frontlines to testify to the importance of both organizations continued support:

> Death is very close to the soldiers now, and this makes them very serious. Each battle serves to drive away superstitions that have filled their minds. . . .
>
> Throughout the whole of the war the Bible has always been eagerly read. Think of the great assistance which has been rendered by you. The books you have contributed were indeed the *most effectual spiritual medicine on the field of battle*.[42]

The acknowledgment of such spiritual medicine proved further effective in loosening the purse strings of many American Protestants because it seemed to be evidence of an understanding of the utility of faith. Beyond all spirituality, pragmatism often reigned supreme in this new century. If the Japanese citizenry were prepared to accept Christianity for its utility, if not for its spiritual promise, that still

41. KFA: Rev. H. Loomis. "Among the Sick and Wounded." *War Time in Japan No. 3*, 5–6, 4. Loomis was also a prominent member of the American Bible Society in Japan.
42. Ibid., 11. Italics were from Kano's letter.

garnered "prestige and momentum," as Galen M. Fisher noted, "that will be worth incalculable sums of money and numbers of men in the Christianization of the Far East." Japan was an investment. And it was one that the YMCA was eager to see pay off.[43]

Pragmatism had also come to shape the attitudes of many of Japan's political and bureaucratic elite with regard to Protestantism in general, and, often, the YMCA in particular. Loomis excitedly reported at the end of the war that Ōkuma Shigenobu, former prime minister of Japan and founder of Waseda University, whom we have met above, was invited to give the commencement exercises at the American Methodist Mission's Aoyama Gakuin College, where he proclaimed:

> I believe that Protestantism is the most advanced form of Christianity. There is a possibility, I think, that the centre of civilization will come round to the Far East when this advanced religion [Christianity] has rightly been interwoven into the thoughts of the nation and the nation has progressed with the times. I believe any nation that makes an antiquated faith its state religion will soon cease to exist. Therefore I hope that you will endeavor to live up to the teaching of Christ.[44]

To view Ōkuma as a "Pseudo-Christian" would be an overstatement, perhaps, but, as a shrewd politician, he was well aware of the opportunities for both the nation and for his own political career if he were to align himself with charitable efforts in the military and in education, two of the main pillars of Japan's ever-increasing might. It is fitting that, despite his praise of and association with Christian organizations, he never became a Christian. He could be a YMCA supporter, but he could never see the need for his own "endeavor to live up to the teaching of Christ."[45]

The association could not afford to let the distinction bother it. Again, this sense of utility was not lost on the leaders of Japan's YMCA associate national secretary V. W. Helm, who had reported to the home office, as early as the beginning of the Russo-Japanese War, that the association representatives in Japan "need to be so able to work with others and through others that those best able to do without us may desire our presence for what we may be able to do with and through still others. In the future our tenure here may be assured not so much by the official positions we occupy as by the personal equation of our lives and our ability to fill a real need."[46] With such a raison d'être, the association continued to seek ways to ingratiate itself with the upper echelons of society in the years following the Russo-Japanese War.

Without a war, however, the YMCA found itself in need of a new task that would make it as invaluable to the government and to its military allies as its military work had done previously. This was more difficult. The YMCA had, in some sense, been associated with war since its earliest American activities. In the Civil and Spanish-American Wars, the YMCA had established itself, under its own name

43. KFA: Galen M. Fisher. "The Mother of the Japanese Army."
44. KFA: Rev. H. Loomis. *War Time in Japan*. No. 3, 31.
45. Some may argue that he was, in his own mind, a Christ figure unto himself.
46. KFA: V. W. Helm. *1903–4 Foreign Secretaries Reports*, 221.

or that of the United States Christian Commission, at the forefront of American military assistance.[47] Yet, in America, by the turn of the century it had parlayed its work for the armed forces during times of peace, as well. So, to follow the model set by their counterparts across the Pacific, the men and women of the YMCA in Japan sought a niche that would allow them to maintain the amity of Japan's elite garnered through their war work. They needed this continued goodwill, as the war effort had brought in significant donations from the Japanese themselves, allowing for at least a facade of self-sufficiency and moral entrepreneurial success. As stated in the 1905 pamphlet *The Young Men of the Sunrise Kingdom*, "the Association has won the approval of cautious non-Christian men of wealth, as is shown by the fact that the MITSUI family, Baron IWASAKI and MURAI Brothers, all contributed liberally to it last year. Perhaps even more striking is the fact that a non-Christian millionaire has offered to give as high as $2,500 for an Association building in Sendai, if citizens of that city will give $1,250."[48]

With such reward from the war effort, YMCA members sought, in essence, to follow the military men into the cities, where the missionaries tried to continue their interrupted lives in schools or at work. Having the background in early English education that many of Japan's missionaries had utilized at the beginning of Meiji, they returned to assist at the elite colleges and universities in ways equally conducive to learning and to moral edification. Here, these men, assisted by their pupils, established student branches of the association, often dedicated as much to social interactions as to Christ. Under the watchful eye of the secretary, young men could live, eat, play, and learn in these dormitories and buildings erected with donated money, much of which came from patrons impressed with the association's war work. G. S. Phelps excitedly proclaimed that "the social side of the work is one of our greatest opportunities."[49]

In many ways, it was. Certainly, it continued to maintain goodwill among much of Japan's political and bureaucratic elite. In protecting young boys from moral vices and in promoting their studies, the association had assisted the government's efforts to foster the next generation of Japan's successful leaders. In his annual report for 1906, Kyoto secretary G. S. Phelps trumpeted that under his watch the Kyoto association had maintained the sense of utility that he and his peers had fostered during the Russo-Japanese War:

> There has been no change in the favorable attitude of PUBLIC OPINION towards the Association. Indeed the success of the evening school and the splendid record of the Army Department, with the Imperial recognition of the work, have greatly enhanced the reputation of the Association. TWELVE PROMINENT BUSINESS

47. Mjagkij, 53; Putney, 186.
48. KFA: *The Young Men of the Sunrise Kingdom*, 3. There is, sadly, no indication of whether the citizens of Sendai were able to offer that large of a donation, or even if they attempted to do so. In any case, the sentiment of the millionaire was almost as worthwhile as his money.
49. KFA: G. S. Phelps, 237.

> MEN have become legal sponsors for the Association. Two leading NEWS-PAPERS have endorsed the work in editorials. We are more and more becoming acquainted with shop boys and merchants. I enjoy the privilege of being a member of the COMMERCIAL CLUB of Kyoto, to which two hundred of the leading merchants belong.[50]

While this new role did not sit well with everyone, the association had found its next contribution to Japan's prosperity. Indeed, Phelps also reported that his biggest detractor, the editor of the *Kobe Chronicle*, had, despite his vociferous denunciations of the association, failed to garner any real following:

> There has been some open criticism of our work in the "Kobe Chronicle", the leading English paper in Japan, in point of circulation. Its editor is rantingly anti-Christian never losing an opportunity to show his dislike. He has several times attacked the Association this year but as he chose the wrong time and spoke with great ignorance of our Association it has not done us much damage. We have sent our army reports broadcast to his constituency and drew largely from Kobe people for Army work funds. He acknowledged defeat when he complained that he could not understand how we got so close to the government and he went so far as to declare that it was unconstitutional for the government to grant us such favors![51]

Much to the editor's dismay, the government's infatuation with the association showed no signs of abating.

Interestingly, the YMCA's social work did not require members to visit potential converts in their homes or neighborhoods. Instead, the association chose to build community centers most often in more pleasant surroundings, including close to the dormitories they had previously constructed on or near college campuses.[52] With its meeting hall, classrooms, and athletic facilities, the buildings became literal beacons for bored men of the urban centers, which in Tokyo was, as Colonel Alfred Eliab Buck, former US minister to Japan, was quoted in a 1905 American fund-raising pamphlet, the building that "stands more prominently before the general public as an index of organized Christianity." This was quite an accomplishment for a Christian building in general, and certainly for one that was not affiliated with a particular sect or one easily recognizable as a church, cathedral, or tabernacle. Yet, as Buck maintained, Tokyo's own YMCA building was the "recognized center of many kinds of educational and benevolent work, which I am confident exert a strong influence for good."[53]

But for the YMCA members social work was an evangelism built upon pleasant interaction and positive relationships, and it was with this moral method that the organization became associated in Japan. Secretary of the Tokyo association C. V. Hibbard, under whose leadership the city's YMCA building was erected, embraced

50. KFA: G. S. Phelps. Annual Report of G. S. Phelps for the year ending Sep. 30, 1905 (Kyoto), 2.
51. Ibid., 216.
52. Sasamori and Kingsbury, 36.
53. KFA: *The Young Men of the Sunrise Kingdom*, 1905.

this evangelistic niche. Under Hibbard's leadership, the association would not only use its facilities for this specific brand of "social" work, it would expand them. With the assistance of his Japanese counterpart, Secretary Yamamoto, but primarily with (mostly foreign) donations, Hibbard added a "game room," equal parts a gymnasium and an area to play popular, less physical games, as well as a nine-thousand-square-foot annex to the already fairly imposing building. In it, Hibbard envisioned a "basement with lavatory, baths, barber shop, etc. and a roof garden suitable for basket ball, hand ball, light apparatus, or restaurant and open air meetings." But it was difficult to discuss Christ's divinity while playing basketball. As the association's leadership tried to justify their work as purely religious teaching, it soon became obvious that the association's work, while spiritual and moral, was considered by many of their attendees to be less about faith, and more about fun. Hibbard could report to the home office that "now . . . as never before the public both Christian and non-Christian looks to the Association in Japan as the effective agent of the church united to execute important social and religious work," but the nature of the work was rarely social or religious. Nonetheless, it was for this reason that the YMCA became as popular as it did, particularly with Japanese politicians. Hibbard, in the same report home, acknowledged this fact, albeit without identifying the contradiction:

> As previously reported the late baron General Kodama looked to the Association to fill the long felt want for wholesome recreation and sound moral instrustion [*sic*] in the army. The minister of war expressed himself similarly. The minister of Education in conversation with our secretaries expressed his confidence in the Y.M.C.A. by asking that we supplement the activities of the Educational Dept. by the establishment of dormitories. In a recent interview the primier [*sic*], Baron Saionji, and the prominent statesman and educator Count Okuma evidenced their interest in what we are trying to do for the moral and social welfare of the students [such] that they offered counsel or such other assistance as they might be able to render.[54]

Other regional leaders, however, were quick to point out the disparity between the association's mission and its Japanese missionizing. Galen M. Fisher, general secretary for the YMCA, desperately wished to remedy the inconsistency, taking the opportunity presented in his 1906 annual report to call attention to it:

> A fourth difficulty is to raise ourselves, as well as our Japanese brothers, to anything near an adequate vision of the spiritual, no less than the social, possibilities of our movement. Who can overdraw them in view of either the student, the city, or the

54. KFA: C. V. Hibbard. "Annual Report for 1906." Tokyo. p. 2. In another report by Galen M. Fisher, then general secretary for the YMCA in Japan, the minister of education is quoted as telling association officials that his peers "were greatly distressed about the moral condition of students and the low character of the ordinary lodging houses and shall welcome whatever you can do to help solve the problem." The quote is followed by a request to the home office for $20,000 to build dormitories for the two imperial universities alone. There is, of course, no mention of expenditure on the part of the Japanese government (KFA: Sept. 30, 1906 Report, p. 3).

> army field alone in Japan herself; or in view of the channels carrying our influence all over Asia; or in view of the approaching World's Student Christian Federation Conference, already casting its light before it round the world? The forceful presentation of Christ to the student body of 140,000 boys and men has never been more than half attempted. The deep plowing of the spiritual life of our membership is the first thing in our policies but often the last thing in our practice. I feel myself to blame for not a little of this. I am driven over and over to the conclusion that all other difficulties head up here. God help us to be more and to do more to solve it than we have had faith to try this past year.[55]

To resolve this discrepancy was also to risk alienating the support of much of Japan's population, particularly when faced with the cessation of war, and thus, of war work, which had won that support originally and had undergirded the association's efforts and success. In the following year's special report of statistics from the Nagasaki association, Secretary J. Merle Davis noted that the association was facing "falling membership due in part to not holding [the] interest of young men who joined 'eagerly' upon the opening of the new building," but also acknowledged that much of the appeal of the YMCA was the novelty of it. Moreover, by abandoning the fresh and attractive aspects of its work in Japan, Davis knew that its utility to Japan's political elite would be diminished, and would be completely obliterated were the association to reverse its course, as Fisher desired. To illustrate as much, Davis recounted an anecdote in his 1907 annual report concerning Ōkuma's YMCA endorsement:

> Last February Count Okuma told an American missionary during a conversation upon the problem of Christianity in Japan, that he believes the type of religion that will gain a permanent hold and general acceptance in Japan is that which [expr] esses itself in practical service to society *without placing dogmas or sacraments in the front of its creed.* He cited the Salvation Army and Young Men's Christian Association as the two leading exponents of this kind of religion. Without criticizing the veteran stateman's [*sic*] estimate of our work and the type of faith it represents, the fact remains that to this practical, critical people the religion that alleviates and ministers to moral intellectual physical need presents a powerful appeal.[56]

Christianity in general and the YMCA in particular were in danger of being pigeonholed as either a novelty or a utility, or both, a trend that continued throughout the Meiji period. Without a war, the association lacked a truly captive audience, and had failed to find a modicum of success in its urban, academic efforts, a fact that was not lost on Japanese politicians and bureaucrats, and yet was also considered

55. KFA: Galen M. Fisher. Sept. 30, 1906 Report, p. 3. Whether this disparity was unique to Japan is not mentioned. Certainly, Japan presents a challenge to evangelists in East Asia as the only country not subject to colonial or semicolonial regulations, thereby making the government of Japan one of the few whose autochthonous leadership controlled all aspects of national life.
56. KFA: J. Merle Davis. Special Report of Statistics, Nagasaki Association. Oct. 5, 1907, p. 1; KFA: J. M. Davis. Annual Report. Nagasaki. 1907. Oct. 5, pp. 4–5. Emphasis in original.

wholly positive by such men, unlike the possibility of public health efforts. Tokutomi Sohō, having long denounced his association with the religion, noted in his periodical, *Kokumin Shimbun*, in 1909 that "Christianity is already a powerful factor of moral and social culture in Japan," for the "Christmas festivities are now very popular in Japan and conducted even in non-Christian families. Christian music is very fashionable in Japan. Pianos, violins, etc., are now manufactured in this country and kept in many families." Similarly, he wrote, "Though not necessarily observed as sacred days, Sundays have been holidays in Japan since 1876," which should, added to the popularity of Christmas, have made the Christians, both foreign and Japanese, terribly happy, and despite, as he later noted, the fact that "the actual converts in Japan at present are less than 200,000." The article was included in the annual publication *The Christian Movement in Japan*, a substantial tome distributed worldwide announcing the successes of evangelism in the nation that past year in the hope of obtaining more funds among their coreligionists. The 1909 issue, in which Tokutomi's article was highlighted, was edited by Ernest W. Clement and Galen M. Fisher, the latter being the general secretary of the YMCA, and, as seen above, concerned about the role of Christianity in Japan so beautifully illustrated in Tokutomi's article. Yet, had he not cited Tokutomi's words, Fisher recognized that all that Christians in Japan, not merely just the YMCA, would have to show for decades of hard work and dedication was the conversion of significantly less than a hundredth of the population. Instead, he embraced it in its entirety, including Tokutomi's conclusion that "on the whole, the prospects of Christianity in Japan are very bright, and there is and will be ample room for foreign workers to assist their Japanese co-workers."[57]

If assistance without doctrine was the best inroad for Japanese Christianity then there could be no conflict with the mission, particularly since, in the 1906 Second Japan YMCA Convention, the National Committee had insisted that it would be able to become wholly self-sufficient in its ability to raise 50,000 yen before 1917, domestically and abroad. In truth, what had previously been the most successful aspect of the work of the association was also its current roadblock. After the wars of the middle and late Meiji, even with the war work undertaken by the YMCA, Westernization's sheen had worn off . Japan had already succeeded in becoming a world power, many politicians and intellectuals believed. Moreover, with disappointment over the Triple Intervention of 1895 and the terms of the Treaty of Portsmouth of 1905, it was beginning to seem silly to admire or fear a "West" so

57. *The Christian Movement 1909*, 463–64; A longtime resident of Japan, Clement (1860–1941) served as an evangelist, teacher, interpreter, editor, correspondent, and author, and was awarded the fifth class of the Order of the Rising Sun (Rogala, 36). The population of Japan at the end of 1909 was estimated at 51,742,565 following the previous census the year prior. Using 200,000 as the number of converts at this time, the exact calculation lists that 0.003865 of the total population of Japan was Christian, or fewer than four in a thousand. It is also interesting to note that, by the same calculations, the cities (where the YMCA was active) contained only 11.52 percent of the population in 1909, with rural areas housing 88.48 percent of the nation's subjects ("Japan in 1909," 1139).

rife with contradiction and failure. The revision of the unequal treaties and the alliance with Britain at the opening of the twentieth century proved that Japan was in no danger of following Asia into the future as a Euro-American colony. And Christianity, too, seemed more trite; after all, did the Protestant ethic really require Protestantism?[58]

Nevertheless, as their industries grew and their influence spread, many of Japan's business and political leaders recognized that Christianity continued to play a role in international relations, and, more important, that it was unnecessary to convert to reap the benefits of this role. While the Second YMCA Japan Convention provided lofty goals for the association, it allowed ample opportunity for the local businessmen and politicians to garner positive press and, at times, to connect, even indirectly, to men like John Mott and John Wanamaker.[59] Such was the case following the conference in Tokyo, when many of the leaders of the international YMCA traveled to Osaka, and thus were "brought forcibly to the attention of the governor, mayor and other officials and leading business men of Osaka" who were eager to take advantage of the opportunity. As George Gleason, secretary of Osaka's YMCA, reported, "the mayor's greeting at the station and his dinner to Messers. Woodward, Sleman and Mott were unprecedented in conservative Osaka. The governor's carriage, one of three such vehicles in our big city, was for a day and a half at their service."[60] Such politicking was not limited to local dignitaries, Galen M. Fisher, the general secretary, noted, as the conference had served national leaders as well:

> We can soberly accept the estimate of Prince Ito that "the Conference will ever remain one of the most memorable events in the history of Japan" and of The Japan Times, edited by a Japanese, that "so passed into history one of the most memorable events this country has witnessed in the course of its foreign intercourse." But they assessed it for its international political and moral value. We can say the same of it because of its religious power.[61]

The religious power that Fisher vehemently believed the YMCA possessed in Japan was debatable at best, but the power it held over other evangelical organizations was more pronounced, at least in the minds of the YMCA's leadership in Japan. As Phelps reported, the humanistic bent of the native churches and the lack of political connections among the other foreign evangelical groups meant that "in

58. Y.M.C.A. shi, 27; Fujio, 55–56. Max Weber's failure to understand nuances of Asian countries and cultures was not limited to Japan. Indeed, China, despite his groundbreaking work on its sociology, bore the brunt of his assumptions, as many a chagrined Sinologist will tell you (van der Sprenkel, 348).

59. Wanamaker, a longtime member of the YMCA, was also one of its greatest philanthropists. Though perhaps not as identifiable today, Wanamaker, a businessman and politician, was as well known as Rockefeller or Macy during his lifetime and assisted in constructing missions and businesses abroad (Appel, 404).

60. KFA: Report of George Gleason for Quarter April to June, 1907. East Northfield, Mass. Aug. 24, 1907, pp. 1–2. Gleason's report on the conference was submitted fairly late. As it turns out, this was due to his nervous breakdown, which also is part of the reason that the report was dispatched from Massachusetts, not Osaka.

61. KFA: Annual Report of Galen M. Fisher for the year 1906–1907, p. 1. Prince Ito is Itō Hirobumi, former prime minister of Japan and later resident general of Korea, one of the most significant figure in Meiji politics.

the future practically the only foreigners who will find a large place in the Christian work in Japan are the Association secretaries. For obvious reasons it will be seen that I write this statement very confidentially." Through its utility, the YMCA had pushed itself to the vanguard of Japanese life, even if that vanguard was far more political than spiritual or salubrious.[62]

But, of course, a vanguard was hardly the entirety of the population, and the forefront here ignored the remainder of Japan's society. Thus, among the perceptive members of the YMCA, the work the association had performed remained incomplete, both religiously and socially as it lacked condign attention to the problems of the poor. Fisher sensed this lacuna, and tried to bring it to the attention of his peers and superiors:

> There is not a little danger that our very prestige and success in certain great movements, such as the Army work in Japan . . . will make it easy for us to overlook the great unmet need of the thousands of men in our membership and the millions more who are properly within our field of work, but whom we are making no systematic nor adequate efforts to influence. . . . the glamour and success of the great movement which we are providentially called to lead in will make it impossible for us to do thorough and deep religious work.[63]

It should seem an obvious choice to concentrate on the impoverished. After all, the Judeo-Christian ethic values the least of us, and Christianity in particular has the example of the Good Samaritan. Yet this pillar of Christian morals seemed to evade many in the organization. Unlike Fisher, Phelps was a bit clearer in identifying a specific point of ignorance of his organization, perhaps because his position was somewhat more focused on Kyoto specifically. In any case, his 1908 report reminded his peers of the importance of assisting those without political influence and clout:

> Kyoto harbours one of the three great slum districts in Japan. Almost as near the sacred Imperial Palace reserve on one side as is the most respectable residence district of the Empire on the other, it presents one of the most deplorable and neglected open sores in the world. This great "Nishijin" region is full of spinning factories and private weaving establishments operated by child and woman labor that would make the worst sweat shop in the ghetto blush. One Japanese physician told me that the year before last his Maternity Hospital had attended one thousand charity cases of confinement among the young girls of this district, not more than ten per cent of which were legitimate. This the result of packing young boys and girls indiscriminately into small, unsanitary sleeping rooms.

62. KFA: Annual Report of G. S. Phelps for year ending Sept. 30, 1907. p. 4.
63. KFA: Annual Report of Galen M. Fisher for the Year 1907–1908. p. 5. Fisher's assessment that thousands of men among the ranks of the association go unnoticed is a bit hyperbolic, but there were certainly millions in the same cities occupied by YMCA city associations who desperately needed assistance, though perhaps not necessarily of a religious kind.

Had Phelps' peers followed up, they would have discovered, as anthropologist Ronald O. Haak did some sixty years later, that Nishijin was a region in desperate need of social work, with or without the religious education that would have provided the backdrop for such assistance from the YMCA. Haak's fieldwork introduced him to an elderly weaver whose family, having long been involved in the textile industry of Nishijin, vividly recalled "the old days when children were sold into Nishijin, where they often incurred TB and were sent home to die. He also knew of children who'd been sold out of Nishijin into brothels, where they dropped from sight, their fathers drinking and gambling away the money."[64]

The dire needs of the poor notwithstanding, by the next year the YMCA in Japan had returned to its base of support: the opening of an archery range and the introduction of a billiard table in the urban centers, which J. Merle Davis noted, "gives an idea of how the work is branching out to touch groups of non-Christian young men, who for the first time since the building was opened, are beginning to apply for membership because of the appeal of popular amusements." The work of the table surpassed that of Davis' colleagues, as it "is doing a signal service by showing the youth of this conservative city that Christianity is broad enough and human enough to encourage the most popular game in Japan." Moreover, "early in March a series of four cinematograph entertainments illustrating the life of Christ" were shown to "probably more than two thousand different Japanese for the most part non-Christians, [who] were held spell-bound by the beautiful pictures depicting the story of Christ's life and sufferings."[65]

Billiards and cinema had pushed the YMCA to Japan's evangelical forefront, both in the eyes of domestic politicians and foreign contributors, as inclined by the requisites of the moral enterprise, and no amount of subaltern need would alter either. The latter read about increased attendance, and donated, as in 1909, when Fisher noted that "within a few months, we have reason to believe that the building fund will be entirely subscribed in America, as Mr. S W Woodward has already put himself down for $15,000," a report that was appended with a note requesting that information remain confidential, and warning his colleagues "not [to] publish for the present, unless the fact gets into the press some other way first."[66]

The YMCA's ultimate failure to establish effective industrial work or medical assistance within Japan's slums had delineated the association's work. As Fisher relayed in February of 1922,

> There is some danger of the Associations in Japan becoming a middle class movement, out of touch with the common people, especially the manual laborers. The phenomenal uprising of the common people during the past three or four years

64. KFA: Report for the year ending September 30, 1908. G. S. Phelps, p. 2; Haak, 44.
65. KFA: Quarterly Report April 8, 1909. J. Merle Davis. p. 1.
66. KFA: Annual Report for the year ending Sept. 30, 1909. Galen M. Fisher, p. 4. The concern with funds is evident, as successful fundraising required the illusion of need, to which precedent (i.e., previous contributions) was a close second.

> and their organization into labor unions and kindred movements is a fact to be taken account of by every statesman and especially by Christian leaders. It would be a thousand pities if the Church and the Association should fail to give to this uprising of the people unselfish, discerning leadership.[67]

But many of Japan's statesmen, as Fisher recognized, appreciated the YMCA's emphasis. If the association refocused its efforts on the "labor unions and kindred movements," fears of a Christian-led insurrection would plague many of Japan's politicians. If the YMCA could not convert politicians, at least it could, as Davis reported in 1908, "cultivate the friendship of more prominent citizens."[68] Soon after, the YMCA began counting among its supporters Baron Gotō, the minister of communications; Baron Kikuchi, president of Kyoto Imperial University; Y. Arakawa, governor of Nagasaki-ken; Ōkuma Shigenobu, "the eminent statesman and founder and head of Waseda"; Baron Shibusawa Eiichi, "the dean of Japanese bankers"; Hattori Kintaro, "the highest tax payer in Tokyo" and founder of the Hattori (later Seiko) clock factory; Baron Sakatani Yoshio, former mayor of Tokyo; Tominaga Ko, mayor of Nagasaki City; Baron Takahashi, president of the Yokohama Specie Bank and vice governor of the Bank of Japan; Count Makino Nobuaki, imperial household minister; and Prince Tokugawa.[69] But these advocates seldom offered the sort of support that was commonly associated with eleemosynary organizations. Rarely did these men offer funds, land, or even connections. The support most often bestowed was recognition, and it was recognition that peppered the association's secretaries' reports from the field. Generally, the support was greater when the YMCA continued as a bourgeois movement, as this was far less political than work among the subaltern. Nevertheless, this pattern shifted in times of great national need, as during wartime or, as the association soon realized, after a natural disaster.

On September 1, 1923, life in Japan changed within a handful of minutes during lunch when a massive earthquake struck Japan's eastern seaboard. At the beginning of the year, total expenditures for the YMCA in Japan outstripped income at both Japan's city and student associations. After September 1, the association was deeply in the red.[70] But Japan's politicians were sensible of their own debt for the outpouring of assistance at the behest of various evangelical organizations in the country,

---

67. KFA: "The Young Men's Christian Association of Japan." Galen M. Fisher. Feb. 2, 1922, p. 59.
68. KFA: Annual Report, Oct. 1, 1908. J. Merle Davis, Nagasaki. p. 8.
69. KFA: Report of G.M. Fisher for first quarter 1909. p. 1; Report of G.M. Fisher for the second quarter of 1909. p. 2; KFA: J. M. Davis, Secretary, Nagasaki, Japan. Report for the quarter ending Mar. 31, 1910. p. 1; KFA: 1911 Reports. Galen M. Fisher: "Waseda University." p. 2; KFA: Annual Report for the year ending Sept. 30, 1911. G. M. Fisher, National General Secretary for Japan. Nov. 2, 1911, pp. 1–2; KFA: Annual Letter Tokyo City Associations. J. Merle Davis. Nov., 1919, pp. 15–21; KFA: Annual Report of the Senior Secretary for Japan for the Year 1927. Phelps. p. 4; KFA: Nagasaki 9/1/27; KFA: From J. Merle Davis to Mott (1/15/10); KFA: Fisher to Mott 6/6/11. p. 1; Phelps to Fisher (4/20/21); KFA: "A Flash from Japan." Fletcher Sims Brockman. Shanghai. Mar. 1, 1923. p. 2.
70. KFA: "Statistics for 1923: National Committee of Young Men's Christian Associations of Japan." G. S. Phelps. Mar. 30, 1923. p. 2; KFA: "Japan Under Affliction." *Association Men*. Arthur Jorgensen. Mar., 1924. p. 3. It is difficult to estimate the expenditures immediately after the earthquake, as most of the records were destroyed.

including the YMCA. The earthquake and the subsequent conflagration razed Tokyo and Yokohama and the surrounding area. "If it be measured by the havoc wrought," mathematician and geologist Charles Davison wrote, "the Japanese earthquake of 1 September 1923 is probably without a rival in the history of the world."[71] But from the ashes rose a unified evangelical Christian movement for recovery.

Not only to help themselves but also to assist their neighbors, the association managed to organize a massive fund-raising effort, as their Christian colleagues aided on the ground. The gutted interiors of the YMCA's buildings in Tokyo and Yokohama became "havens of rest and centers of relief work. There food, clothing, medicines, advice, and spiritual comfort were freely given. . . . Besides these 'villages' tents were erected in thirteen places where refugees were congested and in these were offered the services of employment bureau, land survey, legal advice, information, post-office, library, free barber, play grounds, song services, and milk depots for babies and the sick." Meanwhile, one group, under the direction of Kagawa Toyohiko, insisted on caring for the industrial areas for which the earthquake was one of a number of devastating blows.[72] The association, meanwhile, managed to accomplish a "miracle" in "raising a total of ¥3,275,389.30, of which amount more than one-third was raised in Japan itself, the balance being contributed by loyal friends in Canada and the United States."[73] While the majority of the funds did come from North American associations, the YMCA was happy to announce that "never in the history of the Association in Japan has its work received such hearty support from government officials and business men as during the past year. . . . This is pleasing evidence that the work of the Association is becoming more and more indigenous and that its ministry is winning more and more recognition."[74]

For the YMCA, the earthquake's devastation also brought it the same legitimacy that its war work had done almost twenty years earlier, a moral entrepreneurial success. However, it also squelched the association's industrial work yet again and, further, on its erstwhile desire to pursue medical missionary work as others had done (both within and outside the Japanese empire). The wisdom of this decision was debated, but that debate remained mostly outside the ranks of the association in Japan. Robert Grierson, a medical missionary in Korea from the Canadian Protestant mission reported that foreign evangelists in Korea remained terrified of following their colleagues in the archipelago, informing the readers of *The Christian Movement in Japan, Korea and Formosa* that one "old and experienced Bishop earnestly exhorted the Korean missionaries to avoid the 'mistake' which had been made in withdrawing from medical work," as they had in Japan. Grierson allowed the open debate on "whether the Church in Japan has gained by

---

71. Davison, 41.
72. G. S. Phelps, "Young Men's Christian Association," p. 308.
73. KFA: "A Report to Friends in North America on the Rehabilitation of the Young Men's Christian Association of Japan Following the Great Earthquake of 1923." Tokyo. June, 1931.
74. Phelps, 309.

the financial economy effected by its surrender of healing agencies to the government," but reminded his readers that "one of its [Japan's] most experienced Bishops is on record to the contrary."[75]

The association's leaders in Japan disagreed. They had built up a successful and considerably well-regarded organization, if not necessarily an evangelizing one, resting on their martial, student, and fund-raising work. And the YMCA in Japan had cited medical missionary work as a possibility in its earlier iteration, and, indeed, had claimed cooperation and fellowship with medical missionaries when it suited its purposes. Noted evangelists from William Elliot Griffis to John Cuting Berry, Rudolf Teusler to William Vories to Kagawa Toyohiko all had some association with the association, whether they were physicians or caring Christians, and very rarely did they feel co-opted by the YMCA. Often, in fact, they exhibited the same "moral entrepreneuring" that J. E. Nelson highlighted between the Salvation Army and Japan's government jockeying for enough morality and legitimacy for all parties.[76] It was a fine balance, reflected in the YMCA's decision essentially to farm out medical mission work since there was little profit there, as the majority of the work would be for the poor. Now more than ever, the association was focused on the utility of its fund-raising. As Jorgensen wrote to Herschleb, concerning the effects of the earthquake, "the whole stratum of middle class people, among whom lies the strength of Christianity in Japan, has been dealt a very severe blow from which it will require years to recover."[77] By assisting these individuals, the YMCA could continue to survive in Japan. Thus, it was troubling to Japan's foreign secretaries when their Japanese counterparts insisted on tipping this balance by acting

> somewhat impulsively, it seemed to us . . . welfare service were not discussed with Government officials. The result was that the Y.M.C.A. found itself on about the 15th of September working in thirteen centers, feeding babies, housing refugees, giving out information and comfort and legal advice, carrying on organized play, conducting day and Sunday schools, transmitting messages, hunting up information regarding the safety and welfare of Association members and their friends and what not, without a cent of money to pay the bills.

Faced with rapidly diminishing funds, a number of the association's Japanese secretaries, without acquiescence from their foreign counterparts, sought to borrow funds from Japan's aristocracy under the assumption "that America's millions would be given . . . by Dr. Mott for distribution," inadvertently creating a pyramid scheme when those millions were not immediately forthcoming, and, worse, embarrassing the association in Japan tremendously.[78] But the support that did come from America helped to solidify relations between the Japanese populace and the

75. Grierson, 380; 382.
76. Griffis 1904, 269; Ozawa, 60; Nelson, 52.
77. KFA: Jorgensen to Herschleb. January 2, 1924, p. 1.
78. KFA: W. R. F. Stier. "Report on Work Done by Y.M.C.A. Secretaries during the Earthquake and Fire in Tokyo and Yokohama." November 20, 1923, pp. 4, 6.

American representatives in their country, which was particularly gratifying for the association as they watched American opinions of the Japanese betrayed by the passage of the Johnson-Reed Act, the act of 1924, banning Asian immigrants. But in Tokyo, George Swan reported, "the streets were lined with thousands of people frantically shouting Banzai and above the throngs a multitude of flags of the Rising Sun and the Stars and Stripes were mingled."[79]

Yet, while the Japanese subjects had warmed to the Americans, often embodied by the YMCA in Japan by 1926, the end of the Taishō period, these evangelists sensed that the earthquake had affected the government differently. "The powerful conservative reaction which has followed in the wake of the catastrophe" had made the association's leadership in Japan wary of the new Japanese government and the new Japanese leadership wary of the association.[80] However, the new government was not afraid to readjust the moral enterprise for its own good. The YMCA's leadership feared that this, often one-sided, renegotiation would jeopardize its legitimacy within the recovering nation, as it found many among Japan's conservative cadre ready to "try to monopolize situations for their own exclusive advantage. Association privileges are not exempt from risk in this respect. . . . In the orient where resources are limited and the law of diminishing returns has long been operative men raise barriers about that which they can control and let in only those whom they desire."[81] Nevertheless, the association in Japan soldiered on, managing to recoup their building fund by 1927 and, according to their reports, maintain relatively steady membership. The former success caught the attention of many in Japanese politics more than the latter, allowing the continuance of YMCA work into the Shōwa period.[82]

Unfortunately, this all came at a cost—namely, industrial work and, particularly germane to present purposes, the care and treatment of those afflicted by tuberculosis. However, the YMCA was hardly alone in its inadequacy in dealing with the epidemic. Despite proclaiming in *Kaitakusha*, the organ of the YMCA in Japan, that the evangelical organizations were the only ones working to combat the growing scourge, Allen K. Faust, a well-known minister and educator of the Evangelical and Reformed Churches, acknowledged for a different audience that few of these were making much headway.[83] Most were involved in educational assistance, which, while needed, did little to offset the spread of the disease. Indeed, the misinformation spread might have countered the progress made. Faust reported to the American

79. KFA: Geo. D. Swan. November 15, 1923, p. 2.
80. KFA: Arthur Jorgensen. "Japan Under Affliction." *Association Men*. Mar., 1924, p. 294.
81. KFA: George Swan. "Japanese Life and Association Objectives." Feb. 16, 1924.
82. KFA: 日本基督教青年會同盟青年會情勢一覽. 昭和二年十二月現在. p. 27; KFA: Tominaga Ko et al. "To the Foreign Committee of the National Councils of the Young Men's Christian Association of the United States and Canada." Nagasaki, Japan, July 8, 1927; KFA: Konosuke Yasuda. "Letter from Mayor of Kyoto." July 15, 1927; KFA: Tomiyoko, S. "Testimonial of Governor of Kyoto Fu."; KFA: Chiba Yasuke. "Testimonial of the Chief Counsel of Kyoto Municipality."
83. Rogala, 58; Stirewalt, 43; NCY: 日本キリスト教歴史大事典 (*Nihon kirisutokyō rekishi daijiten*), p. 1185; NCY: Faust, Allen. "福音と肺結核 (Fukuin to haikekkaku)." 開拓者 (*Kaitakusha*). Jan., 1912.

National Tuberculosis Association that while overcrowding, inadequate nutrition, and overwork were among the causes of the disease in Japan, so, too, was "the use of alcoholic drinks and the cigarette habit; blowing the cigarette smoke through the nose, common; sexual excesses," in addition to "other causes that might be termed psychological. For instance, the habits of Old Japan are sedentary rather than active. The people love nature dearly, but they prefer to see the beauties of nature from their back room, to climbing mountains."[84]

Whether they enjoyed mountaineering, and whether they believed the myths surrounding contagion, the people of Japan did prefer to keep their female factory workers alive, at least judging by the latest Factory Law of 1911, which had finally taken effect after strong resistance from factory owners. Now, children under twelve were prohibited from working in factories, and the majority of factory workers were limited to twelve-hour shifts. Yet the law was hardly stringent. Herbert S. Sneyd, a YMCA secretary in Yokohama, noted that "it admits of exceptions. The law was passed five years before it went into effect. Public sentiment has improved tremendously toward the rights of labor and we believe that Japan will soon realize the necessity of more strictly conserving the strength of her laborers, especially the female and the young."[85]

This increase in public sentiment to laboring conditions in Japan, moreover, was due more to economic conditions and yellow journalism than to Christian charity and humanitarianism. The war in Europe had led to an economic boom in Japan, as the world looked to fill the void left when workers on the continent were sent to the trenches. While this would end soon after the armistice, Japan's factories were consuming increasing numbers of young girls. Young women in these conditions had become the subject of a number of exposés since the start of the decade.[86] While many factory owners continued to work under what an 1891 editorial in the *Tokyo keizai zasshi* deemed a "time-honored custom and moral principle," in which "our employment relations are warm and peaceful because employers and workers share common moral sentiments, undefined but every bit real," journalists were investigating the nature of these relations.[87] *Mainichi Shimbun* journalist Yokoyama Gennosuke pioneered these muckraking accounts at the turn of the century with his *Nihon no kasō shakai*, which illustrated the plight of the urban poor.[88] Much to the delight of Christians throughout Japan, such accounts proved popular with the

84. Faust, 354–55. It is hardly surprising that Faust highlighted the role of outdoor activity, as the progressive era was marked by the fresh-air and open-air movements. Of course, the Japanese who could afford to do so were more than happy to indulge in mountaineering. The Japanese Alpine Club had been in existence for almost a decade.
85. KFA: Annual report of H. S. Sneyd, Yokohama, Japan, Sept. 1, 1917, Oct. 9, 1917. p. 1.
86. Minami, 385.
87. Taira 1970, 89 (from Sumiya Mikio's *Nihon Chinrodoshi Ron*. Tokyo: University of Tokyo Press, 1955).
88. Sorensen, 70. Government reports, though unread by most outside of the political sphere, also had begun to acknowledge the connection between the factories and the epidemic, although many of these were downplayed by the politicians who had not researched them. These will be discussed later in this volume.

percentage of the upper class in Japan who saw social welfare as a cause célèbre. As Davis reported,

> One of the most striking and hopeful movements of the year in Japan is the rapid development of a social conscience. As with the other great nations, the war is bringing the working man of Japan to his own. The fortunes which the war is creating are being won at so high a price in industrial congestion, over work, inefficient labor, infant mortality and other ills resulting from social misery and economic unrest that government leaders and capitalists and factory owners are increasingly alarmed... A wave of popular interest and concern over these social and industrial problems is sweeping through the country. The daily press, magazines, books and societies are keeping the subject before the public.[89]

Yet, as in so many causes célèbres, many felt their humanitarian work complete after having read the magazines and books then in vogue. A month later, Davis, so hopeful for the future of the social conscience, lamented that "the slums, small factory and red-light districts of the depressed 'East Side' (of Tokyo), comprising one-third of the area and two-fifths of the people of the city . . . form a separate world, totally removed from the thought and progress of the better parts of town."[90] In his letter to Mott, George Gleason concurred, noting that the popularity of humanitarian literature had not led to Gleason's logical conclusion:

> Some people have the mistaken idea that Japan is nearly Christianized. On the contrary, a few plain facts should convince anybody that Japan is still in awful need. There are in the Empire almost exactly 100,000 licensed prostitutes and geisha, for whose services men are paying $27,250,000 a year. The number of these licensed women of degrading influence equals the total Protestant Church membership. The number languishing in prisons, 56,000, is more than half the Church membership. The deaths from tuberculosis are 81,000 yearly. There are 1,200,000 Eta, or people who still belong to the degraded group of almost outcasts. The 2,000,000 laborers and the tens of thousands of morally ill-prepared young women thrust out into commercial and industrial life, and the confessed irreligion of the industrial workers of the nation is another appeal. The Japanese consume per capita fifteen quarts of liquor per year. While prohibition has been making gains in the countries of the West, in Japan the production of saké, the native rice wine, has increased twice as much in the last two years as in the previous twelve years. Money is flowing in, but where, except in Christianity, is the moral guide to be found to make this wealth a blessing and not a curse?"[91]

Year after year before the war, scant mention was made of the industrial effort, save for the assurance that the investigations continue and that "a good start was made."[92] Still the public, perhaps by not embracing Christianity, had not overcome

89. KFA: Annual Letter Tokyo City Association. J. Merle Davis. Sept. 1, 1918, pp. 4–5.
90. KFA: Annual Report of the Tokyo City Association. J. Merle Davis. Oct. 1, 1918, p. 3.
91. KFA: Annual Letter to Mr. Mott. George Gleason, Osaka, Japan. Vladivostok, Sept. 21, 1918, pp. 8–9.
92. KFA: Annual Report of the Tokyo City Association. J. Merle Davis. Oct. 1, 1918, pp. 12–13.

its inertia. And still the YMCA lamented its own inaction. For years a handful of Japanese Christians had recommended that the association establish industrial branches in Japan's major cities. However, for just as long, the secretaries convinced themselves that the association needed to "postpone its own long-deferred industrial work venture."[93] In 1918, the belief remained that next year's policy would surely include plans to "Open the Industrial Branch."[94]

In 1919 those plans finally came to fruition, albeit nominally. In Tokyo, Japanese association secretary Arakawa arranged to rent "a ten-room house with half an acre of land in the heart of the industrial district of Kameido, East Tokyo . . . and (be) fitted up as a club house for workers," Davis happily announced.[95] A month later, however, Davis believed that it was for naught. "The Japanese do not know how to do such work," he lamented. Moreover, "the foreign missions are too busy with long established lines of educational and evangelistic work to feel the call. It remains for the Young Men's Christian Association, which first discovered this field and studied its needs, to demonstrate by a model social welfare equipment the solution which Christianity can offer to the sorest problem of the city."

The YMCA in the city still lacked a viable industrial branch, one that would minister to the urban workers. It was not alone. Osaka, too, despite being "primarily an industrial city, the greatest manufacturing centre in Japan," had no YMCA industrial branch. Secretary Guy Converse felt this need strongly, and urged his superiors to "meet our responsibility to the men of the community," noting that "we cannot dodge our responsibility."[96] The responsibility, Davis added, extended to Yokohama, Kyoto, and Kobe as well.

The International Committee, however, saw no need to provide funds for this work, regardless of whose responsibility it was. Beginning in 1918, hardly a report was submitted to it in which the secretaries in Japan did not plead for the funds to establish industrial work, noting the names of various local Japanese notables who pledged their assistance:

> Mr/ [*sic*] Shimoshima, Mayor of Honjo Ward, the largest slum district of the capitol, with 220,000 people, has expressed his interest in our proposed industrial branch. He has promised to help in finding the building site and has given us introductions to other officials. It was only through the aid of this official that we were able to finally secure a site for the W.C.T.U. [Women's Christian Temperance Union] Settlement which is being started on the East Side. The city Police Department, the Factory Inspector, the Provincial welfare secretary for factories, and the Government officials of the Philanthropies and Charities Bureau have repeatedly

93. KFA: Annual Letter Tokyo City Association. J. Merle Davis. Sept. 1, 1918, p. 5.
94. KFA: Annual Report of the Tokyo City Association. J. Merle Davis. Oct. 1, 1918, pp. 12–13.
95. KFA: Annual Report Letter of J. M. Davis, General Secretary, Young Men's Christian Association, Tokyo, Japan for the year ending Sept. 30, 1919, p. 7.
96. KFA: Annual Letter Tokyo City Associations, J. Merle Davis. Nov., 1919, p. 15; KFA: Annual Letter. Guy C. Converse, Osaka, Japan, Sept. 4, 1919, pp. 8–9.

> given introductions, valuable statistics and encouragement, during the last three years, in the studies of conditions which we have made.

But introductions, statistics, and encouragement provided no funds, and few were willing to offer those upfront, the cost of which, in Tokyo alone, were tentatively proposed at over $325,000.[97] Neither was the International Committee eager to invest such an exorbitant sum in a mission that would hardly prove profitable in the future. It was not that the YMCA was against industrial work. In America, such work, while not as widespread as its physical education programs, had been undertaken since the turn of the century, and the entry of the United States into World War I saw a concerted effort to increase that mission. It was only logical to intensify this effort, according to associate general secretary of the YMCA's National War Work Council Charles R. Towson's assessment: "The Y.M.C.A. has always recognized its obligation to the industrial worker, and now that this obligation has been increased by the war we want to do everything in our power to meet it and 'make good.' We have pledged our association to help our country and our allies win the war, both by our work among soldiers in the trenches and the soldiers here at home. We believe that it is just as important to help keep up the morale of the soldiers of industry as it is to keep up the morale of those under fire." The association distributed tellingly titled handbooks to those who would work in the industrial branches: "Among Industrial Workers (Ways and Means)," as if the workers themselves were nothing more than zoological specimens.

Had one studied the handbook, one would quickly realize that industrial work was being treated as a male preserve, concentrating solely on working with "industrial men and boys." Its very mission was to "help to get the undivided message of the association to the more than fourteen millions [(*sic*]) of industrial workers who outside of agriculture compose two-thirds of all the male workers of the land."[98] True, the YWCA existed and had even formed its own inchoate industrial branch, but the factory was a man's world, hardly the place for a woman, despite the fact that in the textile mills of Japan the opposite remained true. Perhaps it was inconceivable to have a female industrial branch, but, even so, the American industrial branch was nowhere near as successful as the production of handbooks might lead one to believe. As in Japan, as politician Monroe Sweetland noted bitterly, "these social agencies have been the private preserve of the rich do-gooders, and labor has had only the oblique association which exists in another field between the guinea pig and the scientist."[99]

As the International Committee sat idly by, the clamor from Japan's secretaries grew, citing both the growth of industry caused by the war and the appearance of

---

97. KFA: Annual Letter Tokyo City Associations, J. Merle Davis. Nov., 1919, pp. 18, 20–21. To put this into perspective, today's equivalent amount would be well over $4 million according to the Consumer Price Index Calculator on the webpage of the Bureau of Labor Statistics (http://data.bls.gov/cgi-bin/cpicalc.pl).
98. "Y.M.C.A. AIMS," 4; *Among the Industrial Workers*, title page, 4–6, 103.
99. Sweetland, 419.

small grassroots initiatives among the workers themselves, including ones associated with Christianity, as indicators of the tremendous need of a service only the YMCA was believed capable of providing. If it was not to assist the workers of Japan, perhaps the committee would be willing to help its employers, facing a sea of the angry proletariat. Fisher, writing on behalf of the National Committee of Young Men's Christian Associations of the Japanese Empire, reminded the International Committee:

> The world wide shortage of manufactured goods has led to an increase in the number of factories even more rapid than last year. In Tokyo, Yokohama, Osaka, Kobe, and Nagoya they have sprung up by the hundred each month. The expansion of manufacturing and trade has had the familiar concomitants of high prices, strikes, high wages, and more strikes. Unrest and self-assertion on the part of the workers and alarm, caucuses and concessions on the part of the employers have brought Japan almost at a bound into the struggle between labor and capital.
>
> Flamboyant wealth next door to grinding poverty, degenerate luxury parallel with unrelieved overwork have stirred up the calloused proletariat. There are ominous mutterings from below. The magician of modern progress in Japan, as elsewhere, has raised some spirits which his art is powerless to appease. It is this situation that makes discerning Japanese look anxiously for relief. Christianity claims to be able to cast out demons. It has succeeded in enough cases to beget confidence.
>
> All this shows how opportune is the intensive study and agitation about industrial work which Secretaries Davis and Arakawa have led in Tokyo. They have aroused the Women's Christian Temperance Union, and some of the Missions and Churches to enter the hitherto neglected industrial wards of the city. They have cooperated with the surprisingly successful Christian Association which has sprung up in the Fuji Spinning Mills. The Japan National Committee of the Young Men's Christian Association have asked the International Committee to send over a specialist on industrial and social work. The urgency of a prompt response is apparent. . . .
>
> The industrial situation clamors for attention. Already there are Japanese Christian men trained in social work, but they, no less than the Japanese National Committee, earnestly desire a man abreast of the latest ideas and methods in America to be sent over, so that the very foundation stones may be well and truly laid.[100]

Perhaps the YMCA secretaries in Japan were hasty. Within the next year, the boom of wartime production busted, and with it numerous factories went under. G. Ernest Trueman, a young secretary in Nagoya who was seen as a possible successor

100. KFA: Annual Report Letter of G.M. Fisher, Honorary General Secretary. National Committee of Young Men's Christian Associations of the Japanese Empire for the year ending Sept. 30, 1919, pp. 3–4, 13. It is unclear why "Association" is plural in this title. One may fairly assume that, in highlighting the cooperation of various evangelical organizations under the leadership or auspices of the YMCA, the previously singular "Association" is made multiple. It is not used again. There is also, of course, a plausible possibility that it is simply a typo.

to Davis, recorded that "in one week in Tokyo and vicinity 154 factories closed down their workmen going to swell the ranks of the unemployed."[101] Without extra funding from the International Committee, the local YMCA branches in Japan provided the social work they could for the newly unemployed. But without a national division of factory work (and factory unemployment), policies varied. Nevertheless, no local branches provided sufficient factory health care. Instead, the YMCA workers did what they had perfected over the years in Japan—English classes, physical education, and entertainments. All of these were fairly acceptable to many factory owners and employers, a few of whom offered the association assistance. Davis assured Mott that, even without financial support from the center, the work was successful and worthwhile:

> The Industrial Department has made progress during the Winter. The educational classes for factory men and boys, conducted six days a week have been well attended, a Bible group of twenty is held one a week and some forty neighborhood children are gathered on Sundays for Bible instruction, singing, and games.
>
> Three times a week these children are led in organized play and calisthenics by one of our physical instructors. A monthly moving picture entertainment and lecture for factory men and women has crowded our tiny quarters to capacity. I have been asked twice to speak to large groups of spinning and weaving operatives on their semi-monthly holiday in the Mill assembly rooms. ¥3,200. in gifts have come from factory owners and people interested in the betterment of industrial conditions, and in this way we expect to make the department stand up-on its own legs.[102]

But success and worth did not make for any amelioration in industrial conditions, and the secretaries continued to push for financial assistance to assist socially. In anticipation of Mott's impending visit to the nation, the secretaries provided him with a number of confidential reports on the state of the country, including its social and industrial conditions. The exodus from the country to the city continued, and in the city these workers "find bad air in homes and factories; food poorly cooked and of inferior quality; low, damp floors in houses situated on flats which are flooded with every heavy storm; sanitary conditions which breed contagion and dangerous sickness; long hours of work; standing from twelve to sixteen hours at high powered machines [despite factory laws]; unhygienic factory conditions, with dust and chemicals ladening the air; overcrowding of dormitories; night work for women and girls; child labor, with the stunting of growth." Physically and physiologically, factory work was difficult, and "the moral conditions of the dormitories for girl workers in some factories, especially certain spinning mills, are extremely bad."[103] As Gleason pointed out in his pro-Japanese polemic *What Shall I Think of*

101. KFA: Quarterly Report—April, May, June, G. Ernest Trueman, Nagoya, Japan. July, 3, 1920, p. 1.
102. KFA: Davis to Mott (4/1/21).
103. KFA: "Social and Industrial Conditions." *Confidential Notes on Japan*, pp. 11–12. Mott's tour was postponed due to the 1923 earthquake. He would visit Japan in 1925.

Japan?, "The long hours of labor, regularly eleven in cotton mills and fourteen or even sixteen in the silk mills, the low wages, the lack of care of employees" remained. But Gleason was positive that they would soon change:

> Why a paternal government like Japan should wait for the evils of child labor, woman's labor, long hours, unsanitary factories, congested houses and slums to show themselves has been a puzzling question. But this seeming lack of foresight is plainly due to the conviction that the people can be sacrificed for the nation. . . . Now Japan is a creditor nation and the surplus population has been cared for, the Government is turning its attention to the welfare of the working man.[104]

However, the domestic politicians rarely offered such monetary assistance either politically or directly to the organization, but their moral support of the enterprise, or the perception of this support, was often just as beneficial. Unfortunately for the association, this continued to mean a yielding of principles. And, as the Japanese empire grew, so too did the amount of concessions necessary to the increasing numbers of Japanese politicians and bureaucrats. For many in the association, the cost was questionable. In a report, Fisher maintained that the YMCA had successfully broken into the inchoate Japanese field in Manchuria through the South Manchurian Railroad, in which the "directors of the company adopted all our recommendations and will erect buildings and support an extensive work covering the whole system." He reported this as a measure of success, despite the fact that, as he privately admitted, "this work will not be connected with us and will not bear the name 'Christian.'" Nevertheless, because of the business advice provided by consultants in the YMCA, Fisher felt he could publicly declare that "the railway which is the very backbone of all progress in Manchuria, will be more or less permeated by the Christian spirit, and direct Christian work will be facilitated."[105] The work in Manchuria was left under the leadership of C. V. Hibbard, whose work in the area with the Japanese army during the Russo-Japanese War had allowed him early access to authorities heading up the work on the railroad. Despite his ties to the South Manchuria Railway Company leadership, Hibbard noted that, while the leadership had a "favorable attitude" to YMCA work, "these men honestly believe that this social and moral work will be more effective if done without the name of Christianity." Moreover, Hibbard, added, the railway's leadership "have accordingly proposed to us that we bring in our methods and our men to work as employees of the Railway but under our general direction. To my mind this arrangement would take the men and the work out from under our control without freeing us from responsibility." The entirety of the work with the railway, despite being lauded by the association as another success, would, assuming it worked, actually "be a barrier to the establishment of regular association work." For the YMCA, therefore, the

104. Gleason, 228.
105. KFA: Annual Report for the year ending Sept. 30, 1909 Galen M. Fisher, p. 4.

definition of success in Japan was being altered, and it was being altered at the hands of the nation's leaders.[106]

But the YMCA was still not addressing tuberculosis. Nevertheless, as the Meiji era closed, steps were being taken by Christian medical missionaries to combat the poverty and disease of Japan's slums. These actions, though not directly instigated by the YMCA, were being taken, in turn, both out of context, and for their own interests, by the YMCA's secretaries to have been performed under their aegis. In fairness, the lines between missions were often blurred, and certainly were hazy under an association claiming allegiance from all Protestant sects. Nevertheless, the YMCA had already established its niche primarily in war work, recreation and urban education, none of which had yet been terribly affected by the underside of Japan's modernization. As the association continued its work, a handful of Japanese Christians reconfigured the White Cross Society (Hakujūjikai) in Tokyo in 1911 ostensibly to combat the tuberculosis epidemic rampant in the city. Indeed, the society did found a small hospital in Kamakura, but its mission was primarily to bring pressure to bear on the government to prevent the spread of the epidemic. It is interesting to note that the following year foreigners in Japan founded "the Anti-tuberculosis Society of Foreigners in Japan." Although mostly comprising missionaries (indeed, it had been established at a missionary conference), the organization itself was meant to protect the foreign population of Japan from the scourge that had already spread throughout the country. Needless to say, it was not particularly successful. Unfortunately, no further information on this organization is available.

But conditions were no better than before the enactment of the Factory Law, and Japan's association secretaries remained trapped. Beyond the economic woes, tuberculosis had spread to its ranks, forcing the association's hand. Verling W. Helm had fallen victim to the disease in 1907 at the age of thirty-three. He was soon followed by Phelps' wife—as well as Guy Converse; Gleason's daughter, son, and wife; a Japanese secretary; Murakami; and the son of another association secretary, H. S. Sneyd. As Phelps noted, "We have certainly been hit hard during the past six months." These illnesses actually occurred over the span of a quarter century, but Phelps' sentiment is understood. Helm left behind a family, including a son who had been born barely a week before he died. Phelps' wife, Mary Ward Phelps, was sent to Attleboro to convalesce, while Converse (suspected of having the disease) traveled to Beijing to the Rockefeller Hospital. George Gleason's wife "who seems to be suffering from tuberculosis" took her husband out of commission. Murakami is most likely Sophia University professor and author Murakami Naojiro. The obituary of Karl Sneyd, H. S. Sneyd's son, listed his cause of death as bronchiectasis, which is

106. R. Morse, 476; KFA: Report of C. V. Hibbard for the Year 1909, pp. 2–3. Hibbard would become secretary of the International Committee of the YMCA and, later, director of the National Japanese American Student Relocation Council, whose work ensured that imprisoned Japanese American college students could continue their education outside the internment camps to which they had been restricted. (OAC: Letter from C.V. Hibbard, Director, National Japanese American Student Relocation Council, to Remsen Bird, Mar. 21, 1944.)

frequently caused by tuberculosis. In this case, Karl was most certainly afflicted with tuberculosis.[107] Thus, if the International Committee would not agree to funding for a sanitarium for Japan's factory workers, perhaps it would be amenable to building one for its secretaries in Japan. G. Sidney Phelps responded to a questionnaire on mission sanitariums in East Asia to former general secretary of Tsinanfu (Jinan) Charles A. Herschleb, then stationed at the International Committee's New York office, stating his emphatic belief that "a sanitarium should be established by mission boards in Japan." He noted that "such an establishment would undoubtedly be of marked value in promoting the maintenance of health and lessening the number of breakdowns. In our own group I believe that such an institution, if properly equipped and managed, would have saved us money and considerable efficiency." Phelps ruled out Korea as a possible location, despite its ameliorative climate, reiterating the importance of establishing this institution in Japan proper:

> It should be carefully organized and adequately financed, providing a staff which would include a good surgeon, a second physician who could make stated trips to the large missionary centres for the purpose of giving advice to missionaries, a dentist who would be in Karuizawa during the summer, or preferably spend a few weeks at each of the missionary summer resorts and who would also itinerate among the chief mission centers during the winter. At least two trained nurses should be in attendance and the institution should be open summer and winter. In fact we feel great need of a suitable winter rest resort which could be run something on the lines of the Battle Creek Sanitarium which welcomes and provides for guests who simply need a chance to rest and to secure healthful recreation under comfortable conditions and at reasonable expense.

Phelps reported that there had been tentative plans for a similar institution under the auspices of the American Episcopal Mission, but he noted that "there is considerable dissatisfaction among the missionaries with both Dr. McSparren and with Dr. Teusler of that mission, not so much on the grounds of their professional qualifications . . . but rather because of their lack of sympathy and courteous consideration of the sensibilities and perhaps foibles of their patients."[108]

---

107. KFA: *Verling Winchel Helm: A Christian Man*. The Secretaries in Japan of the International Committee of Young Men's Christian Associations. Tokyo, 1907. "The Last Days" by G. S. Phelps, p. 41, 69; KFA: Phelps to Brockman (12/13/26), p. 3; KFA: Phelps to Herschleb (4/21/23); KFA: From Gleason to Walter M. Wood of Philadelphia, 3/31/10; KFA: To Mott from Fisher (9/12/11), p. 2; KFA: "Foreign Personnel" Spring, 1922, p. 23; KFA: Sneyd to Herschleb (3/3/27), p. 1; KFA: "Foreign Personnel" Spring, 1922, p. 23; Draper, 306; Salkin, 577.

108. Xing, 44; KFA: Phelps to Herschleb. Nov. 24, 1922, pp. 1–2. Interestingly enough, Phelps rules that the "frequency of sprue within the missionary ranks in Korea suggests caution in taking missionaries from Japan to that country" to establish a sanitarium. "Sprue," more commonly recognized today as celiac disease, does seem to predispose a person to a greater risk of acquiring tuberculosis (Ludvigsson et al., 23). Dr. Joseph L. McSparran was the head of Osaka's St. Barnabas Hospital, while Teusler headed Tokyo's St. Luke's Hospital. As it turned out, the Episcopal Church also had problems with McSparran, though not Teusler (*Churchman's*, 211).

In addition, in 1913 a number of Japanese medical and business elite, as well as a few former politicians, formed the Japan Anti-tuberculosis League as an NGO that sought to educate the public about prevention of the disease and to continue the push for public health care of the tubercular. Unlike the evangelical organizations discussed in this chapter, the league, as pointed out by William Johnston, "did not cite the human suffering that tuberculosis caused or the right of the people to lead healthy lives as justifications for its establishment." Instead, the continued prosperity of the Japanese nation was the sole purpose for the league's combat against the epidemic.[109]

As discussed previously, far more Japanese Christians were willing to challenge the government in ways the foreign Christians were not. The White Cross Society, however, had little problem with the connection the YMCA forced by identifying the work of the former under the auspices of the latter when it served the purposes of the association. Further, this approach of political appeasement of the YMCA meant continued support from American philanthropists, including Rockefeller. While these funds rarely trickled down to the White Cross Society, it did bring an awareness of both the organization and the issues addressed to an international audience. Not surprisingly, therefore, G. Ernest Trueman, Nagasaki secretary, noted that by permitting the YMCA to continue to perform fairly innocuous social work "the Japanese seem at last to have realized that there is a better use to put the foreigner to than to make him the butt of their wit or the basis of their envy."[110] A few within the association continued to struggle with the outsourcing of significant social work. George Gleason noted, "Throughout the country the idea of social service is in the air. During the last year in Osaka a Smoke Prevention Society and an Anti-Tuberculosis Society have been formed. . . . It is the time for the Association to undertake more active social work. The need for such work is evidenced by the report that people in Osaka on the average die ten years earlier than in the country at large."[111] Yet such work continued to elude most of the association's leadership. Gleason himself, despite being one of the most aware among the YMCA's secretaries of the need for such work, managed to distribute merely "several hundred booklets on tuberculosis prevention . . . to the educational department students," for whom he organized one lecture.[112]

The emphasis on student work was not wholly misguided. As the vast majority of the leadership of the association continued to place tuberculosis at the bottom of the agenda, Japanese undergraduates in the Christian student societies embraced work with the tubercular and with the victims of other diseases afflicting the residents of

---

109. Johnston 1995, 235; NCY: 日本キリスト教歴史大事典 (*Nihon kirisutokyō rekishi daijiten*), p. 1105; Hagen, 204; Johnston 1995, 237–38. For more information on the Japan Anti-tuberculosis League, please see Johnston's work.

110. KFA: G. Ernest Trueman, Secretary, Nagasaki, Japan. Annual Report for the year ending Sept. 30, 1910, p. 1.

111. KFA: Annual Report for the year ending Sept. 30, 1913. George Gleason, General Secretary, Osaka, Japan, p. 5.

112. KFA: Annual Report of George Gleason, Osaka, Japan, for year ending Sept. 30, 1914, p. 2.

the cities' slums. This surprised a number of the association's foreign leadership, as "social service by students in Japan is made extremely difficult on account of the crowded curricula, many students having twenty-five to thirty hours of lectures a week. Medical students are among the busiest." Nevertheless, these students made time for such social work as the YMCA's directors in Japan had still failed to undertake. Fisher, as general secretary, nonetheless reported their efforts proudly under the aegis of the association, with whom they had only vague association:

> It is therefore especially encouraging to note that the Christian medical students in Kumamoto have for years been the mainstay of a Christian dispensary conducted under the guidance of Dr. Fukuda, an old student volunteer of the University of Edinburgh; and in Kyoto more recently the Christian medical men have been doing likewise. There has also been some visiting of hospitals. I have twice spoken to students on the need of reforming factory conditions and they showed the keenest interest. The time is not far distant when this interest will find outlet in personal service and in legislation fathered by students who will join the growing group of Christian university graduates in the Imperial Diet. Secretary Davis recently published a careful study into conditions among industrial workers in Tokyo which reveals a great need for Christian and social service among this neglected class.[113]

Davis was a natural choice for this task. Not only was he based in the capital, a city with 2,174 factories and within which lung diseases were the most prominent of the city's almost thirty-nine thousand deaths yearly, but his Japanese was also advanced enough that he was able to "have prepared and delivered in Japanese the first two of a course of five lectures on Social and Industrial Problems and the Church before the Theological and upper college students of Aoyama Gakuin." Following the lecture, the students

> voted to gather and distribute Christmas bundles to the very poor of the slums as their special Christmas service . . . 121 bundles containing clothing, underwear, socks, mittens, tracts and booklets, were made up, each labeled with a pointed Scripture verse and practical motto of good cheer and advice. These packages were loaded into hand carts and pulled by the boys three miles into the industrial slums. Then followed a house to house distribution with a word of greeting to each family. I am hopeful that the interest aroused by one of these classes which is connected with one of the most prosperous Congregational Churches in the city, may result in establishing a point of contact between that church and the slums.[114]

For those whose work on tuberculosis prevention was not as direct, it proved far easier to offer exposés on the slums, often in the hopes that others would pursue what the current YMCA leadership would not or could not undertake, and, further, that they would do so in such a way that this leadership could benefit.[115] The first

113. KFA: Annual Report for the year ending Sept. 30, 1914. Fisher, National General Secretary, Japan, p. 7.
114. Hitchcock, 44–45; KFA: Quarter's Report Tokyo City Association. J. Merle Davis. Oct. 1 to Dec. 31, 1917, p. 4.
115. KFA: Annual Report of George Gleason, Osaka, Japan, for year ending Sept. 30, 1915, p. 9.

decade of the Taishō period saw a preponderance of such muckraking, particularly in Tokyo. "*THE TIDE OF INDUSTRY*," as Davis referred to it, had entered Tokyo, encircling the city "by a belt of industrial suburbs, marked by towering chimneys, murky atmosphere and wretched slums, whose population has increased during the last decade by over 300 percent and today numbers 800,000 people." As the slums of Tokyo grew, the conditions of their residents worsened. Moreover, as historian Ishizuka Hiromichi maintained, the government's attempts at urban renewal often were aimed solely at fire prevention, and did little to curb the spread of epidemics or the social conditions rampant within these areas.[116] Having unloaded industry onto the zaibatsu, the industrial workers who populated the slums were not currently the government's charges, if they ever were. But neither were they yet the YMCA's, as Davis continued to lament in print:

> Across this wide stream tower the foundries, leather mills, linen, muslin and cotton mills of the city, and here on flats reclaimed from the sea, averaging only four feet above high tide, and subject to annual floods, live in great congestion and poverty the 500,000 people of Honjo and Fukagawa wards, a population in itself greater than any other city of Japan save Osaka. It is a safe estimate that 1,000,000 people including families are working in factories, mills and small industrial enterprises. This vast city within a city has been up to the present virtually neglected by the Christian movement and by any form of social agency. It forms a factor of the city's life that must be speedily reckoned with by the Young Men's Christian Association if it is to be instrumental in solving the social and spiritual needs of this nation.[117]

For the Japanese government, if not the entire populace, the YMCA had managed to establish itself as an influential force within the cities. Although not necessarily successful evangelically, the association's efforts in Japan were considered, according to prominent missionary Rev. Albertus Pieters, "one of the most successful forms of [evangelical] work" in Japan. A leader in the Reformed Church Mission in Japan, Pieters acknowledged that "it is far easier to raise large sums of money for it than for the regular evangelicalistic work," and it was this fact that allowed it to remain relevant. Nevertheless, Pieters noted, "the Salvation Army is to many persons the ideal of pure evangelism," and "the work of the Y.M.C.A. and of the Salvation Army . . . [lie] at opposite extremes from each other in character and methods."[118]

But without government subsidies and without funds from the factory owners to improve and supplement the lives of their laborers, the task of assisting and aiding the factory girls of the textile industry fell to the private sector, to organizations in

116. KFA: Annual Report Tokyo Association 1915 and 1916. J. M. Davis, Oct. 1916, p. 6; Ishizuka 1981, 190.

117. KFA: Annual Report Tokyo Association 1915 and 1916. J. M. Davis, Oct. 1916, p. 8. Emphasis in original. The "wide stream" to which Davis refers is the Sumida River. Across the river from Fukagawa-Honjo lies Sanya, an area still considered to be a slum district today. Postwar, however, Fukagawa-Honjo was able to rebuild itself as a residential area (Gill, 84).

118. Pieters, 131.

the larger society, a society which depended on the goods these women dedicated their lives to making. Certainly, the factory and the slums surrounding it proved a visible site to focus attempts to ameliorate some of the more obvious problems, including the spread of tuberculosis. That said, it remained easier to overlook these public health conditions than to improve them. The task was too great, and its uncertain results might not have justified a massive governmental effort. As John Merle Davis, head of the Tokyo branch of the YMCA noted, despite it being "a safe estimate that 1,000,000 people including families are working in factories, mills and small industrial enterprises" along the Sumida River in Tokyo, nevertheless "this vast city within a city has been up to the present virtually neglected by the Christian movement and any form of social agency." Like Davis' organization (as we shall discuss in the next chapter), the Salvation Army noted the neglect of the "industrial suburbs, marked by towering chimneys, murky atmosphere and wretched slums" throughout the country. Yet, both these evangelical groups identified different problems within the community, and focused on those solely. While this certainly improved some conditions, it addressed only a handful of the myriad issues that years of industrial employment had wrought. Even for evangelists, it was difficult to justify work without gain, although monetary gains from their enterprises were rarely expected. Nevertheless, the hope of saving souls still fueled efforts. If life could be made more comfortable for the women of the factory, why could their afterlife not be improved as well? Thus, for the YMCA, the emphasis beyond soteriological work was in part cosmetic. As noted in an English-language brochure, *Osaka: The Factory City of the East, Some Facts and Some Comparisons*, the association in Osaka had assisted in work that "relieved the distressed from two great fires . . . and is an active force in the recent activities of citizens for opening public playgrounds" within the slums of the industrial district.[119]

So, too, was there an attempt to offer Christian religious education. Sadly, however, this did little physically to improve the lot in life of the women of the factories, but was meant to assist them in coping with all of the murk, tubercular miasma and wretchedness of their surroundings. Galen Fisher, one of the more social work-oriented secretaries of the YMCA in Japan, questioned this emphasis:

> Can we be satisfied to see churches open for services only on Sunday and on one or two other evenings? What effect are these services having over the neighborhoods immediately around the churches? Are they meeting the vital needs of the wage-earning class? In industrial and wage-earning communities, where opportunities for recreation, for self-improvement, and for good-companionship are lacking, *is it right that churches should continue to offer only religious instruction a few hours a week?*

119. KFA: "Annual Report Tokyo Association, 1915 and 1916." J. M. Davis, Oct. 1916. p. 8, 6; KFA: *Osaka: The Factory City of the East, Some Facts and Some Comparisons*. Jan. 1913, p. 1.

In many cases, the simple fact of attention was thought to be more beneficial than social improvements or religious instruction. As Fisher maintained, theirs was a "merely humanistic social settlement that ameliorates, but does not cure." The cure, therefore, was to come from other sources, presumably Christian. In a document that was not to be published, the association admitted that in spite of the attempts to improve conditions or to offer religious instruction such as those they had undertaken, urbanization around industrial output had accelerated and "over one-half, and in many cases *two-thirds, of the employees [of the new factories responsible for this growth] are girls*." Thus, it was hoped that others would take up the mantle of the YMCA and pursue the work that it had not. Ideally, Fisher noted, these missionaries should have "special training and adaptability." In fact, they should be "*younger missionaries with command of the language*." In other words, they should be Japanese, not foreign, Christians. Despite proclaiming their desire to help, the YMCA hoped to transfer this work to their domestic counterparts.[120]

As their counterparts within the association had, a handful of members of the Salvation Army had seen both the need and the potential of ameliorating the social and epidemiological aspects of factory work, which we shall consider in the next chapter. As early as 1902, pamphlets noted that "every place where a large number of people work together is a precious mine and factory for The Army," and determined that, unsurprisingly, the best of these spiritual mines and factories were, in fact, actual "mills, factories, and mines." But the reality of assistance and utilization proved as complicated for the Army as it had the YMCA.[121]

Even with its roots in the slums of London, the Salvation Army's work in Japan was still fairly removed from the life of the subaltern. In her 1919 remembrance of her brief alliance with the Salvation Army, during which time she accompanied some of its officers to a factory site, socialist and political labor activist Yamakawa Kikue recalled her anger at what she saw as the ineptitude of the officers. In the factory, the officers taught the female workers hymns that lauded the notion of labor for salvation and preached the message of work blessed by god. Yamakawa was ashamed of both the callousness and futility of the visit:

> I wanted to leave the platform where I sat with the other visitors (from The Army) and join the factory girls. I wanted to apologise to these women. I wanted to prostrate myself before them. I wanted to do this because I was tormented by the guilty feeling that I—we—are the ones who have corrupted them, who have cheated them, who have trampled on them. So I wanted to apologise to them, to tell them that I was their friend. Instead, I sat on the platform with their enemies. From the heated platform, I looked down on them, as they knelt, barefoot, in the unheated hall. I have never forgotten those feelings of guilt and distress.[122]

---

120. KFA: "Social Problems and the Christian Movement." *Forward Steps in Mission Policy*. Galen M. Fisher. 1917, pp. 6–7. Emphasis in original.
121. SANA: "Catching and Keeping the Crowds: II.—Mills, Factories, and Mines." *The Field Officer of the Salvation Army*. Vol. 10, no. 10 (Oct., 1902), p. 445.
122. Shima, 94; Mackie, 96.

A supporter of the Army's work on prostitution, Yamakawa had hoped that the visit would have done something to ameliorate the situation she had found in the factories, wherein the girls "looked to be twelve or fifteen years of age, but they lacked the vitality of the young. They looked pale and tired as if they were sick." In fact, Yamakawa knew they were sick, and so did, she suspected, the Salvation Army. These girls, in spite of repeated halfhearted attempts at labor laws, "would have to work through the night again. . . . They would lose weight during a week of night work and fail to regain it in the following week when they went back on the day shift." The fact that these women were unable to acclimate to a steady work schedule was responsible, in Yamakawa's opinion, for the poor health of these workers. In her view, this caused "the textile workers to develop tuberculosis at a rate three times that of other women, and to suffer an extremely high death rate."[123]

Yamakawa's statistics were not far off. As Ishihara Osamu, a doctor commissioned by the Meiji government's Ministry of Commerce and Agriculture to investigate what had long been obvious to almost anyone with a connection to the industry, discovered that of the two hundred thousand new workers within the industry his staff surveyed 2.2 percent of those women were forced to return to their villages within a year, sick with severe tuberculosis and "tuberculosis-type illnesses," a category created to comprise a disease with a number of variations. Of those who died of any illness, tuberculosis and its variants constituted over 70 percent.[124]

Both the major evangelical organizations, the YMCA and the Salvation Army, appeared to be confounded by the larger issues prevalent within the factory system in Japan—the conditions, the maintenance, the priorities of the factories and mills offered far too many problems to tackle aside from just the spread of tuberculosis. A narrow focus on just some of these problematic manifestations—prostitution, social unrest, and political upheaval—proved more profitable to the organizations. Indeed, it was not until the involvement of the medical missionary groups or the medical missionary departments of such organizations as the Salvation Army, that some progress was made in combating the disease.

Unremedied by evangelical groups, the government, or the factory owners, there remained something in the factories and mills that caused their workers to fall ill with tuberculosis. Owing to its multifactorial causation, the disease persistently resisted attempts at amelioration. Without a cure for the bacillus itself, medical science was impeded, but two causative variables remained—the worker herself and her environment. Those women whom Yamakawa had seen prostrating themselves in the freezing hall proved ripe breeding grounds for the bacillus. And in the hall itself, the cold compromising the workers' health, as well as the conditions in the workrooms and the crowded dormitories, assisted tuberculosis to spread through the ranks of workers. Yamakawa could only watch in horror.

123. Yamakawa, 896.
124. Tsurumi, 169; Kagoyama, 20; Ishihara, 53.

7

"The Soldiers Must Have the Real Fighting Spirit"

The Salvation Army

Although the Salvation Army arrived later than the YMCA, the soldiers of the Army believed that its late arrival could help it avoid some of the pitfalls the YMCA had experienced in Japan. The Army had already established itself in opposition to the association, a distinction mirrored in nomenclature. While the YMCA was a somewhat loosely organized fraternal alliance, the Salvation Army prided itself on its rigid structure and discipline. Less than fifteen years after its founding, the organization transformed itself in 1878 into a "Salvation Army to carry the Blood of Christ and the Fire of the Holy Ghost into every corner of the world." Based on its relatively unchanging vision ever since, the Army was "prepared for a war," and, by the end of the nineteenth century, it had stepped onto Japan's battlefield.[1]

On September 4, 1895, less than fifty years after Perry had sailed into Uraga Harbor, the first fourteen officers of the Kyūseigun (lit. "save the world army") landed some thirty kilometers from Perry's site. These men and women, led by Colonel Edward Wright, were an international crew of Americans, Australians, New Zealanders, Britons, Scotsmen, and Irish. Yet they held to a strict "native policy" to ingratiate themselves with their new charges. Within Japan, they would be Japanese:

> We shall adopt Japanese means, Japanese dress, and the Japanese mode of life. We shall live in native houses, and eat native food. We had not come here to live as English people, with a good house and two or three servants; it is our intention to live as the common people of Japan live.[2]

As it turned out, within Japan, they would be a laughingstock. The kimonos they had commissioned to wear were meant for home use only, and, thus, as later recounted by the *Japan Advertiser*, when they marched off the ship, drums in hand, "their appearance one bright morning in these clothes naturally created considerable amusement and interest." Their first public sermonizing was equally unsuccessful, as the curious Japanese subjects in attendance "roared with laughter in spite of themselves." The New York edition of the Army's *War Cry* celebrated the fortieth anniversary of the Salvation Army's entrance into Japan by recalling the words of

1. Begbie, 403.
2. Ion 1993, 75; F. Coutts, 101; Akimoto 1, 3; Yamamuro 1906, 432; Baggs, 4–5.

one attendant: "Those Westerners were so strange! It was an evening's entertainment to go to one of their meetings and watch and hear the flagrant breaches of the simplest rules of Japanese etiquette. The audience paid much more attention to the shortcomings of the officers than they did to the message."[3]

But the Army had come, in part, at the behest of a young Japanese Christian, Ishii Juji, a former police officer and medical student, who claimed to have begun his own branch of the Army, the "Oriental Salvation Army" among the wards of the orphanage of which he was the superintendent. Under Ishii's guidance, the Okayama Orphan Asylum founded the first Japanese branch of the Army in 1891, although this branch remained unknown to those outside of the orphanage until Ishii informed his peers in San Francisco of its existence in 1893. Upon learning of these young soldiers, San Francisco officers felt that the time was ripe for a foreign presence to guide the native population, who, according to Ishii's testimony, were clearly ready for evangelization. "The Army idea appears to take a favorable hold of the Japanese mind," proclaimed the editor of the San Francisco edition of the *War Cry*, a sentiment echoed by officer Clara Howard when she noted that "there is a valiant regiment waiting to welcome, and fall in line, with those whom General Booth shall send to needy Japan, (D.V.) to hasten and prepare for the coming of the King."[4] It seemed wholly reasonable, therefore, to suspect, as the editors of the Army publication *The Field Officer of the Salvation Army* had, that in Japan "the people are very sympathetically disposed towards Christianity, very hospitable and warm hearted. No doubt the Colonel and his comrades will receive a hearty reception. Our methods will suit their taste and the love of our officers will win their affections, so that undoubtedly a future of great victory awaits us there."[5]

Unfortunately for the Army, it would take more than the invitation of one man leading a ragtag children's army and the perception of national hospitality to establish the group within its new nation. Japan had no shortage of evangelists, and, to many, the officers of the Salvation Army were—despite their odd entrance onto the scene—indistinguishable from other foreign missionaries. Yet the Army had seen success throughout the British Empire, Europe, America, and various countries in Africa and South America, and had managed to set itself apart from its coreligionists. Its work in Japan would be no different.

The Salvation Army had, from the beginning, established itself as a champion of England's poorest individuals. In his so-called "Cab Horse Charter" (found in his polemic *In Darkest England and the Way Out*), William Booth, the founder and general of the Army until his death in 1912, expounded on his reasoning for ministering to these men and women as "a very real illustration of poor broken-down

3. Rightmire, 16–17.
4. SAR: "Japan: A Sketch of J. Ishii, His Orphanage and Native 'Salvation Army.'" *War Cry*. San Francisco. May 19, 1894, pp. 8–9; "The Past Year," 360.
5. SANA: "Our Foreign Field. Japan." *The Field Officer of the Salvation Army*. Vol. 3, no. 3. Mar., 1895. p. 86. D.V. is most likely "deo volente" or "god willing."

humanity." The horse that pulls the cab in the street, Booth believed, was cared for better than the same humans who walk in those streets:

> When he [the cab horse] is down he is helped up, and while he lives he has food, shelter and work. That, although a humble standard, is at present absolutely unattainable by millions—literally by millions—of our fellow-men and women in this country. . . .
>
> The first question, then, which confronts us is, what are the dimensions of the Evil? How many of our fellow-men dwell in this Darkest England? How can we take the census of those who have fallen below the Cab Horse standard to which it is our aim to elevate the most wretched of our countrymen?
>
> The moment you attempt to answer this question, you are confronted by the fact that the social problem has scarcely been studied at all scientifically.[6]

However, Booth wanted to move beyond the science of poverty to counteract the results of that science, whether poverty was its consequence or its object. And it was a science with which he was well acquainted. Although by no means wealthy, Booth lived relatively comfortably until his father's decline and death, when Booth, at age thirteen, was forced to leave school and find employment by which to support his mother and sisters. Such a task was difficult for any child, but was made more difficult by the fact that Booth remained a pawnbroker's apprentice for "six or seven years," during which time he "had scarcely any income as an apprentice, and was so hard up when my father died, that I could do next to nothing to assist my dear mother and sisters, which was the cause of no little humiliation and grief."[7] This experience, and the fact that his apprenticeship pressed him into contact with men and women who were forced to part with their possessions to make ends meet, focused Booth's efforts away from mere monetary gain. Having converted to Methodism, Booth worked his way up the ranks of the Reform Church but was drawn from his comfortable pastorate to an open-air evangelism among the nation's urban slums. Thus, turning from the clergy and prelature, Booth embraced the call of evangelism and the establishment of an independent lay ministry who would concentrate more on ministering to their poorer peers than to marketing God to society's affluent. He was soon joined by his wife, Catherine, herself a powerful evangelist, and by the growing flock who assisted the Booths in their burgeoning social work.[8]

That Catherine Booth was an integral part of Booth's following would play a major role in the organization of the Salvation Army worldwide. The Army was one of the few evangelical organizations that allowed women within its ranks, let alone permitted them to hold high rank in the mission. Whereas other evangelical groups limited women's roles, when allowed at all, often relegating them to auxiliary groups, the Army allowed women to "hold any position of authority or power in The Army, from that of a local officer to that of the General," codifying the consideration

6. W. Booth, 1890, 19, 20.
7. Railton, 5.
8. Briggs, 698.

of them "as being equal with men in all the social relations of life, whether it be as mothers, wives, sisters, or comrades." It could be pointed out, however, that for a considerable length of time, the Salvation Army, when it was led by both men and women, was firmly within the hands of the Booth family. From its inception until 1939, the command of the Army was only outside their lineage for five years, having been overseen by William, his eldest son, and, later, by his daughter Evangeline. In addition, Catherine, as previously mentioned, played a significant role in the Army's leadership, as did William and Catherine's son, their granddaughter and Catherine's namesake, and their son-in-law.[9]

In raising the role of women to positions of equality and even prominence, Booth and his officers were undermining the hegemony of the clergy on faith and the basis on which these men deemed individuals worthy of both assisting and converting, a fact that may seem promising in medical missionary work in the slums of Japan. The poor and the indigent, while requiring assistance, had little to offer a church in terms of charitable donations or social prestige. Yet these were the people among whom William and Catherine Booth had staked out a niche. The inclusion of women, both within the Army's ranks and among those whom it sought to assist, was seen originally as ridiculous by the establishment in the days of upper middle class women's auxiliary clubs and church bazaars. Women would remain unsullied by both the streets and by the masculine task of preaching, and those who were already in the streets could, at best, be an individual cause célèbre discussed at salons and auxiliary meetings, but, despite such notoriety, never assisted directly. The so-called hallelujah lasses, like Catherine Booth and her daughters, who had risen from lower class backgrounds and seemed determined to return to them, were as unfeminine as bluestockings or suffragettes. Thus desexualized, they were regarded by other religionists as an affront to God's intention. In Melbourne's Wesleyan *Spectator* periodical, one Reverend George Daniel reminded women (and the men who loved or ruled over them) that "the laws of nature and of the Bible undoubtedly determine this [the home] to be woman's place. Her power in the world and in the church is the exercise of influence, and not the exercise of authority."[10] The hallelujah lasses, however, had no interest in minding their place, if for no other reason than, being from lower-class households, they had never been spared from labor to mind the home as their wealthier counterparts had. Many echoed Catherine's admission to her mother that she "felt quite at home on the *platform*—far more than . . . in the *kitchen*." Where Catherine led, the lasses followed, benefiting from her trailblazing and creating new types of ministry where only she had the platform. Playing on their still-unique position as female evangelists, these

9. Taiz, 222; Besant, 286; Walker, 289; P. Wilson, 254–55.
10. From "Woman's Place in the Church." *Spectator*. Oct. 21, 1884 (from Swain, 68). For an insightful analysis of the role of women in the early evangelist movement in Australia, see Shurlee Swain's article "In These Days of Female Evangelists and Hallelujah Lasses: Women Preachers and the Redefinition of Gender Roles in the Churches in Late Nineteenth-Century Australia."

women pushed their novelty still further to attract an audience, often employing a type of guerilla theater to entertain and to enlighten.[11] As exemplified by Eliza Haynes, the woman who walked around her neighborhood with "streamers falling from her unbraided hair," playing fiddle, and wearing a signboard proclaiming that she was "Happy Eliza," promoting her future preaching engagements, these evangelists could leverage sensationalism to draw a crowd. If a receptive audience was not forthcoming, General Bramwell Booth later noted, "we had better send lasses."[12]

But the involvement of women proved less controversial than the Army's emphasis on social welfare among the downtrodden, at least beyond the clergy, another fact that might predispose them to work in Japan's slums. In fact, Booth's polemical *In Darkest England and the Way Out* met with consternation from somewhat surprising sources. The Charity Organisation Society of England, a group established in the wake of the Poor Law to ensure that England limited its assistance to such actions as would empower individuals to assist themselves, feared that too much of the Army's effort was being spent on providing for the undeserving, the criminal and the vagrant. Moreover, the fact that many minor organizations existed to assist the poor made the society wary that the wrong sorts among the indigent were taking advantage of the lack of communication between these organizations to avail themselves of every possible outlet for funds without ever bettering themselves.[13] After over twenty years of work, Booth's pronouncement of the guiding principles of his Army seemed the antithesis of the society's efforts. While admitting that Booth "has shown great powers of organization and great zeal and devotion in a good cause," and that, because so many of his officers come from the ranks of the poor, he had employed some of the "most effective *aides* to charitable work which he desires to undertake," the Society's Council of London publicly remonstrated Booth, whose principles it felt would fail to fulfill the spirit of both England's Poor Laws and its belief in public welfare. As explained by the secretary, C. S. Loch, Booth's "plea is that he can reform those who are out of work," which Loch identified as Germanic socialism in its belief. Furthermore, Loch warned, "You will not help men from the point of view of employment. Our rejoinder is that want of employment, in nine cases out of ten in which the plea is used, is not the cause of distress. It is as often as not drink." And even if Booth was able to combat alcoholism as a cause of poverty, Loch continued,

> General Booth lays no stress on the progress already made, and now being made, and he pours contempt on thrift and all manner of preventive methods which have reduced our dependent classes to continually smaller proportions. He would relieve all who asked. First feed, he says, then preach. But food to all, with the task of work,

11. Walker 1998, 294; 296. Emphasis in original.
12. Walkowitz, 75; Walker 2001, 197–98. The equal inclusion of women in the Army's leadership was also utilitarian, as the organization's marriage policies mandate that an Army officer can only marry another officer, or face expulsion.
13. Hall, 130; Roberts, 49.

> and prospects of what may follow, will create applicants by the hundreds—many more than he can provide for. Men will come for what they can get, and go when they are tired, or have earned a little. From one shelter they will go to another. The relief to be had freely and without many necessary safeguards may aid a few, but it will help to make vagrants of many, or at least not raise them out of their vagrancy. . . . General Booth does not begin at concerted action amongst refuges, but by displacing them. He will add to the disorganization and not remove it.[14]

Loch was by no means reserved in his analysis of Booth and his Army, but both faced more stinging criticism from a somewhat surprising source. Thomas Henry Huxley, Darwin's so-called bulldog—who proclaimed upon reading Darwin's work, "I am sharpening up my claws and beak in readiness for defense of the 'noble book'"—had taken great offense at Booth's doctrine.[15] It was not with Booth's religion that Huxley took issue, per se. As previously discussed, the nature of Darwin's theories on evolution were not antithetical to religious belief. John Gulick, a colleague of Huxley, remained affiliated with the YMCA and a staunch proponent of Darwin's theories. Huxley, a steadfast agnostic, was not averse to discussions of faith.[16] Rather, Huxley attacked Booth in the press with the tenacity of a bulldog for acting as the despot of "mere autocratic Socialism, masked by its theological exterior."[17] The exterior proved to Huxley to take the "form of somewhat corybantic Christianity" that claimed to be "a desirable and trustworthy method of permanently amending the conduct of mankind."[18] In extended correspondence to his pupil and colleague Michael Foster, Huxley maintained that his editorials "have their little game spoilt," and gleefully reported that "you can't imagine the quantity of letters I get from The Salvation Army subordinates thanking me—and telling me all sorts of stories in strict confidence—the poor devils are frightened out of their lives by headquarters spies—Some beg me not to reply as their letters are opened."[19]

Though beset from all sides, Booth's Salvation Army weathered this criticism and continued to grow, particularly overseas. The class and ideological struggles within the British clergy were not particularly damning abroad, especially in countries not rooted in the Judeo-Christian tradition. Thus, within Japan, the jockeying for position among evangelical groups occurred beyond the attention of much of the populace, regardless of class. Indeed, even the perceived "socialistic" tendencies of the Army were considered by many Japanese politicians and bureaucrats as politically impotent, at least until the early Shōwa period.[20] As both the society

14. Loch, 12; 51; 71; 89–90. Emphasis in original.
15. Clodd, 100.
16. Huxley, in fact, is often credited with introducing the term "agnosticism," and responded to calls that he would be better classified as an atheist or an infidel with the following riposte: "I say of agnosticism in this matter, '*J'y suis, et j'y reste*'" (Barr, 253; Huxley 1889, 30).
17. White, 165; Huxley 1891, 7.
18. Huxley 1891, 53–54.
19. Foster and Huxley, Letter 316.
20. Ion 1993, 75–76.

and Huxley were condemning the Army, the dean of Canterbury, Frederic William Farrar, had noted that the officers of Booth's Army “will sing their way around the world in spite of us.” Music did play a large part in the Army's evangelical repertoire, but often was accompanied by guerilla theatrical techniques, even beyond those employed by “Happy Eliza.” Every issue of *The Field Officer of the Salvation Army* included new music, often appropriated from popular melodies, but employing spiritual lyrics, and suggestions of various preaching methods to capture the public imagination. For instance, various issues from 1904 introduced the details of a mock children's auction held by the Army, of preaching from a casket or in chains, and of dressing as a herdsman while proselytizing.[21]

But Farrar, though facetious, was incorrect in attributing the Army's success to its musical prowess. The importance placed on social work among the poor by the Salvation Army's officers after the publication of Booth's polemic was enhanced some three years later, half a world away. There, in India, twenty-year-old officer Henry J. Andrews (or Harry, as he was known) established a small dispensary in his bathroom. Though he had no medical training, Andrews treated numerous patients until finally convincing Bramwell Booth, then the commissioner, to institute an actual medical mission in place of his bathroom. Andrews received the training his aptitude merited and, as Booth recalled, “returned to India a fully qualified man, and was placed in charge of our then largest hospital.” His was to be the first of many such institutions under the administration of the Salvation Army.[22]

The emphasis on medical missionary work, though begun in earnest with Andrews, was not far from the minds of the Booths. As a young man, William Booth was afflicted with “a violent attack of fever.” For Booth, this experience was an epiphany: “My life was in danger, but God mercifully restored me to health, and I went out to devote my spared life to the work of saving souls.” Sadly, the power of faith did not save his young colleague. Booth's friend and coreligionist William Sansom fell ill soon after Booth's recovery, a recovery Booth also credited to Sansom's news that he had managed to continue organizing open-air evangelical meetings during Booth's days as an invalid.[23] While Booth had to contend with a fever, Sansom had little hope against tuberculosis. Despite his family's attempts to aid him, Sansom succumbed to his illness, in Booth's very presence.

Tuberculosis was not unknown to the area in which Booth and Sansom worked, and, indeed, Sansom's final days corresponded to those of a young convert to Booth's group, also dying of tuberculosis, a woman whom Booth had “comforted . . . in her last hours of pain.”[24] Unlike the doomed convert, Catherine Booth had survived her own bout with tuberculosis as a young woman. No less serious than

21. Farrar, 904; SANA: *The Field Officer of the Salvation Army*. Vol. 12, no. 3, Mar., 1904, pp. 90–94; vol. 12, no. 10, Oct., 1904, p. 388.
22. B. Booth, 95; Searle, 187.
23. W. Booth, 2005, 9.
24. Begbie, 87; Bennett, 48–49.

the convert's, Catherine's suffering was recorded in her diary, as on June 13, 1847 when she recounted a trip to the church, "but felt very poorly with faintness and palpitation." She tried to return later that night, but continued to have difficulty:

> At evening I went again and stopped to receive the sacrament, but was so ill I could scarcely walk up to the communion rail, and was forced to hold it to keep myself from sinking. Mr. Heady, the minister, saw I was ill, and held the cup for me. I afterward came home, supported between Mr. Wells and another gentleman. The pain was so violent I had to keep stopping in the street. The cold sweat stood on my forehead.

Yet her belief comforted her, as it had her future husband.[25] Whether delivered from suffering by grace or by death, the effect of illness on the Booth family and on their Army was profound.

The experiences of the Booth family in London's East End created a precedent for the Army's action throughout the world. Relatively unhindered by borders, Booth saw his brand of evangelism as assistance—not merely in the salvation of the populace, but also in its physical, emotional, and mental health. In a famous moment from Booth's last public speech, the general, despite the Army's "native policy," emphasized his focus on individuals, not nations:

> While women weep, as they do now, I'll fight; while little children go hungry, as they do now, I'll fight; while men go to prison, in and out, in and out, as they do now, I'll fight; while there is a drunkard left, while there is a poor girl lost upon the streets, while there remains one dark soul without the light of God, I'll fight, I'll fight to the very end![26]

In truth, the emphasis on the individual was not antithetical to the "native policy." In immersing the officers in their environment, forcing their compliance with national standards, the Army hoped to ensure that these men and women

---

25. Wilson, 21; Booth Tucker, 54.
26. Woodall, 218 Booth's affirmation calls to mind a more well known, albeit later quote, that of the protagonist Tom Joad in John Steinbeck's *The Grapes of Wrath*:

> Wherever they's a fight so hungry people can eat, I'll be there. Wherever they's a cop beatin' up a guy, I'll be there. If Casy knowed why, I'll be in the way guys yell when they're mad an'—I'll be in the way kids laugh when they're hungry an' they know supper's ready. An' when our folks eat the stuff they raise an' live in the houses they build—why, I'll be there. (Steinbeck, 419)

Steinbeck, a staunch New Dealer, was undoubtedly aware of Booth's words, if only because he viewed the Salvation Army with distrust. This lack of confidence permeates *The Grapes of Wrath*, although the Army is only mentioned twice; this was not as offhandedly as casual readers might think. Both times, the Army appears as a hypocritical organization, a religious group that Joad acknowledges had "come an' done us good. . . . They was bein' nice to us." However, he cautions, "If one of us tried to walk out (of the hall), we'd a-drawed solitary. That's preachin'. Doin' good to a fella that's down an' can't smack ya in the puss for it" (ibid., 94). The Janus face of the Army also occurs to the character of Annie Littlefield, a woman who represents government assistance, who reports that when her family was starving, she went to the Salvation Army, where "they made us crawl for our dinner. They took our dignity. They—I hate 'em!" (ibid., 316). Steinbeck's distaste for the Army has been noted by scholars (Bullivant, 246; McDannell, 134, 136), but the parallels between Steinbeck's semantics and style and those of Booth has not.

would be able to relate better to their presumed charges. Of course, it seems naive, particularly in light of the fact that the Army only managed to look ridiculous. Moreover, the fact that the officers had limited to no Japanese linguistic ability might also be considered a negation of the "native policy." Whether the desire to integrate successfully reflected an equally strong desire to undermine accusations of cultural imperialism proves a moot point, better described by Jack Nelson's theory of moral entrepreneurship, but it did mark another early difference between the Army and the association.

This difference was not lost on the Japanese. While the Army did appear comical at first, there were a few in Japan to whom the Army spoke effectively. One of the most famous, and certainly the biggest Japanese asset to the Army, was a young printer's assistant named Yamamuro Gunpei, a name that would eventually become synonymous with Japan's Salvation Army. Having traveled to Tokyo in the hope of one day attending the Imperial University, Yamamuro became lost in the slums populated by the capital's working class, with reference to which he recalled that his "surroundings were horrible. Of my two hundred fellow-workmen nearly all spent their earnings in riotous living, and more than one of them finished his life in disgust by committing suicide." He would have been wont to join them save for the Christianity he happened to encounter in that same environment.[27] An adherent of the maxim "heaven helps those who help themselves" and to *Self-Help*, Samuel Smiles' didactic work that championed it, Yamamuro dreamed of assisting his neighbors understand a religion that seemed to them to be out of touch with their lives. Christian converts in Japan had come primarily from the middle and upper classes, and it was to these classes that foreign evangelists had preached. But to Yamamuro, hardly coming from such a privileged background, Christianity seemed to address how even impoverished life had meaning, and in which suffering was not for naught. As he recalled, "*Self-Help* showed that the power of Christianity lay in its applicability to the practical needs of everyday life."[28]

As he helped himself through school, Yamamuro became acquainted with the Salvation Army before its arrival through a series of interesting coincidences:

> A well-known social worker in Japan, Mr. Ishi, fell sick; and while lying helpless in hospital he employed a friend of mine to read to him an English book which was greatly written about at that time in the Japanese newspapers. It was The General's wonderful book: "In Darkest England and the Way Out." The hospital in which Mr. Ishi lay was near the college, and I accompanied my friend to take such notes upon

27. SANA: "Men and Things That Have Influenced Me: No. III.—Staff-Captain Yamamuro, Editor of the Japanese 'War Cry.'" *The Field Officer of the Salvation Army*. Vol. 12, no. 8, Aug. 15, 1904. p. 302.
28. Smiles, 13; Best, 179–80; Lord, 5. It is interesting to note, as Rightmire does, that Yamamuro requested he be baptized by the Tsukiji church of the Evangelical Association of North America, an evangelical group which had been in Japan for over a decade. The Association refused him. Yamamuro claimed that this was due to the fact that he was young and impoverished, although Paul Eller reported in his *History of Evangelical Missions* that the Evangelical Association welcomed many underprivileged converts in Japan (Rightmire, 24–25; Cary 1909a, 137; Eller, 204).

> the book as Mr. Ishi wished to keep for reference. The book made a deep impression upon my mind, and filled me with longing to learn more of this wonderful Salvation Army, which, however, I knew at that time only as a Social Agency.[29]

In the interim between his note taking and the Army's arrival, Yamamuro had dedicated himself to his new "life's ambition and consecration—the preaching of the salvation of God to the common people."[30] Although he admitted to struggling with his faith, Yamamuro contacted the Army soon after its arrival, and, despite cultural and linguistic barriers, Yamamuro discovered among the officers a number of kindred spirits. In its literature, Yamamuro found an analogue to *Self-Help*. In its ideology, Yamamuro believed he found the best application of Christianity in the quotidian. For him, the Army "told clearly what character one saved by Christ and living for God's glory should have, what sort of life he should undertake, what business he should engage in, how he should serve God and man, and how he should strive for the salvation of the world."[31] Whether the Army had saved any souls in the three months before Yamamuro's entrance is unknown, but it is undeniable that the marriage of the Army and Yamamuro proved just as beneficial to the former as the latter claimed it was for him.[32]

Within a few years, Yamamuro had produced one of his most famous works, and one of the biggest boons to the Army's movement in Japan: 平民之福音 (*Heimin no fukuin*), or *The Common People's Gospel*, was published less than four years after Yamamuro joined the organization, and quickly became one of its best sellers. Written "for the sake of this truth," *The Common People's Gospel* tried to convey the essence of Jesus' teaching in a manner comprehensible to a wide Japanese audience, including those whose literacy was more limited; written colloquially, it included *furigana* (syllabic transliterations) of every kanji.[33]

The publication of Yamamuro's first work was not the only accomplishment of the Army in Japan by the turn of the century. The Salvation Army's periodical *Toki no koe* had been published since its arrival, and was helmed almost as early by Yamamuro.[34] In addition to literature, the Army focused its work on the urban poor, so that, by 1900, it had attempted to marry labor reform and fire prevention to its proselytizing.[35] The emphasis on cities, shared with the Young Men's

29. SANA: "Men and Things That Have Influenced Me: No. III.—Staff-Captain Yamamuro, Editor of the Japanese 'War Cry.'" *The Field Officer of the Salvation Army*. Vol. 12, no. 8, Aug. 15, 1904. p. 304.
It is highly likely that Mr. Ishi is Ishii Juji. The discrepancy in the spelling of the surname is due to Yamamuro's article being transcribed from an interview.
30. Ibid., 304.
31. Rightmire, 34–35; SANA: "Chats with Missionary Officers: VI.—Lieut.-Colonel Yamamuro, Japan." *The Field Officer of the Salvation Army*. Vol. 25, no. 9, Oct., 1917. p. 640.
32. In his dissertation, Baggs maintains that the Army had not managed to gather any converts before Yamamuro (Baggs, 56). In addition, the Army itself would later claim that Yamamuro was the first (SANA: 心は真に手は人に [Serving God and man], p. 4). It hardly matters, of course, as Yamamuro became the perfect embodiment of a Japanese Salvation Army officer.
33. Yamamuro 1901, 6.
34. SANA: ときのこえ. 1996, 11/15, no. 22252. p. 1; Lord, 13.
35. SANA: 心は真に手は人に (Serving God and man). p. 4.

Christian Association, would prove central to the work undertaken, but removed the Army from a significant base, particularly due to the poverty of the countryside. Nevertheless, while Yamamuro laughingly reported that, after life in Tokyo, he "could no longer tell a melon from an eggplant," he believed, as did his colleagues, that the "rural customs are unspeakably ridiculous," to the point that attention to the countryside was perhaps worthless.[36]

The emphasis on the urban population had long precedent in the Salvation Army. So, too, did the emphasis on women, as noted above. In Japan, the importance of women's roles in the Army led to an awareness of social issues affecting females specifically. Thus, the greatest undertaking of the Army around the turn of the century utilized both the organization's involvement in Japan cities and its position at the forefront of women's issues. Prostitution in the nation's cities saw a marked increase after the Meiji Restoration, and one not necessarily in keeping with the rise in population therein. Moreover, by the turn of the century, the industry had established a tight control over its wares in the passage of the Rules Regulating Licensed Prostitutes, so that, in 1900, the Nagoya District Court discovered that "there is scarcely no difference between their treatment and that accorded to convicts."[37] It was to these women, many still girls, that the Salvation Army turned its attention at the dawn of the twentieth century. As then territorial commander Henry Bullard recalled upon his retirement, that within a year of his arrival in Japan, the Salvation Army had undertaken "the great Social Agitation." As described upon Booth's visit to Japan seven years later, "a certain class of Japanese girls were then not merely shut into that dreadful life to which they had generally been sold, but the police were used rather to prevent than to assist the escape of any girl who might wish to lead a better life."[38] These women, Bullard reported, were "gathered into districts, and each [brothel] house was licensed by the Government." Within Tokyo,

> The chief of these Licensed Quarters, the "Yoshawara," were 5,000 female inmates, given up to vice. . . . All the women had to be licensed and registered with the police. When once this had been done, it was practically impossible for them to give up their life of sin, whatever might be their disinclination or even physical disability. It was a penal offence to encourage them to leave or to harbor them if they escaped, through the system was abhorred by the best spirits of the Japanese Empire.[39]

---

36. Baggs, 62.
37. Garon 1993, 713. For an excellent analysis of prostitution in early twentieth century Japan, please see Sheldon Garon's article, "The World's Oldest Debate? Prostitution and the State in Imperial Japan, 1900–1945," in *The American Historical Review*.
38. SANA: "'Reminiscences of Early-Day Fighting: SA History Viewed from a Personal Angle' VI.—Commissioner Henry Bullard (Retired)." *The Officers' Review: Incorporating 'The Staff Review' and 'The Officer.'* Vol. 2, 1933; SANA: "Our Present Standing." *The Field Officer of the Salvation Army*. Vol. 15, no. 6. June, 1907.
39. SANA: "'Reminiscences of Early-Day Fighting: SA History Viewed from a Personal Angle" VI.—Commissioner Henry Bullard (Retired)." *The Officers' Review: Incorporating 'The Staff Review' and 'The Officer.'* Vol. 2, 1933. Technically, the quarters to which Bullard refers is the "Yoshiwara" (吉原). Presumably, the "best spirits" of the Japanese Empire are Christians, although, considering how few Christians there were in the Japanese Empire,

Although regulation of licensed prostitutes (and the criminalization of unlicensed prostitution) became the purview of the imperial government in 1900, and debt slavery of much of the country's prostitution had become illegal over a quarter of a century earlier, the system remained far too unjust and immoral for the Army, who continued to see within it a vicious cycle of indentured servitude, in part because the girls trapped therein were ignorant of the victories of late that had been made on their behalf.[40] To bring attention to this issue both internationally and within Japan's brothels themselves, the Army "decided to make an organized endeavour to help these women, whatever the consequences." With a rescue house established under the care of Yamamuro and his wife, both captains in the Salvation Army, the officers set off for the licensed quarters of Tokyo with "a special Rescue number of our Japanese 'War Cry,' proclaiming our willingness to protect any girl who came to us." Although the Army in Japan "had then not more than a dozen Corps and between thirty and forty Officers in the country," a small band of "Officers and Soldiers . . . marched singing, with Flag flying and drum beating, through the main entrance to the notorious Yoshawara Licensed Quarter, where we . . . distributed the special Rescue 'War Cry' among the girls who flocked out to see what was happening, and whom we invited to forsake their life of sin and come to our Rescue home." No sooner had they begun their preaching than they "were violently attacked by crowds of men who had gathered around. They smashed our drum, tore up our Flag, and beat and wounded all members of our little band, who escaped with difficulty."

Yet, despite the violence, the mission was considered a resounding success, since it created a public relations nightmare for the brothels:

> This apparent defeat was what we had anticipated, and gave us the publicity we required. The principal newspapers were full of details of our attack, and advertised the establishment of our Rescue Home. With scarcely an exception they took sides with us and urged that the law should be changed so that any woman or girl in the licensed Quarters might be free to return to the paths of virtue. The Tokyo papers began the issue of two and even three special editions daily, a quite new venture for Japanese journalism. The agitation stirred the nation to an extent to which it had never previously been stirred on any social subject, and throughout which Government officers and police rendered us constant and invaluable aid.[41]

---

it seems a rather limited view of the number of Japanese subjects opposed to the district, particularly if one considers how many unwilling residents of that district were not terribly pleased to be employed therein.

40. Garon 1997, 92; Garon 1993, 714; Baggs, 86; Ramseyer 1991, 97; Ramseyer 1996, 112. J. Mark Ramseyer offers an interesting reassessment of prostitution from the end of Meiji until the war in much of his work, including the two works cited above. Certainly not conducive to the Army's interpretation, Ramseyer's investigation offers an alternative to the belief of the helpless girl coerced into prostitution with no agency of her own. An interesting perspective for those researching prostitution in Japan, most of his work remains outside the purview of this dissertation.

41. SANA: "'Reminiscences of Early-Day Fighting: SA History Viewed from a Personal Angle" VI.—Commissioner Henry Bullard (Retired).' *The Officers' Review: Incorporating 'The Staff Review' and 'The Officer.'* Vol. 2, 1933.

Journalists proved worthy allies, as did the Nagoya-based American Methodist evangelist U. G. Murphy. Murphy, an associate of Bullard, had been studying Japanese law, and had succeeded in suits to free young prostitutes from their servitude based on the 1872 legislation. Although hindered by the police, Murphy's actions, like Bullard and his officers, garnered significant press coverage.[42] Murphy himself later reported one instancc in which a young girl, groomed for a life of prostitution, sought refuge at an office of a national newspaper:

> A girl thirteen years old, sold to a brothel in Tokyo as a prostitute in training, heard of the efforts that were being put forth for the release of women of illfame, and escaping from the Yoshiwara quarters found her way across the city to the *Mainichi* news paper office, six miles away, and begged that she be protected. She said that while she was not yet a prostitute, yet she hoped it would be possible for the paper to help her, as only a few years intervened between her and ruin. The interest aroused in the girl's case by the fiery appeals of the editors spread nearly all over the empire, and in order to quietly settle the matter the keeper readily agreed to let the girl go for a few *yen*.[43]

In appealing to the *Mainichi Shimbun* the young woman had made a wise choice. Shimada Sabūro, the paper's editor, was also a member of the Diet, a Christian, and a man Yamamuro once called "the oldest and truest friend of the Salvation Army in Japan." As both journalist and politician, Shimada railed against the failure to enforce self-emancipation within brothels, which he deemed a "humanitarian issue," and unequivocally condemned "the perpetrator of this rape, this prostitution against the holy reign of Meiji," whom he noted "must be judged to be the Home Minister."[44]

But while the newspapers sought to engage the public, the Army tried to address its literature to a very specific audience. Because the majority of Japan's young, urban prostitutes lacked higher levels of education, Yamamuro tailored the Army's words, as he had his *Heimin no fukuin*, to be comprehensible to them. While

42. F. Coutts, 103; Baggs, 86.
43. Murphy, 104.
44. Akimoto 2, 8; Baggs, 133; Huffman 1997, 255. This would be neither the first nor the last time that Shimada used such strong language to denounce the injustices he witnessed in Japan. Perhaps more famous were his fulminations about the pollution of Japan's largest mine, the Ashio copper mine, not far from Nikkō, an act that certainly annoyed the many politicians and bureaucrats (including Mutsu Munemitsu and Shibusawa Eiichi) with whom the mine's owner, Furukawa Ichibei, was friendly—although both Mutsu and Shibusawa acknowledged that not all Furukawa mining actions were wholly acceptable (Huffman 1997, 183; Stone, 386; Nimura, 134). Indeed, for this purpose, Shimada is credited with coining the term *kōgai* (公害), commonly used to represent "pollution," but also carrying the connotation of what Neil Waters called the "destruction of the public interest, or of communality" (Waters, 21). In representing the public interest, therefore, Shimada's yellow journalism ensured that the pollution from the mine, and the various issues it wrought, would not go unnoticed. In a six-month period bridging 1901 and 1902, the *Mainichi Shimbun* published an average of two articles a day on Ashio (Stone, 397).

    The Ashio case is a fascinating study, and Nimura Kazuo's work offers a detailed study of the mine (and particularly of the 1907 riots of the mine's laborers), although sadly he does not mention the work of Shimada and other muckrakers.

he wrote of the evils of prostitution ("the world's most shameful, bitter, sorrowful, and, above all, evil occupation"), Yamamuro also included practical information to assist these women:

> If you really want to quit, you can do so legally. The law of this land says clearly that no person has the right to force you to keep on at your work, no matter how sunk in debt you may be. No one can use you cruelly as so many pawned humans. Submit to the police an official 'notification of cessation of business' and you can be free again! Naturally, the brothel keepers will not let you quit if they can help it. They will do all within their power to stop you, and they may even hire hooligans to frighten you. But if you are determined, do not lose heart, and press on, you certainly can expect to win your freedom in time, for the law is on your side.

Should the women fear they were alone in this fight, law on their side or no, Yamamuro was quick to suggest the assistance of his organization as they embraced their new lives:

> You probably are thinking what good would it do to become free when you would have only the rags on your back, and have no idea from where your next meal would come. . . . An organization called the Salvation Army is ready to help you . . . Its main office is located in Tokyo . . . There you can ask for advice and receive every kind of aid in helping you get started in new lives. If you have any fears or worries about visiting this place, forget them. The Salvation Army thruout [*sic*] the world is dedicated to working with all its might and main to save unfortunate women like yourselves. We cannot stand idly by and watch your misery, because all of us like all of you are sisters in the eyes of the one true God. We want you to know that we care. It is up to you to decide once and for all what you will do with your lives.[45]

Marking the success of this campaign, a significant number of women did decide that they wanted to leave the brothels. And the brothels did attack, although they mostly attacked the Army—much to its jubilation. Violence attracted more press, and concretized the Army's battle. In having what Salvationist John Coutts deemed "a tangible social evil," the Army was able to point to analogues between the desire for human rights and the desire for salvation.[46] In fact, this was one of the Army's greatest strengths. Where the YMCA (at least in peacetime) counted on its extracurricular activities to draw people into the physical sphere of the association, the Army sought its battles in the thick of social injustices. This dichotomy was cultivated by the latter and, more important, was witnessed by Japan's urban dwellers at all levels of society. As these men and women discovered, the Army was working within Japanese society to improve it (even if improvements were undertaken in the name of a god), and to improve it along lines that the Japanese politicians had already determined. The organization's acceptance of society, as evidenced by the Army's involvement in it, and even, though perhaps laughably, by the officers' attempts to

45. Baggs, 90–91.
46. J. Coutts, 85.

assimilate through a native policy, became a hallmark of the Army's work in Japan. So, too, did its emphasis on the individual, foremost in Booth's ideology, become an accepted and acceptable part of Army work in Japan. This, then, proved as palatable to many on the right as it had to their colleagues on the political left. By virtue of accepting Japan and seeking to assist individuals within the workings of Japanese society, the Army preempted conservative criticism. Indeed, as Baggs maintains, conservatives had to acknowledge that "the Army could perform a useful function in a Japanese society where, unlike Western society, no tradition of extrafamilial social welfare service existed."[47]

On the strength of this social agitation of 1900 and of famine relief in Japan's Tōhoku region after the Russo-Japanese War (the latter being one of the few forays into the countryside, although the work was based in the region's largest city), as *The Field Officer of the Salvation Army* recorded, "The Army has been recognised as a great force for righteousness and the good of the people of Japan. We have now 37 Corps and 143 Officers." It was to view the progress that his Army had made in the country that William Booth visited Japan as part of his world tour of Army outposts in 1907.[48] As it underscored for the organization worldwide, *The Salvation Army Year Book* stated that, for both Booth's soldiers in the Army and for those subjects of the emperor for whom his soldiers sought to care, "quite the most important event in Army affairs during the month was the meeting of His Imperial Majesty the Emperor of Japan and our beloved leader, The General." It is hardly surprising, therefore, that the editor of *The Year Book* refused to limit such a momentous occasion to a fleeting sentence:

> Perhaps the most striking tribute to The General as a benefactor of the race was the audience which His Imperial Majesty the Emperor of Japan accorded him on Saturday morning, April 20th, at Tokio.
>
> When The General entered into the presence of the Emperor, His Majesty beamed upon his guest, and at once expressed his pleasure at meeting him. He then proceeded to ask the usual questions respecting The General's health, the length of his visit to Japan, and when he intended to leave, with the expression of a hope that he might enjoy good health.
>
> The General thanked His Majesty for the audience, expressed his gratification at the warm welcome he had received from his subjects, and the hope that his people might be privileged to help in advancing the highest interests of His Majesty's Empire.

---

47. Baggs, 123. It is interesting to note, as Baggs does, that Buddhist social welfare groups were hardly known before the arrival of their Christian counterparts, most failing to pursue such work until after the turn of the century (and then in response to such Christian evangelical groups as the Army and the YMCA—hence the arrival of the YMBA, the Young Men's Buddhist Association) (Addison, 336; Saunders 1922, 72).

48. K. Watanabe, 83; SANA: "Our Present Standing" *The Field Officer of the Salvation Army*. Vol. 15, no. 6. June, 1907.

> The Emperor expressed his sympathy with the efforts of The Army on behalf of the suffering poor, and after further conversation cordially bade The General adieu.
>
> Thus, with stately ceremony, The Army's Leader, in the Providence of God, received in this remote part of the world a recognition similar to that which drew the attention of the work at the other extreme, Buckingham Palace, in 1904, and in Scandinavia last year.

Although brief, the meeting was a watershed and was gratifying for both sides. According to journalist (and one-time Christian) Tokutomi Sohō, only two foreign visitors made an "outstanding impression" on the emperor during his long reign; Booth was the second.[49] More significantly, however, the meeting represented significant shifts for the organization and for the nation. For Booth, it not only legitimized his organization to the rest of his Army in its first East Asian nation but also served as validation to some of those who had previously viewed the Army as naive or disingenuous. For the emperor, the coverage of the meeting in both the Salvation Army's publication and in the international press recognized Japan as a civilized nation worthy of comparison to those of Europe.

More than that, however, Meiji later discovered that Booth, according to his officers in the Emperor's nation, "suggested that The Salvation Army in Japan should investigate the possibility of medical care for indigent tuberculosis patients." Booth donated to the creation of his future sanatorium, but neither he nor the emperor would live to see the end result.[50] Obviously, it was not that Meiji was unfamiliar with the disease, as it had touched his colleagues and even members of his family.[51] But for many both in government and in the Army, nursing the poor and indigent seemed a logical responsibility of the Army. Certainly, the Army's work with the indentured servants of Japan's brothels had offered the organization a glimpse of the medical state of the nation. As one prostitute wrote to Kyoto's prefectural office, who notified Yamamuro, the woman's presumed tuberculosis had become another burden in an already-difficult life:

> Recently I went to the police to get permission to leave the brothel. For some reason the police did not allow me to leave. The reason I want to leave the brothel is my poor health. For this reason, I cannot please the customers or satisfy my master. I am thirty-three and am alone in this world. I do not have any parents or brothers. I am all alone, so my master treats me brutally. Recently one of my co-workers, Yuki, was kicked downstairs from the second floor. She died as a result of that fall. Because of this I have come to fear my master even more than before. So please,

49. SANA: "Looking Back." *The Salvation Army Year Book*. 1908. p. 5; SANA: "Royal Recognition." *The Salvation Army Year Book*. 1908. p. 10; Bullard, 45; SANA: "Memories of the Founder I.—By Lieut.-Commissioner Gunpei Yamamuro, T. C., Japan." *The Field Officer of the Salvation Army*. Vol. 48, no. 2. Feb. 1929. p. 117.
50. SANA: "History of the Salvation Army Kiyose Hospital and Hospice."
51. Chakraborty, 9; Keene 2002, 832.

> please allow me to quit the brothel. You can verify the truth about my master's cruelty by asking around.[52]

It is telling, of course, that being a prostitute and being abandoned by one's family were seen as more socially acceptable than being tubercular, as indicated by the woman's willingness to divulge the minutiae of her position, but not of her disease, which, as it reads, could be almost anything—even venereal.

But tuberculosis, though not uncommon in Japan's pleasure quarters, was far more widespread in its factory and slum districts. Normally, the involvement of Japan's labor force in the work of any organization, domestic or foreign, set much of Japan's political elite on edge, since it smacked of socialism. These, of course, were not unfamiliar charges for the Salvation Army, but in Japan, at least, the organization had distinguished itself as being apolitical, whilst creating "thirty-nine Corps and Outposts, and . . . Rescue Homes, a Home for Dicharged [*sic*] prisoners, Cheap Food Dépôt, Lodging-House, Labour Bureau, etc."[53]

All of this was made possible, in part, by the Army's annual Self-Denial fund. This fund, common throughout the Salvation Army's branches worldwide, as originally conceived of by Booth, was meant "to raise money for the spreading of Salvation and relieving the necessities of the poor. This is done by going without some form of luxury—in many cases the devotion of lovers of God causes them to go without or to postpone even necessities."[54] From its start in 1886, the fund, the result of which took place annually over the course of only one week, had "grown in popularity and in results." More important, however, "in every country the impression produced by the knowledge of such acts has been far more widespread than the effort itself, or its cash results would indicate." Indeed, the involvement of every individual, not merely wealthy philanthropists, proved to be a boon not only to the Army's coffers but to its public relations, and the additional role of women, particularly in Japan, where many women took a secondary role in charitable work, both physically and financially, seemed to assist the women as much as the Army:

> In Japan, ladies who never before labored personally have managed by sewing or other work to earn money, just as so many of our Soldiers do elsewhere, to add to the result. There has been thus a world-wide awakening to the old idea of a personal self-denial for the good of others, and we expect more of that every year.[55]

Nevertheless, sewing was slow going, and while Japan's self-denial brought in funds fairly consistently (each year's income exceeding the last's, in most cases), the necessary amount for construction of the sanatorium did not keep apace with the rising number of tuberculosis cases near the Army's headquarters. Nor did the

52. Hane, 216.
53. SANA: Lieutenant-Colonel Charles Duce. "For Foreign Service: VI.—Japan as a Mission Field." *The Field Officer of the Salvation Army*. Vol. 18, no. 6. June 1910. p. 233.
54. SANA: "Self-Denial." *The Salvation Army Year Book*. 1916, pp. 65–66.
55. SANA: "What Self-Denial Means." *The Salvation Army Year Book*. Ed. Colonel Theodore Kitching. 1913. p. 79.

estimated budget for the International Salvation Army provide enough funds for such an expenditure, the entire sum dedicated to field work in Japan, Korea, Java, and the evangelization of "Native Races in Africa and the West Indies" constituting less than 9 percent of the £173,000 budget.[56] It is clear that eking out enough funds to combat the scourge would be a hard sell. Still, as Japan's corps scrimped and sewed, soldiers used the interim to continue to educate themselves and their charges courtesy of the Army's publications, which reminded them that of utmost important should be "the prevention of disease in every form:"

> This very specially applies to Salvation Army Officers, and more particularly to those doing slum work. The constant mixing with all conditions of life in the close and crowded streets, and still more close and crowded houses; the close contact with the very poor, and not always very clean, masses of the people in The Army meetings; the frequent visitation by Officers to sick and dying men and women in close, unventilated rooms and dark and dingy dens, the so-called "homes" of the stricken poor—all make it very important that a general and more or less special knowledge of how to protect themselves against contagious and infectious diseases is exceeding desirable to all those who thus spend their lives.

The tract continued exhorting the magnitude of "gaining of a knowledge of how to deal with the dangers of contagion and infection—to fight these enemies of activity and personal safety."

> As a demonstration of this point, the following incident of real life may be useful. Some years ago a healthy family moved into an empty house, which was comfortable and well situated, and seemed in every way suited to their needs. They never had any special tendency to ordinary ailment, and considered themselves quite strong and robust. Two young men, who were specially strong and active, where [*sic*] given a room with a bed in which they both slept. About six months after they took possession, these young lads began to cough, and nothing seemed able to stop it. At first there were no signs of any cause for the coughing, and they were puzzled and anxious regarding the matter. Then the boy began to lose flesh, to get wearied and languid, and at last, after careful examination, his lungs were found to be suspiciously affected. This continued, and got gradually worse, until at last it was found necessary to to [*sic*] advise his removal from the city.
>
> After this the other members of the family remained right, until, a few months after the young man had left home, his bed-fellow of the previous months also began to cough, and within a like time became affected much as his brother had been. Then he also was sent off to find health, if possible, in a warmer and drier climate.
>
> The Usual Popular Explanation of such incidents was either the catching of a cold which had been neglected, and so brought on lung trouble, or a hereditary transmission from some distant progenitors a qualified visitation of God which could not be averted.

56. SANA: "Why So Much Money?" *The Salvation Army Year Book*. 1914. p. 15.

Not surprisingly, this was insufficient. Rather, the "real explanation" was as follows:

> In this house, and in this particular bedspace, for some months before this family took possession, a young woman lay dying of tubercular disease of the lungs—consumption—and when she was carried out there were left behind colonies of those active germs which cause lung disease. The contagion or infection was patiently waiting until a favourable soil for their active development was found, when again the process of disease and death would go on. This is a very good object-lesson of how danger may lurk around anyone. It explains the great need of ordinary knowledge of the processes that are going on around a case of consumption, and it also gives the indication of how such dangers may and can be avoided, even under the most difficult circumstances. . . .
>
> I have taken up this special form of infectious disease because I have again and again been consulted by Officers, some in the early stages, some in the later, suffering from it, and many of them having evidently contracted it in the course of their daily duties. I have also had experience of such cases amongst hard-working Officers, where the affected one was sleeping constantly with the other, and no care or provision was being taken to protect the healthy one from the infection. I do not think this is done carelessly but ignorantly, and therefore I have tried to show how much depends on knowing something about the risks and dangers of the disease which is now known to be preeminently infectious. . . .
>
> I have tried in this short paper to indicate the importance of the infectious nature of this sad disease, a disease preeminently of the young, a disease which is responsible for the deaths of hundreds of thousands each year in our country, and also to give a clear idea of what the danger consists of and the means to be adopted to avert it.[57]

Still, not all of the information from Headquarters was wholly devoid of common myths about public health:

> Gout, cancer, and nervous diseases, such as the many forms of insanity and epilepsy, are examples of hereditary tendencies. So, also, is consumption, though this dread malady is contracted by many who do not belong to consumptive families. . . .
>
> Where the consumptive taint is suspected, close, impure and damp atmospheres should be sedulously avoided. The food should have a generous proportion of fats, while an abundance of fresh air—particularly early morning air—and exercise is an absolute necessity. . . .
>
> If a plant bends too much in one direction, a great philosopher has said, it needs to be bent just so far in the *opposite* direction. So let the highly-strung, nervous, and over-active individual have plenty of rest and sleep in a quiet, dark room, while those of the lymphatic temperament with consumptive tendencies,

57. SANA: "Ailments of Army Officers. Prevention of Contagion in Sick Visiting by 'a Glasgow Physician.'" *The Field Officer of the Salvation Army*. Vol. 12, no. 10. Oct., 1904; SANA: "II.—Prevention of Contagion in Sick Visiting." *The Field Officer of the Salvation Army*. Vol. 12, no. 11. Nov., 1904.

> rise early, drink in the life-giving morning air and seek plenty of exercise, living, as far as possible, in a dry, healthy climate.[58]

Certainly, though particularly helpful to teach the nature of contagion, particularly in such a stigmatized disease as tuberculosis, the literature nevertheless reflected the health fads of the period. The rise of the open-air movement and the emphasis on hearty and rich food for those believed to be afflicted by consumptive "tendencies" were mirrored in the medical advice of the day:

> Consumption, or tuberculosis, is an infectious disease caused by the presence of germs called the tubercle bacilli. These germs may affect different parts of the body, e.g. the lungs (consumption), the joints, especially the hip and knee; the bones, especially the vertebrae, where you get a deformed condition as seen in hunchback; the bladder and kidneys; the covering of the brain, when the disease is known as tubercular meningitis; the glands, especially those of the neck.
>
> Consumption is not hereditary, but a child may be born with a tendency to the disease which may be overcome by strict attention to the ordinary rules of health. Some predisposing causes of consumption are: Insufficient food, indulgence in alcohol, bad air, dusty occupations, etc. Consumption germs are spread by the sputum (spittle) and other discharges from the patient. The following precautions should be taken:–
>
> Consumptives should always sleep alone, as the fine spray coughed out often contains germs. The phlegm of a consumptive should be received on to pieces of rag (never on a handkerchief) which should be burnt immediately, or a suitable spittoon, containing a solution of 1 in 20 carbolic acid, should be used. The consumptive should never spit on to the ground, as the sputum after a time dries up and is blown about.

Indeed, the advice of the Army often mixed valid theory with popular conjecture, as below:

> Every means possible to improve the general state of health of delicate children and adults, especially those with consumptive parents, should be taken. Fat bacon, butter, dripping, cream, etc., should form a prominent part of the diet. They should have plenty of pure pasteurized milk, fresh air and sunshine. Late hours and smoking and drinking should be avoided. A cold should never be neglected, and chills should be avoided. The bedroom windows should be kept open night and day, and healthy outdoor occupations indulged in.[59]

For many in the evangelical community, Salvationists notwithstanding, disinfectant, fresh air, and heavy foods were assisted by faith. Theotherapy and faith healing were promoted within the Army as requisites of mens sana in corpore sano:

58. SANA: "Combating Diseases." *The Field Officer of the Salvation Army*. Vol. 15, no. 2. Feb., 1907. p. 50.
59. Bryder, 85; Snedden, 629; SANA: "A Course of Instruction in Home-Nursing by 'London County Council Instructor.'" *The Field Officer of the Salvation Army Year*. Vol. 24, no. 7. July, 1916. p. 482.

> Theories of Faith Healing have been pushed to such extremes by fanatics that many thoughtful people, as well as the timid, have come to look with suspicion upon any teaching related to this subject. But when God bestows some special blessing upon His children it is not His will for them to become fanatical in any sense. Therefore, I have been careful since my experience of healing to keep first things first—spiritual health before physical health—for I am sure God is more concerned about our being delivered from sin and fired with love for Himself and precious souls than anything else.

In the personal testimony of one Mrs. Peacock, whose recovery was lauded in Japan, God's salubrious nature testifies to this:

> In November, 1913, I had a breakdown in health. . . . I fought against the weakness but finally had to give up, and a specialist pronounced my illness to be tuberculosis. Following this another lung specialist was consulted who also said my lungs were badly affected and advised me to go to a sanatorium right away. I continued to become weaker and finally was compelled to take to my bed. After a period of careful nursing I rallied a trifle, and the doctor arranged for me to go to a sanatorium. On my arrival there I was put through a severe examination, and the diagnosis of my case agreed with that of the physicians who had previous examined me. Seeing the many poor souls there who were stricken with the dreadful disease, I felt very discouraged. I had a conviction that God could heal me but had not sufficient faith to step out on His promises as I did not have a clear understanding of God's plan with regard to the question of Divine healing. But His Holy Spirit was leading me. One night, not being able to sleep, God's voice spoke to me out of the stillness of the night quite audibly, "Go home and I will heal you." I could not doubt God's voice, and next day had some one phone to my husband.

Mrs. Peacock reported that she convalesced at her home under the care of a nurse. However, when the nurse proved cost prohibitive, she was, presumably, forced to recover alone:

> One morning about 5 o'clock I heard a voice over my bed saying these words:–
>
> Ye fearful saints fresh courage take,
> The cloud you so much dread
> Is big with mercy and shall break
> In blessing o'er your head.
>
> God's Word
>
> I listened and was very quiet for some time, realizing it to be the voice of God. I prayed that He might speak yet a little clearer message from His Word. Later in the morning I opened "The Soldier's Guide which was on a table by my bed. It opened to these words:–
>
> "Is any sick among you? let him call for the elders of the church; and let them pray over him, anointing him with oil in the name of the Lord: and the prayer of faith shall save the sick, and the Lord shall raise him up; and if he have committed sins, they shall be forgiven him" (James v. 14–15)

Mrs. Peacock not only endured, but prevailed, thanks to what she believed was divine assistance:

> A Crowning Witness
>
> My faith began to grow and during the day I prayed God to send me some one who would help me to accept the healing God offered me in His previous Word. Two days later a lady whom I had met during the summer called my husband over the phone at his office and said she would like to come and see me. She came and talked with me about Divine Healing, telling me how wonderfully God had healed her and encouraged me to believe that God could do the same for me if I would accept His gift. I asked her to pray with me, which she did, and praise God I was instantly healed. . . .
>
> On the second day after my healing I started to help with the house work as I had done previous to my illness. When my neighbours saw I had taken my curtains down and was cleaning house, they said poor Mrs. Peacock must be losing her reason now. But, praise God, I was a new woman, body, soul, and spirit, because with the physical healing came a spiritual blessing and vision such as I shall never be able to describe.
>
> When the doctor made his usual call, I told him what God had done, thanked him for all his attention and interest in me, and said that I would not need his services any longer. He was astonished, but as he could find no trouble in my lungs, he said he honoured my faith in God, but added that I should never do any hospital visitation, or attend Meetings in crowded Halls, etc. Since my healing God seems to have called me to do more hospital work than ever before, and whenever I have the opportunity, I am, in the strength of the Lord, able to conduct Meetings.[60]

While the fate of Mrs. Peacock after her testimony is unknown, it, of course, behooved the Army to promote the role of faith in convalescence and recovery. The notion of theotherapy, perhaps more than the verity of faith healing, legitimized for the Army and other medical missions the addition of the mission to the medicine. Furthermore, it proved valuable to foster a global belief in faith healing, as it honored evangelists by proclaiming theirs to be a divine medicine, to the likes of which those who felt themselves thus healed often dedicated themselves, and vice versa:

> Eighteen years ago a young woman, now an Adjutant here in Australia, was gradually pining away with consumption in the State of new South Wales, says Lieutenant-Colonel Graham, of Australia. For two or three years she had been so ill as to be unable to be out of doors after sunset, for the doctors told her that one lung was entirely gone and the other affected by that deadly disease consumption. About this time, however, the poor sufferer met The Salvation Army and occasionally attended the Sunday afternoon Meetings.

60. SANA: "'How I Was Cured of Tuberculosis' by Mrs. Major Peacock, Chicago." *The Field Officer of the Salvation Army*. Vol. 32, no. 3. Mar. 1921. pp. 266–67.

> While at home one day she casually remarked to her unsaved sister how much she would like to be a Salvation Army Officer. There was great depth of feeling beneath the expression, which possibly the sister, although unsaved, felt, for she replied, "*Why don't you ask your God to heal you, then?*" Though she made no comment the invalid sister thought over the suggestion for a moment or two and then said, "Well, He can—if He wishes."
>
> The sick girl did not at first pray *definitely* for physical healing, perhaps thinking herself too far gone for recovery, but she did pray that God would deal with her as He saw best, ready to accept His will for her—whether it might be to heal her or not. Very shortly after this she began to realize that she was getting a bit better and on being fully convinced that such was the case, she proved her faith by venturing out after sunset (the first time in three years) and went to an Army Meeting. She went again and again, felt better for so doing and eventually was enrolled as a Soldier in a Corps in my Division. As she launched out in work as a Soldier, she became stronger physically and spiritually, and ere long applied for officership. . . .
>
> Her case proves undoubtedly that God does grant health and opportunity to some who honestly and earnestly desire to work for Him and win souls. Maybe you are one to be thus honoured.[61]

True, theotherapy was not necessarily in keeping with the medical education of the day. However, for many lacking in medical education, the belief in "germs" or "viruses" was as much a leap of faith as that in faith healing itself. Thus, many intelligent individuals saw in their recovery evidence of both. Kagawa Toyohiko, himself a "consumptive," believed fervently in the healing power of the divine:

> The fullness of God's power in the universe is wonderful. Even in illness, there is a healing process. The mentally ill may be cured. . . . Even those with lung trouble may get well. The sick can be healed.
>
> All my life I have been ill. While in the second year of middle school, I had to stop because the apex of one lung had become tubercular. I began to have hemorrhages when I was seventeen years old, and two years later I was so seriously ill that I had to rest for a year. For four or five years the fever did not leave me. At twenty I hardly weighed seventy-six pounds; I now weigh more than one hundred and forty. So when you are told that you have tuberculosis, you need not worry. Sickness has to do with the spirit. When the spirit is healed, the physical sickness will go. If you say, "I have consumption, therefore it's hopeless," you will not get well. . . .
>
> Tuberculosis is an internal injury of the body. If you injure the outside of the body, even though the blood flow [*sic*], you will get well. So why not believe that an internal injury may be cured, also? . . . We do not get well by taking the doctor's medicine only. The regenerating power of the God of heaven, helping as it works through a person, is the real doctor.[62]

61. SANA: "More Remarkable Testimonies to Divine Intervention." *The Field Officer of the Salvation Army*. Vol. 24, no. 8. Aug., 1916. p. 540.
62. Saunders 1931, 311.

The editor of *Toki no koe*, too, questioned why the power of faith—"as with medicine, as with doctors"—was not credited with healing powers when it had, in his experience allowed the sick to rise. It was hardly the opinion of a handful of radicals: Army officer James J. Cooke concurred with Kagawa and Yamamuro, who had proclaimed that "God grants healing to the sick." However, Cooke also recognized the potential difficulties in addressing theotherapy. Though prayers for healing within his family had presumably gone unanswered, he countered that "the Lord will not willingly heal us if we do not YIELD OUR WILL absolutely to Him. Our body is the temple of the Holy Ghost. . . . The conclusion to which I am brought with respect to Divine healing is—'*God answers the prayers that He inspires.*' Truly we know not how to pray as we ought, till the Holy Spirit leads us."[63]

In time, however, the Army raised the funds necessary to assist Kagawa's regenerating power of the God of heaven. In 1912 the Army reported that the wait was over, and that the groundbreaking ceremony for medical work had "finally passed." Under the watchful eyes of Yamamuro Kieko, Gunpei's wife, and Dr. Matsuda Sanya, the Army's first doctor in Japan, the Army's Japanese medical mission began to take form. From the laying of the foundation to the appointment of staff, work proceeded rapidly. In addition, Matsuda had undertaken the establishment of a general hospital, a clinic for day laborers, and a "slum visitation team," which, in "giving medical aid to thousands of people living in crowded conditions, brought to light an alarming number of tuberculosis cases." Indeed, in the Army's publication's series on the quotidian activities of the Salvation Army Hospital for the Poor, the focus stayed consistently on "the horrifying tuberculosis and venereal diseases (*osorubeki kekkaku to karyūbyō*)."[64] Still, the vast numbers of tuberculosis' victims continued to shock many of the Army's oldest foreign soldiers in Japan. As Lieutenant Commissioner Charles Duce, one of the original band who sought to combat forced prostitution in the Yoshiwara, noted at the Army's International Social Council in 1921, "One would think that consumption ought not to exist in Japan, with its beautifully clear air and warm sunshine, with houses that open out to every breeze that blows, and with comparative absence of smoke." The misconception of contagion notwithstanding, Duce amended that "from my earliest experiences in that country, going back no[w] nearly a quarter of a century, I can remember how struck we all were at the large number of capable men in leading circles who were cut off before the age of forty by this dread disease." For this reason, Matsuda, a tireless advocate for Japan's stricken poor, who had given up a lucrative medical career that befitted

63. SAR: "Byōshitsu no beddo no ue de kanja no hi wo toritsu aru." *Toki no koe*. June 1, 1924; SAR: "Shippei to shinkō." *Toki no koe*. June 1, 1925. p. 5; NDL: Yamamuro Gunpei. *Byōjō no ian*. 1936. p. 46; SANA: "The Blessed Fact of Divine Healing." *The Field Officer of the Salvation Army*. Vol. 25, no. 10. Nov., 1917. p. 680.

64. SAR: "Kyūseigun byōin naru." *Toki no koe*. July 15, 1912. p. 4; SANA: "History of the Salvation Army Kiyose Hospital and Hospice." P. 2; SANA: "Conquering Tuberculosis in Japan." p. 1; SAR: "Kyūseigun byōin no jigyō." *Toki no koe*. July 15, 1914. p. 4; SAR: "Kyūseigun byōin no kangofuchō." *Toki no koe*. Aug. 1, 1912. p. 7; SANA: "Conquering Tuberculosis in Japan." p. 1; SAR: "Kyūseigun byōin no ichijitsu." *Toki no koe*. Apr. 15, 1913. p. 7.

his standing as a Tokyo Imperial University graduate, toiled to assist not only the nation's afflicted but also their peers who had stigmatized them:

> The Salvation Army opened its general Hospital for the poor in 1912, and the staff there soon found that about half the medical cases were sufferers from consumption. In order to deal with this a Consultation Bureau for consumptive patients was established at the Hospital in 1913, the first such Institution to be set up in Japan, although many have now followed the Army's example.

Duce elaborated on the duties of the Bureau thus:

> 1. The early detection of consumption.
> 2. Examining patients and supplying medicine.
> 3. Determining the most suitable means of treatment and of disinfection; advising with regard to the patient's marriage, the rearing of sickly children or babies, and the feeding of children in the natural way.
> 4. Facilitating entry into Hospital.
> 5. Advising in regard to the patient's chances with nursing or disinfecting.
> 6. Medical visitation of patients.
> 7. Rendering assistance in connection with nursing or disinfecting.
> 8. The distribution of comforts to the patients.
> 9. Leading patients to Salvation.
> 10. Assisting with funeral arrangements.
> 11. House-house medical visitation of consumptive patients in the slums.
> 12. Giving advice by correspondence.
> 13. Giving lectures on consumption and its treatment, when opportunities present.

That evangelization was not a high priority is a testament to Matsuda's commitment to his career, and is certainly not an indication of the intensity of Matsuda's faith.[65]

Though a trailblazer, Matsuda, too, was following examples of previous medical missions. As the Bureau for Social Work within the Home Department acknowledged in its outline of national social work for foreign audiences,

> The oldest medical relief agencies in Japan are "Dōaisha" and the Charity Hospital Estalished [*sic*] by a Frenchman, both of which were opened in the 12th year of Meiji (1879). Then come the Tokio Charity Hospital, the Japan Red Cross Hospital and St. Barnabas' Hospital in Osaka established by an American. These were all founded before the 20th year of Meiji (1887).[66]

They did not, however, act as sanatorium.

As the Army was aware, Japan was not without its religiously unaffiliated hospitals, but the majority of these, too, were private, and, in this case, expensive. More significant, sanatoria specifically for the tubercular continued shy of government

65. *Social Problems*, 207–11.

66. The *dōaisha* was founded by Takamatsu Ryōun, who, moved by the impartiality of the International Red Cross, treated casualties on both sides of the Battle of Hakodate. Though he would not establish the Japanese Red Cross, his association worked under the same principles (Miyazaki, 440).

responsibility. This was, of course, by design. Estimated at well over one million afflicted, and increasing each year by twenty to thirty thousand (as the Bureau for Social Work calculated based on the death rate), this was a rather foolish way to calculate an accurate portrait of the nation's tubercular. To begin with, tuberculosis can progress very slowly, so extrapolation from the mortality rate yields only a fraction of those afflicted or carrying the disease (where immunity is possible or the infection remains dormant). Perhaps more significant, however, many patients and their physicians were well aware of the stigma that still faced those condemned to a diagnosis of tuberculosis. Thus, to spare them the indignities and discrimination that accompanied such a diagnosis, many doctors, family members, and patients would euphemize the disease, describing it as any number of other less feared ailments. For these reasons, it is likely that far more people were afflicted than were enumerated. Regardless, the Home Department (to which the bureau belonged) periodically passed legislation to combat the disease, but often merely placed such work out of its hands and its budget. Beginning in 1904, the department issued an ordinance to prevent tuberculosis, and another ten years later to state the need to establish sanatoriums. Finally, the 1919 Tuberculosis Act was meant to convey the importance of prevention, but enactment was spotty, and fairly optional. By these acts, the Home Minister "may order in the cities which have a population of above 50,000 or if necessary, he may order any public body to establish a tubercular sanitorium." Nevertheless, only "one six [*sic*] to one half of the expenditures of the above sanitorium are met by the National Government." (Technically, by the department's legislation, the national government could provide no more than half of the public sanatorium's expenditures.) However, despite supposedly mandating the establishment of sanatoriums in at least nine cities throughout the archipelago, only five were scheduled for construction.[67] Nevertheless, the bureau was eager to count the Army's own hospitals, and those of other evangelical groups, among the resources that the government was providing.[68]

It was not a wholly one-sided exchange. While the government, as an entity, did not provide any funds for the public health work pursued by private interests (who acted in part to fill the lacuna in social work), it certainly saw no reason why individual members of the government should be discouraged from assisting. Indeed, for the moral entrepreneuring to continue, there needed to be an exchange of currency, in this case, qua legitimacy. And legitimacy was easily supplied by the government. Beginning in 1914, and continuing annually from 1918 until 1941, His Imperial Majesty, the emperor, provided a small sum in recognition of the Army's social work. Although the total of all grants was likely between thirty-five and forty thousand dollars, which covered very little of the organization's expenses (as Baggs

67. In 1920, Japan had forty-one cities with a population significantly over fifty thousand, fourteen of which had populations over one hundred thousand. This meant that, at best, in 1922 the Home Ministry had fulfilled slightly more than a tenth of the work it had legislated ("Dai 10 hyō" [First census, 10]).
68. Bureau for Social Work, 44–45, 48–50.

pointed out), the amount was unimportant. Rather, the prestige of being one of the few organizations granted the imperial commendation provided the Army with the cachet to merit its continued relationship with and legitimization by the government.[69] In part, too, cachet, legitimacy, and imperial recognition came from the Army's reliance on its native officers, not the least of whom were the Yamamuro family, Gunpei, Kieko, and their children, including Buho and Tamiko.[70] Few other foreign evangelical organizations were led primarily by autochthonous members. This also meant that those in harm's way were Japanese. From beatings by brothel keepers to death by disease, Japanese officers were, if not the leaders, then side by side with their foreign peers on the frontline of the Army's work. This, then, perhaps more than any prior work in the nation, ingratiated the Army to its self-appointed charges.

The growing reality of the sanatorium on the outskirts of Japan's capital, too, allowed the Army to experience an appreciation for its efforts on every level of society, from the slums to the Imperial Palace.[71] Certainly, the work was timely. Japan now faced a two-front war—one in China, which the government was eager to pursue, and another on the home front, in which (or perhaps because) the casualties far outnumbered those fighting abroad, the government was loath to involve itself directly.[72] Thus, although the bacillus Calmette-Guérin vaccine[73]—limited in effectiveness though it was—still had not been discovered, and streptomycin's isolation was another twenty years in the future, Matsuda's institution was still deemed a "necessity." If nothing else, his staff could control the spread of the disease through an effective quarantine, while still maintaining the humanity of his patients, allowing them to convalesce in a literally healthy environment.[74]

The beds filled quickly. Outside, no village or town with more than ten thousand people was free from the disease, and the region around Japan's major cities saw an exponential increase in the death rates. And, as Matsuda's patients flourished (or at least subsisted) under his care, the mere existence of the sanatorium, to say nothing of the Army's educational outreach based therein, proved an effective avenue for the organization's attempt to remedy the pernicious rumors and stigma

69. Baggs, 169–70.
70. SANA: "Who's Who." *The Salvation Army Year Book*, 1913, p. 101. That Yamamuro merited mention in the yearbook's short list of important figures a year before the (foreign) territorial commander, to whom Yamamuro was then second in command, indicates not only Yamamuro's vast influence and power but also the respect and position accorded Japanese officers of the Army.
71. SAR: "News of the War." *Toki no koe*. May 15, 1913, p. 8.
72. NDL: "Meiji 39nen yori Taishō 3nen ni itaru (=ōkyū kenen**unsure of reading: 住九ヶ年) jinkō goman ijō no shiku ni okeru shibō sen ni tai **對 suru kekkaku shibō hirei." *Kekkaku shibō tōkeihyō [dai 1satsu]: Meiji 38 shi Taishō 3nen*. p 29; Knibbs, 204.
73. An antituberculosis measure first used in humans as a vaccine in 1921.
74. Yamamoto and Yamamoto, 331; SAR: "Ryōyōjo setsuritsu no hitsuyō," *Toki no koe*, Feb. 11, 1916, p. 8; Pope, 329. Moreover, the establishment of the sanatorium on the outskirts of Tokyo provided the population with a far more accessible alternative to later medical establishments founded far from both urban centers and transportation.

surrounding the disease.[75] In addition, Matsuda founded various programs for his patients, including a school and a cooperative farm, as the disease, though pernicious, could be a slow one, and his convalescents had nothing but time.[76]

Matsuda's resourcefulness, and that of Yamamuro Kieko, Gunpei's wife, proved helpful to both the tubercular and the throne. The sanatorium had rapidly outgrown its modest beginnings, and required more wards, yet building materials proved expensive. To cover costs, Yamamuro Kieko had written to the emperor entreating him to provide some assistance. Following the death of the empress dowager, "as is the custom in Japan, a building was erected for her funeral." The lumber, owing to the role it had played in memorializing the empress, could not be put to any "ordinary use." Thus, rather than waste the wood, the emperor "agreed to donate the lumber to The Salvation Army," where it was "used as a Women's Ward of our new Sanatorium."[77] By donating, rather than discarding, the lumber from the empress' funeral, the emperor—and, by extension, his government—could claim a tangible stake in the Army's medical mission. They could also counter accusations of failing to serve a large portion of their subjects. In return, the Army, whose leaders had "long been impressed with the acute need there is in Japan for Sanatoriums for the treatment of tuberculosis," could claim pioneering status, since, despite there having been "large numbers of people [who] suffer from this scourge," previously, there was "no provision for indigent patients, the result [of which] is much suffering and an easy spread of the disease."[78]

Whereas the YMCA had long concluded that China was a more fertile ground for its efforts in general, the Army, due in part to its medical mission, had a bright future in Japan, and one worth emulating—not only in Asia, but throughout the globe. Although it acknowledged that "progress during the early years was comparatively slow," nevertheless, following Booth's audience with the Meiji emperor, the Army experienced such progress as to mark "a new epoch in Christian influence, and the Army has from that period made very noticeable advances, whilst the range of its influence continues to extend." With the establishment of "a fine Hospital," the Army's clout grew as it had "done excellent service under Dr. Matsuda, who is assisted by Captain (Dr.) Iwasa." Under their leadership, the Army's medical mission thrived:

> The latest yearly figures to hand give 4,202 out-patients, with 17,805 return attendances; while Dispensaries give another 6,490.

75. SAR: "Ryōyōjo setsuritsu no hitsuyō." *Toki no koe*. Feb. 11, 1916. p. 8; SAR: "Haibyō chi**illegible kingenshū (**written as shifu)." *Toki no koe*. Feb. 11, 1916. p. 4.
76. The farm also proved a source of income, and also outlasted the sanatorium, as it is still in working order today. SAR: "Ryōyōjo ha gakkōchi." *Toki no koe*. Dec. 15, 1916. p. 3.
77. SANA: "History of the Salvation Army Kiyose Hospital and Hospice." p. 1; SANA: "Salvation Doctors." *The Salvation Army Year Book*. 1915. p. 28.
78. SANA: "Some Features of the Year's Work." *The Salvation Army Year Book*. 1917. p. 7.

> A splendid work is also in progress at the William Booth Memorial Sanatorium for poor tuberculosis patients; indeed, so great is the need that the Government last year contributed £1,160 for the erection of an additional wing.
>
> We look forward to a great extension of this kind of Medical work in Japan, and hope that presently Chosen [Korea], and China, too, may have similar Institutions for the helping of the people and the strengthening and further spreading of the blessed message and ministrations of the One Salvation Army.[79]

More significant, by utilizing the Booth Memorial Sanatorium as both an institution and a symbol, a hospital for the sick and a beacon of successful Army work, Japan's Salvation Army had become a model not merely for other East Asian branches, and not alone for medical missionary work, but for the world's Armies and for the importance of social relief in general. Colonel and auditor general of the Army's East Asian work, Arthur Bates, in lauding the accomplishments of Japan's Army, posed a rhetorical call to arms to its counterparts worldwide, questioning, "Are all the wise people to be found in the East/ [*sic*] Surely among Western nations should be found sufficient consecrated intelligences to meet the needs, not only of their own countries, but of the world."[80]

Nevertheless, as an institution, the Sanatorium could not cure the disease. It could offer palliative care in a peaceful, tolerant environment; it could effectively quarantine the contagious patients from spreading the disease further; and it could offer hope to individuals and to society, but there was still no "silver bullet" for tuberculosis. As much as its members preached divine healing, the supposed variables involved (i.e., the faith of the invalid and the earnestness of the prayer), to say nothing of the ontological issues of a deity to perform or facilitate such therapy, it was difficult to assure patients of the inevitability of healing within the institution. Rates of conversion among patients are unclear, but medical missionary work in general, and work without a tangible result specifically, were hardly saving the masses, physically or spiritually. Without converts, the Army's coffers in Japan were in want of funds. Much of the work was funded or was meant to be funded by cartridges, which were defined in the first issue of *The Salvation Army Year Book* as "an envelope in which is placed the weekly contributions of Soldiers and Recruits, and, in some cases, friends. It is independent of collection monies, and is relied upon to furnish as much as possible of the incidental expenses of the War." By increasing the number of converts, therefore, the Army could, ostensibly, increase its funding, creating a very real need for evangelization beyond the work of merely spreading the gospel. For Ensign Matsunaga of Okayama, the aim was clear and the combination of financial gain from spiritual enlightenment was not at all contradictory:

79. Xing, 44; SANA: "Japan." *The Salvation Army Year Book*. 1919. p. 57; SANA: "Salvation Army Medical Enterprises." *The Salvation Army Year Book*. 1919. p. 33.
80. SANA: "Some Thoughts on Exactitude—Spiritual, Mental, and Material: II.—Mental Exactitude." *The Field Officer of the Salvation Army*. Vol. 23, no. 1. Jan., 1915. p. 29.

> *The Soldiers must have the real fighting spirit.* Soul-saving must be first and foremost. This must come before anything and everything else.
>
> We must get our Converts so thoroughly saved that from gratitude to God and The Salvation Army they cannot help but pay their Cartridge. . . .
>
> No one should be omitted from the paying of Cartridges; it is not only the duty, but the privilege of every Salvationist.
>
> We must exercise care and discrimination in letting the Convert, Recruit or Soldier commence to pay a small amount, and increase it gradually, remembering that each comrade has his own peculiar circumstances and needs. Try to clearly understand the circumstances and means of each, and show full appreciation of what each pays, whether small or large. This is the way to encourage them to pay more.[81]

Matsunaga's explanation was comfortingly simplistic, though in reality it was difficult to balance both the perceived successes of Japan's Army and its call for funds. There was always a fine line between trumpeting victories and persuading donors that the organization was desperately in need of funds. With their marketing attempts, the YMCA in Japan rarely managed to garner such money from its international headquarters, let alone from average citizens, contrasting somewhat to the Army. Ironically, the tragedy of the Great Kantō earthquake managed to bring both funds and attention to the Army's plight, even in the midst of the plight of all the residents of Japan's most populous region.

Clearly, the Army did enjoy both monetary and evangelistic devotion among its soldiers, including those on the frontline of the war against tuberculosis. Nevertheless, the main aim of the Army was not to conquer an incurable disease, despite the efforts of Dr. Matsuda and his assistant, Dr. Iwasa, and their staff. Certainly, under their care, not only did the sanatorium expand but a second one opened across the city.[82] But salvation of the soul still trumped the health of the body, and to a large extent, the former transcended monetary concerns. Practically, however, budgets proved the limiting agent when conversion rates were low and tuberculosis lacked curative treatments.

With two sanatoriums to its name by the end of the Taishō period, the Army certainly had more to show for its medical missionary efforts in combating tuberculosis in Japan than the YMCA. But both organizations discovered that they were limited by the bounds of the "moral enterprise" in which each was embroiled, both between each other and between each and the Japanese government, constantly maneuvering to maintain the appearance of holding the moral high ground while not angering its partner in the enterprise. This negotiation of appearances was rarely one in which the majority of the Japanese populace had much influence, save for the possibility of conversion. Nevertheless, the Japanese people could affect the overall

81. SANA: "Cartridge." *The Salvation Army Year Book*. 1906. p. 54; SANA: "How to Increase the Cartridge." By Ensign Matsunaga, Okayama, Japan. Trans. Lieut.-Col Pugmire, chief secretary for Japan. Vol. 44, no. 6. June 1927. pp. 519–20. Emphasis in original.
82. SANA: "Conquering Tuberculosis in Japan," p. 2.

success of each organization, even without converting, by appearing to accept the assistance, and thus offering themselves as "Pseudo-Christians." The evangelists and, to a lesser extent, the government were still dependent on the population's acceptance of assistance or rule. Where the government had a far greater capacity for ignoring the will of the people (and, indeed, the force to crush it, if necessary), the evangelists had to tread carefully. Perhaps, as Sendai evangelist and linguist Christopher Noss noted, "The missionaries in Japan have had a very hard time and have been much misunderstood by those working in China and other lands where conditions are different," for here, as the adage went, "if you want to have any authority among the Japanese make up your mind not to claim any. If you insist on having authority, you may have it, but you will have nothing else."[83] To claim to have the key to salvation was undoubtedly to suggest a form of authority, but at least the Salvation Army believed that it could also employ its medical missionary work to counteract any potentially negative consequences of this implicit insistence on authority. But this meant that, in a sense, the victims of tuberculosis often became basically currency—a focal point of these organizational relationships, essentially figurative coin of the realm between moral entrepreneurs and a way for the Army to gain the support of Japan's healthy population while still maintaining a semblance of moral authority. In this way, both the epidemic and those within the religious community who sought to end it consumed the tubercular.

83. Noss, 246–47.

8

"The Great Gulf Fixed"

Rudolf Teusler and William Vories

Not every foreign evangelist in Japan remained under both the auspices and the control of a larger umbrella organization like the YMCA or the Salvation Army. Yet the men of this small group, and they were invariably male, were not simply itinerant Christians. Where Christians like Uchimura and Kagawa forged their own spiritual paths from the start, not all of their foreign counterparts remained members of the Protestant denomination to which they originally subscribed. Because they were not beholden to organizations like the YMCA and the Salvation Army, the foreign evangelists who forged ahead independently had greater freedom to perform missionary work as they saw fit and in ways that worked with their own talents and strengths. Thus, where such organizations sought to balance evangelizing Japan with monetary solvency, men like Dr. Rudolf Teusler and William Vories concentrated on what the contemporary Presiding Bishop of the Episcopal Church in the United States and Doctor of Divinity, Henry St. George Tucker deemed "not simply to make all the nations of the world Christian, but also so to Christianize their relations one with another that the peoples of the world may become a brotherhood."[1]

Both Teusler and Vories, though from different backgrounds, denominations, and professions, dedicated themselves to pursuing their goal of international Christian brotherhood through the medical missionary track. Joseph C. Grew, America's ambassador to Japan at the opening of the second Sino-Japanese War, lauded the role of medicine not only in the evangelist's arsenal but also as the embodiment of Christian understanding and values, maintaining that "the departures and developments in science, not only in matters of communication and transit but in a thousand other ways apart from the machinery of war, will constantly and progressively tend to destroy the barriers which today separate the human family." Grew continued:

> And of all the factors of science which must inevitably and increasingly exert their influence in that direction, none can exceed the science of medicine. For medicine best exemplifies the fundamental principles of Christianity: it knows no nationality, no politics, no social boundaries; is unconfined by religious sect or creed. The

1. H. Tucker, xii.

> spirit of the Good Samaritan is increasingly alive today, exerting its healing influence, rising above prejudice or partisanship or dogma; soothing, blending, uniting in our strife-ridden world.[2]

From here, it behooves us to examine each man's contribution to tuberculosis combat individually, though both sought to fulfill their mission as Grew defined it.

Rudolf Bolling Teusler

Medicine may have known no sect or creed, but that certainly never caused Teusler to question his decision to pursue it. Rudolf Bolling Teusler, a postbellum southerner of German descent who earned his medical doctorate before his twenty-first birthday, studied the boundlessness of medicine at a time when it seemed to become comprehensible and comprehensive. As averred by the so-called "father of modern medicine," Dr. William Osler, theirs was a medicine that finally "simplified the abstruse and complicated knowledge of the chemical laboratories, . . . and presented it in a form readily assimilable by the men who have to use it." One of Teusler's classmates and friends, Dr. Charles B. Robins, recalled that "the period when Dr. Teusler and I were at the Medical College of Virginia was somewhat a period of metamorphosis in medicine . . . so that Dr. Teusler's medical birth was about at the dawn of modern medicine."[3]

Though he had a bright future in Virginia and perceived medicine transcending nations Teusler saw fit to pursue his practice in Japan, where he believed that he could heal the body and the soul. From the turn of the twentieth century until his death, thirty-four years later, Teusler, as eulogized by Dr. John W. Wood, secretary of foreign missions for the Episcopal Church,

> Worked as a Christian physician to erect barriers against disease, to heal the sick, serve the under-privileged, and to cooperate with his Japanese friends in the application of modern medicine to Japan's physical ills, though the creation of adequate medical facilities to serve the individual and the community along well tested lines.[4]

Although he was unaffiliated with the larger Christian evangelical organizations like the YMCA and the Salvation Army and ostensibly worked under the broad auspices of the Episcopal Church of America, Teusler drew on the resources of other missions and, without apology or excuses, pursued relations with Japanese physicians who were unrelated to either foreign evangelical or native Christian

2. Lyon, 53; Grew, ix.
3. Osler, xxix; Robbins and MacNaught, 11. Teusler was actually the cousin of Edith Bolling Galt Wilson, the wife of Woodrow Wilson. Unfortunately, the family tie does not appear to have assisted Teusler in his work, save for a handful of lunch invitations. Nor, it turns out, did the rest of his ancestry, which was purported to have included Pocahontas and the Plantagenets ("Obituary," 496).
4. Nakamura, 6; SSC, 1.

groups. Upon his arrival in Tokyo, Teusler was housed by the Methodist Mission and contacted "several prominent physicians—Dr. Kitazato—Dr Sezuki (inspector general of the Navy) Dr Tegami and others." Though he acknowledged to the home office that these physicians were "non believers and one, I know, a professed Buddist, [*sic*]" he enjoyed their "jenuine [*sic*] interest in the plans for opening the hospital and dispensary" and offers of assistance, and felt no need to pretend that these relationships would offer any new converts.[5]

To the home office it soon became obvious that Teusler, though himself a devout Christian and a promising evangelist, was dedicated above all else to his hospital. St. Luke's Hospital existed before Teusler's arrival, but it was Teusler with whom it became synonymous. The Tsukiji Hospital, as it was known previously, despite fairly auspicious beginnings in 1874 as the first institution to introduce Lister's antiseptic system, had since been the victim of repeated unsuccessful attempts at establishing a medical mission, only to be abandoned as a failure. To the head of the Episcopal Church, Bishop McKim, "it seemed to bear a very bad reflection indeed on the work not only of the American Church Mission, but of the American Church at home."[6] Thus, it behooved McKim to allow Teusler his dedication. If nothing else, he could hardly make it worse.

Nevertheless, McKim cautioned Teusler against rushing into a revival of the hospital, a condition to which Teusler, perhaps uncharacteristically agreed, and justified as the opportunity to learn Japanese as well as to continue his relationships with Japanese physicians and his survey of the state of medicine in the relatively recent nation. Like Tsukiji, the facilities he found in Japan were "rather inadequately filled up and run in a ship shod [*sic*] manner, with a poor regard for cleanliness," despite over fifty years of both private and state-funded medical education and practice. Nevertheless, his Japanese counterparts proved eager to welcome a presumably well-funded doctor and, as Teusler was pleased to report, had "promised to send me patients."[7]

As it turned out, Teusler never needed to plead with other physicians to advertise his services. Within his first four months in Japan, despite agreeing to wait a year to open St. Luke's and its associated dispensaries, Teusler reported having received 221 patients, including many in June due to an epidemic of tonsillitis. While it is unclear if these men and women were sent by Japanese medical professionals or came by virtue of their own discovery and of their own volition (not to mention whether these men and women themselves were Japanese), it seemed clear to Teusler that the hospital was not merely an evangelical niche but a medical necessity. Thus, it was hardly surprising that Japanese physicians proved eager to welcome Teusler,

5. AEC: "Letter to Mr. John Wood." Mar. 11, 1900.
6. Whitney, 347; Robbins and MacNaught, 29. Dr. Henry Faulds, the first doctor at the Tsukiji Hospital, and the last successful one before the arrival of Teusler, was also notable as the man who introduced fingerprinting as a form of identification to Japan, if not the world (Herschel, 77).
7. AEC: "Letter to Rev. Arthur S. Lloyd." June 30, 1900; Whitney, 347.

his education, and, perhaps most importantly, his equipment. Teusler brought his surgical tools with him, as well as $150 of the Episcopal Church board's money, in addition to $300 from his own savings, which he planned to employ in "fitting out the two dispensaries and hospital" he had planned. It was in surgery and prescriptions that Teusler envisioned the funds for the work, and even before opening the hospital, he had performed "a few minor surgical operations," and founded two dispensaries around the city. He believed these measures would "make the work self supporting" in time.[8]

With the official opening of St. Luke's on February 12, 1901, Teusler's belief proved prescient:

> There is a fixed schedule of charges for treatment and medicine, and only in cases of direct poverty are these entirely remitted, therefore, although frequently medicine is dispensed at or below costs, of absolute charity we have very little. As there was no regular foreign drug store in Tokyo and our stock of drugs very good, I decided to keep open the drug department of the dispensary as a regular pharmacy, hoping in this way to hasten the time when the hospital can be self supporting. This has proven quite satisfactory.

In less than six months, nearly three hundred patients filled over 1,500 prescriptions.[9]

Teusler's promise of a hospital—if not well-stocked, then certainly partially stocked—and the prospect of a paycheck attracted the attention of some of Japan's finest physicians:

> Dr. J. H. Macdonald, the oldest and last known general practicioner [*sic*] in Tokyo, kindly consented to be consulting physician to the Det. Of Practice, and Dr. Whitney, the foreign occulist [*sic*] here, gives his services as consultant to the Dept of the Eye and Ear. I engaged as assistants two Japanese physicians, Dr Kawase, a graduate of the Boston University Medical School, and a member of the English Church, and Dr. Inakita [?], also a Christian, and for seven years Resident physician to Dr. Whitney's Hospital. To both of these men a very economical salary is paid as they were anxious to connect themselves with a foreign general hospital.[10]

That physicians would want to align themselves with a foreign and previously poorly performing hospital might have seemed odd. Why, after all, would anyone willingly throw in his/her lot with an untested and, more importantly, private, hospital? Yet, as the vicissitudes of politics had made evident, there was little security in a governmental or government-funded position. The continual changing of the guard effected both foreign and Japanese physicians, but foreign physicians were also subject to dismissal paradoxically for having effectively performed their work. Initially invited as consultants and educators, the physicians who had previously filled

8. The Spirit of Missions, 1; AEC: "Letter to Rev. Arthur S. Lloyd." June 30, 1900.
9. AEC: "Report of Rudolf B. Teusler, M.D./Residence Tokyo, for the year ending June 30–1901." July 1, 1901.
10. Ibid.

the upper echelons of their field in Japan were being supplanted by their Japanese students. By the turn of the twentieth century, one correspondent to the American Medical Association noted, though Germans had, decades earlier, comprised the entire medical department of the Imperial University, among the current "medical faculty composed of twenty professors, all the Germans but two, viz., Prof. Erwin Baelz and Prof. Julius Scriba, have been weeded out." Although fairly well regarded in Japan, Scriba lacked the clout of Baelz, both in Japan and among the foreign community. Indeed, the author of the dispatch to the AMA dismissed Scriba's medical prowess, belittling his "technic" as "not what one would have expected from a German as far as cleanliness and antisepsis are concerned," and noting dismissively that Scriba "uses chloroform exclusively as an anesthetic," when ether was evidently preferable. He then denounced Scriba's practice of keeping patients "upright when operating on the face and head, because this position, he says, lessens the tendency to hemorrhage, never hinting at the fact that such a position immensely increases the danger of the patient's dying from the effects of the chloroform."[11]

Regardless of his ignorance of anesthesia, Scriba was savvy enough to situate himself successfully in Japanese medicine at the turn of the century. To Teusler's delight (and, more important, that of the Episcopal Church of America), Scriba required a new opportunity, since he soon fell victim to the government downsizing. For the last few years of his life, Scriba, "the most eminent surgeon in Japan," agreed to send his patients to St. Luke's, "operating on them there, and all fees go to the hospital except his own personal charges to patient. He gives his services as Consulting and Operating Surgeon to the dispensary clinic and the fees for this go to the hospital also." Both his presence and his funds, as well as those of Canadian Methodist Dr. Davidson Macdonald, promised the burgeoning hospital "the confidence of the public, Japanese and foreign."[12]

Scriba's exit from public life was actually somewhat controversial, as it remains unclear whether it was volitional. Contemporary sources maintained that he retired from his position as chair of surgery at the university, either of his own accord or at the request of the government. Teusler's biographers, the Reverends Howard Robbins and George MacNaught, insisted that the sheer strength of Teusler's invitation was enough to wrench Scriba from his comfortable position with the Japanese government. They reported that presiding bishop of the Evangelical Church and then president of St. Paul's College in Tokyo Henry St. George Tucker proclaimed that "the greatest stroke Dr. Teusler ever made was when he got Dr. Scriba as head of the surgical service at St. Luke's. He had a tremendous reputation in Japan, and that was one of the most effective ways to bring St. Luke's to both the foreign and Japanese attention." Teusler himself used his good fortune to request more funds from the church board, pointing out that "Dr Screiber [*sic*] has steadily refused

11. "Medicine," 1238.
12. Nakamura, 17–18; AEC: "An Appeal for St. Luke's Hospital, Tokyo." R. B. Teusler, MD. July 3, 1902. p. 2.

several offers to become consulting surgeon to different hospitals stating to me and others that if possible he wishes all of his work done at St. Luke's."[13]

Scriba's work at the hospital would continue until his death in 1905 and, though Teusler managed a coup of sorts by engaging the talents of Baelz as a consultant, Baelz would provide prestige, but Scriba provided work and funds, as an actual member of St. Luke's. While the AMA might deride Scriba, while praising Baelz as "a fine teacher of clinical medicine and, as a general practitioner, . . . at the head of his profession in Japan," whose success was guaranteed since he served as physician to the imperial family, Scriba remained the more appealing to Teusler. Despite the three decades between them, the two proved good friends. Not only were both avid sportsmen, but, as physicians, both were under no illusions as to the threat of tuberculosis to Japan, despite the fact, as Teusler lamented, that "under the present Law of Japan, the physician is not even allowed to place a patient suffering from one of these (highly infectious) diseases in the buildings (Densenbyo) reserved and designated by law for the segregation and treatment of infectious diseases." Thus, Teusler confirmed, "it is a fact beyond dispute that the hiatus here in Japan, between Research Medicine as such, and its application to the general public, is the crux of the whole situation." Tuberculosis was a scourge, but it was a scourge that required at least acknowledgment. In Scriba, therefore, Teusler recognized a kindred spirit. Certainly, Scriba was derided for almost immediately throwing his lot in with tuberculin which, as noted previously, was ineffective. Scriba failed to note any bacteriological indication for his conclusion, while Baelz once again received the higher praise for his more circumspect findings on tuberculin. Nonetheless, Scriba's optimism meant that he, too, recognized the importance of work on the disease.[14]

Yet no renown, knowledge, or optimism would matter if Teusler's institution deviated from its intended purpose—namely, "to make the hospital to them (the patients) a practical application of Christian Charity . . . to make the teaching of Christianity the prime reason for the existence of the hospital." As long as Scriba was able to work in a well-furnished hospital, the doctor, though not an evangelist himself, was not averse to St. Luke's mission, a fact that Teusler touted both as a beneficial attribute of his physician and as a testament to the necessity of funds to continue advancing the condition of the hospital. For Scriba, therefore, the facts that, within mere months of working at St. Luke's, "already his patients are crowding to him," and that the hospital needed to "be enlarged so as to accommodate from 80 to 10[0] patients," were far more significant than the importance of both its medical and moral mission. According to Teusler, "Dr. Scriber [*sic*] . . . understands thoroughly that the primal reason for the existance [*sic*] of St. Luke's Hospital is that it . . . teach and bring home to the Japanese Christianity, and he in every way feels

13. Bowers, 126; Robbins and MacNaught, 71–72; AEC: Teusler to Lloyd, July 3, 1902.
14. "Medicine of the Far East," 1238; Fukuda 2008, 59; Teusler, 205, 207; Johnston, 204.

his aid to this end and has shown interest in the work from this standpoint," so long as he received his "new addition to the hospital."[15]

Scriba, as it turned out, would have little time to appreciate the addition, since the renowned physician would die of tuberculosis in the opening days of 1905, at the age of fifty-six.[16] Nevertheless, the fact that Teusler (and his supporters in the Evangelical Church) had been eager to employ and assist such a man, even if only for a short time, was indicative of a willingness not necessarily to ignore the hospital's stated mission, but to view the achievement of this mission as more important than any of its components in isolation. If Scriba, whose religious beliefs and affiliation, though Christian, remained largely unknown, was nevertheless established as a key figure in the hospital, there was a clear, albeit tacit, acknowledgement that the medical acumen of the staff was at least as important as their moral leanings in attaining the goal of enlightening Japan's infirmed. While other medical missions tried to maintain a strict denominational bent or clear control within an affiliation, Teusler would continue to employ physicians who, while by no means hostile to his sect, the American Evangelical Church, did not necessarily wholly identify themselves with his denomination or beliefs. Certainly, though the vast majority (if not the entirety) of Teusler's staff was Christian and, of course, evangelical, they did not need to be Evangelical.

This awareness of the importance of personnel ability, rather than belief, was new and would prove both increasingly useful and economical. Where organizations had required adherence to principles— the Salvation Army more so than the YMCA—Teusler (and, as we shall discover later in this chapter, William Merrell Vories) was free to embrace practitioners outside his denomination. With his employment of and partnership with Dr. Scriba, Teusler had determined that, under his guidance, the institution would remain on the correct evangelical path, even if the denomination of his staff deviated slightly. Through this justification, Teusler would prove able to embrace the assistance of Japanese medical professionals in a way that even the nondenominational organizations could not. Where native Christians had joined the ranks of foreign evangelical organizations, some even reaching the upper echelons of domestic leadership, few were able to occupy similarly responsible positions within the medical missions without the direct oversight of a foreign counterpart, and certainly not so soon after the beginning of the group's work.

Nevertheless, the transition was far from smooth even within St. Luke's. Like so many of his counterparts in other missions, Teusler had feared that, without foreign leadership, Japan's physicians, like its Christians, would be unable to cope, let alone work successfully. Upon learning of Scriba's death, Teusler wrote a hasty letter to

15. AEC: Report of Rudolf B. Teusler, M.D./Residence Tokyo, for the year ending June 30—1901. To the Rt. Rev. John McKim. July 1, 1901; AEC: Letter from Lloyd to Bishop McKim. July 3, 1902; AEC: Letter to Wood from Teusler. Oct. 17, 1902.

16. Bowers, 127.

Dr. John Wood, secretary of the Board of Missions, to inform him that "as there is no other foreign doctor in charge . . . things will be largely at a standstill." It had been a sentiment shared by the Evangelical board as well. When Teusler had first acquired the services of Scriba, the latter had recommended two Japanese physicians who might prove useful to St. Luke's work, both medically and morally. It remains unclear whether the board embraced these physicians, though the Tokyo bishop certainly seemed dismissive, referring to them as "practitioners," whose names he was unable to recall.[17]

Despite his assurances to the contrary, like so many earlier foreign evangelists, the religion Teusler hoped to spread through his work was not Christianity in general, but that of his own sect, the American Evangelical Church. Thus, after Scriba's death, Teusler continued to press to expand St. Luke's, and even hoped to do so at the cost of the native congregation adjacent to the hospital's land. These Japanese religionists, all of whom identified themselves as Christian, were considered by Teusler to be interlopers in his appointed mission and, thus, false Christians, as he believed that they failed to consider moving their church for Teusler's good. While Teusler urged his home board to grant them sufficient funds to move their place of worship, he lambasted both sides for detaining his work. Although he tried to reach some reasonable compromise, he viewed the neighboring congregants as having had "no legal claim to the land" and he decried the home board for its intention to "have no connection with the matter, beyond paying the money at a specific time." Teusler railed against his Japanese coreligionists, accusing them and their fellow Japanese subjects, regardless of religion, of continuous "business methods [that] are not honest," and demanded that St. Luke's require "a clear title to the land and the Church off the property." It is hardly surprisingly, therefore, that, as much as American Evangelism, Teusler's was a religion of pragmatism. He would freely work with those whose belief in the numinous differed from his, so long as their professional skills were up to par, but he had no time for anyone, Christian or not, whom he saw as hindering his immediate progress.[18]

The relationship between Teusler and the Japanese, including native Christians, might seem complicated, but was evidence of Teusler's pragmatism. Though willing to work with Japanese as equals, he knew that, in order for St. Luke's to prove viable as both hospital and herald, the institution needed to appear not merely novel but necessary. Tokyo hardly offered a dearth of medical options by the turn of the century—among those noted by Teusler were "a great many small hospitals, run by individual doctors, which are poorly equipped and indifferently conducted." So, too, were there "a few large institutions, notably the University and Red Cross hospitals which are doing a good work and are rapidly becoming well appointed." Of course, for a population rapidly approaching three million, there was still room, Teusler

17. Robbins & MacNaught, 64; AEC: Letter to Wood. Jan. 5, 1905; AEC: Letter from Lloyd to Bishop (McKim). July 3, 1902.
18. AEC: Letter to Wood. June 8, 1905; AEC: Private Letter to Wood. Aug. 11, 1906.

believed, for a hospital like St. Luke's, so long as such a "young foreign hospital must do excellant [*sic*] work to win the confidence of the people and show itself well equipped and enterprising if it really proposes to become a permanent institution, commanding the patronage of all classes." Pragmatically, therefore, "it is not enough that a foreign hospital give them as good as they can get else where, from their own native physicians, but we must give them better, or the people as a whole will not patronize the work." And patronization by the people as a whole was necessary to make the institution self-supporting, the practical goal of evangelical work that supplemented and supported the spiritual goal. Teusler's greatest fear concerning his work in Japan was that St. Luke's would be unable to "justly claim to be superior to those around it." In such a situation, "in place of increasing its usefulness as an adjunct to the work of the Church, it will drag out a few years as a petty dispensary, reaching only some of the poorest classes and depend entirely for its support on the Church at home, finaly [*sic*] to come to an untimely end and die in obscurity."[19]

To combat any slow decline into obscurity, Teusler employed, at least as consultants, the Japanese physicians and surgeons who replaced foreign medical professors like Scriba and Baelz. They included Aoyama Tanemichi, Kitasato's supposed rival, and Satō Sankichi, who would later amputate Ōkuma Shigenobu's injured leg. In addition to Japanese practictioners, Teusler continued to court newly arrived foreign physicians, extending "to both of them the privilege of putting their patients in St. Luke's when in need of hospital accommodation." Though presumably the foreign unnamed physicians were Christian, of the Japanese physicians Teusler employed or with whom he advertised his consultation, only Aoyama "had a strong affinity for Christianity." More significantly, both Aoyama and Satō, had significant (though unbeknownst to Teusler) connections to Ōkuma. Satō's is obvious: having amputated the politician's shattered leg, he had kept the assassination attempt from being successful. Baelz, who witnessed the aftermath, noted that the leg of the then minister of foreign affairs, resembled little more than a "bag of pebbles," and, with Satō's immediate removal of the limb, Ōkuma owed his life to the surgeon.[20] Yet Aoyama, too, enjoyed a favorable relationship with the politician. Although it seems doubtful that his machinations ensured that Kitasato's institute would be transferred to government control under Tokyo University, Aoyama had been a close friend of Ōkuma for many years before the former's association with St. Luke's and the latter's transfer of the institute.[21] St. Luke's ties to such a powerful politician, even through intermediaries, secured the medical mission early attention from Japan's government. Thus, as with other such hospitals, Teusler had been quick to offer the institution to the Meiji war effort during the year's conflict between Russia and Japan.

19. AEC: "A Tokyo Hospital—Being some description of our Medical Mission Work in Japan's Capital: Its growth and development during the past three years." Rudolf Bolling Teusler, MD. p. 1.
20. Bowers, 128; AEC: "St. Luke's Hospital Report: From June 31st, 1904 to July 1st, 1905." Aug. 10, 1905. From Teusler to McKim. p. 3; Mitamura, 165; Bartholomew 2011, 52; Baelz, 92; Bowers, 128.
21. Bartholomew 1989, 184, 203.

For this, he was happy to receive the acknowledgement and gratitude of General Terauchi Masatake, the minister of war, who had also utilized the YMCA's offer to provide army social work during the same campaign.[22]

Nevertheless, even as he built these professional relationships, Teusler still required outside support for his existence and had to sell his business plan primarily to American investors and philanthropists, few of whom cared about the physical health of a nation so far from their own:

> It may be asked why then try to establish Mission hospitals in Japan at all, and the answer to this lies in the counter question:—Do you believe that we as Christians have a responsability [*sic*] to give to the Japanese Nation Christianity? Is it incumbent upon us as consistent members of the Church and followers of Christ, to support both with our prayers and means Missionary effort amongst these people? If your answer is Yes, then to you the reason for maintaining the furthering Mission Medical work in Japan should become at once clear; for in this we have one of the most, if not the most, efficient means of reaching the people, winning their confidence and leading them to Christ.

Yet Teusler was a pragmatist, as well as a true believer, which permitted him a deft hand as a moral entrepreneur, and continued thus:

> There is also an answer from the business standpoint:—St. Luke's has fully demonstrated after three years of work, by actual results obtained, that if a Mission hospital is properly equipped and run in Tokyo, it at once becomes much more than self-supporting. Our Church therefore can, by meeting the present demand for extension, establish an institution which will adequately exemplify the philanthropical and charitable side of Christian Missions, and that at no cost, so far as running expenses are concerned, to the Church at home. From the time of Christ until today, preaching the Gospel and tending the sick and suffering have gone hand in hand, and because for Mission Medical work to succeed in Japan there are certain conditions required, shall we hesitate or doubt its need. If the opportunity now ours in Tokyo is taken full advantage of, we can establish at once and pay its own way from the start. If the opening is allowed to pass it will be very difficult if not impossible for us, because of our inadequate size and equipment, to hold the position we have won.
>
> There still remains to be considered our duty to the native Christians to establish a Church hospital, and the service which the work is daily rendering the large body of Mission workers and other foreigners in Japan. Affording them a hospital near at hand in time of sickness and need, instead of, as has been the case several times already, their having to take long and expensive trips to America in search of treatment at the hands of foreign physicians in foreign institutions. St. Luke's is the only Mission hospital in the whole of the Tokyo Diocese and our doors are open to all, rich or poor, Christian or heathen, irrespective of creed or belief.[23]

22. Robbins and MacNaught, 50; Davidann, 112.
23. AEC: "A Tokyo Hospital—Being some description of our Medical Mission Work in Japan's Capital: Its growth and development during the past three years." Teusler, 1–2.

The hospital depended upon foreign funds, both from America and from foreign dignitaries and missionaries residing in Japan. Thus, Teusler continuously pointed out the merits of maintaining a "well-appointed hospital" at exactly St. Luke's location to render medical assistance to "our own Missionaries and the large body of foreigners in the East," noting that "Tokyo offers a better climates [*sic*] for hospital and surgical work than the cities further south and in China and the Philippines."[24]

But the evangelist doctor feared that all his connections would come to naught economically in the face of what he deemed the lack of philanthropy in Japan. After all, he noted, there was "no board of well-to-do men in Japan who without compensation give their time, money and best endeavors to build up this or that hospital or institution for the general good." Moreover, "when a rich Japanese dies he does not leave his money to charity. . . . Endowment funds are unknown. . . . Charity in Japan begins at home, and up to the present has remained there. A man helps his relatives but goes no further."[25] Yet the institution had, according to Teusler, also served to assist "several members of the Japanese nobility, and men of the highest influence, both in the army and civic life."[26] It was, therefore, his hope that these Japanese notables would ensure that the hospital could not only become self-supporting, but could become truly charitable—assisting those subjects who, up to now, having "little or no money and limited judgement," were forced to visit "Machi Isha," or street doctors, who "have only a very limited medical education and practically no equipment or resources," and whose treatment proves "thoroughly inefficient and in case after case which has come under our observation, the time thus lost has proven the cause of the death of the patent [*sic*]."[27] At the mercy of quacks and chicaners, the vast majority of Japan's ill threatened the health of the nation, both figuratively and literally. With a disease as virulent as tuberculosis, Teusler, who had secretly faced "the possibility of a tubercular infection," and had returned to America to recuperate in 1907, knew that, still without a cure, immediate isolation could save hundreds. However, even as he obtained funds to enlarge his hospital, Teusler still lacked the staff necessary to ensure compliance. To this end, the doctor turned his eye toward the creation of a nursing school for the purposes of supplying the hospital with a constant curative presence, and one that would teach its students to be "comforted in mind as well as body" through knowledge of "the great Physician of Souls."[28] In addition, he requested an assistant, who would be not only a doctor but a Christian and who, Teusler believed, would be "a special kind of man . . . somewhat difficult to find." While the nurses, both the students and their teachers, could be Japanese and, of course, female, Teusler's assistant could not. Although

24. AEC: "A statement of the needs of St. Luke's Hospital, Tokyo." R. B. Teusler, MD. Tokyo, Apr. 2, 1907. p. 4.
25. Robbins and MacNaught, 61–62.
26. CUB: "A church in the capital of Japan: Being some account of the successful work of St. Luke's Hospital in the city of Tokyo." Rudolf Bolling Teusler. *The Spirit of Missions*. Dec. 1904. p. 2.
27. AEC: "A statement of the needs of St. Luke's Hospital, Tokyo." R. B. Teusler, MD. Tokyo, Apr. 2, 1907. p. 2.
28. Robbins & MacNaught, 57; AEC: Letter from McKim to Rev. H. R. Hulse in New York City. Apr. 6, 1907.

he claimed that this bias was not his own, but was strictly a necessity when dealing with Teusler's foreign-born patients, Bishop McKim had noted that the American Evangelical Church had had poor luck when permitting Japanese subjects in "positions of responsibility," as "one of our prominent Japanese Christians, a physician of some years standing and a graduate of the Medical College of the Imperial University" had been made interim superintendent of St. Luke's before Teusler's arrival. The result was "a dead failure. The administration was bad, the place was dirty and always looked down at the heels."[29] Thus, Teusler hoped to find the man he was seeking in America, where "in addition to the usial [*sic*] requirements in regard to character and Christian training," Teusler believed he could obtain "a gentleman in the more restricted sense of the term and a man of some address and bearing. It is better for him to have had hospital training and he must have had a thorough medical education. He must be a man of good judgement and weight. . . . He must not seem too young or immature."

Though since his arrival in Japan Teusler had employed and entrusted a doctor and nurse couple, Dr. Kubo and Mrs. Araki, both of whom had trained abroad and could communicate in English, Teusler was pleased to have found an American, one Dr. Trinder to serve as his assistant. Almost immediately, however, Trinder have proved an overwhelming failure, and had left without a word. As Teusler angrily reported to Wood:

> I was astonished yesterday when I received the cable stating that Trinder had withdrawn. I can find no explanation for his behavior and his method of doing business has upset all of my plans and caused me the greatest amount of annoyance and chagrin. It is now four months since Dr. Trinder applied for Japan and nearly two months since his appointment. All of this time in which I could have gotten some other man he has waisted [*sic*] and I am about where I was last summer. Added to this he has disarranged all of my plans and thrown out of order much of the work in the hospital. I have told all of my patients here in Tokyo that he would be out by February and had even made definite engagements for his two cases. After I received the cable on Dec. 11th advising me of his appointment it never occurred to me that he would develop into a quitter.

Trinder's betrayal smarted, not least because he had not offered to "return the fifty dollars that have been wasted in the cables," and because Teusler was also forced to "countermand an order for his sign which I was having made to be hung up promptly." Yet, despite the added offense of the money and the nameplate, Teusler still could not be convinced to abandon his presumed need for a foreign assistant, even in the short term. Nevertheless, as he would claim, American physicians proved too selfish and too greedy for Teusler's work. After a day of interviewing potential and oft-recommended assistants, Teusler relayed his concerns: "One of the first questions which every one of them asked me was, 'What is there in it for

29. AEC: Letter from Teusler to Wood. Aug. 22, 1908; AEC: Letter from McKim to Hulse. Apr. 6, 1907.

me?' I told them that if that was what they were looking for I didn't want them. There is no place in our work for any man who is looking to see what he can get out of it for himself." Bishop McKim, who had found a Japanese medical missionary so irresponsible and irredeemable as to question the point of employing native Christian physicians in their own country, had, by Trinder's resignation, advised Teusler to continue his vacation as previously planned, "turning over . . . work to Kubo," rather than the now-absent Trinder. Teusler, however, refused.[30]

Dr. Kubo Tokutarō had joined St. Luke's staff six months after Scriba had done so, making him the longest-serving physician working solely at the institution. Beholden to the hospital not merely for his livelihood, Kubo had also met his wife at St. Luke's. Araki Iyo, Kubo's wife, had worked with Teusler longer than her husband had—since before St. Luke's founding. Soon after Teusler's arrival, Araki, a graduate of Kobe's Canadian Church Training School who was working as a private nurse for a patient of Teusler's, became the medical missionary's entire staff. In her short memoir, "The Life Story of a Japanese Nurse," Araki recalled that early on "we had no internes [*sic*], so I worked both day and night and helped Dr. Teusler all I could." For his part, Teusler acknowledged that Araki was "very efficient" and "seems to be very intelligent and to love her work from the purest motives."[31] Quickly, Teusler came to trust Araki with his work, medical, spiritual, and educational. Thus, she was entrusted with the administration as well of Teusler's nursing college, "a training-school for native nurses." While the Japanese Red Cross, which had previously stood at the helm of Japan's recent nursing education, was assisted, Araki recognized, by "the fact that they are under Government control," nevertheless that "nursing throughout Japan, until recently, has been looked upon as a menial occupation rather than a profession." Under Teusler and Araki's administration, and using "standards . . . [that] have been based upon the practice here in the United States," St. Luke's Hospital was to be "the only one in Japan requiring its applicants to be high school graduates and insisting upon a minimum of a three-year undergraduate course." Though in 1918 the position of principal was separated from that of superintendent of nurses, the former going to a female American medical missionary, Araki by then had served as both for sixteen years, since the institution's founding in 1902.[32] Thus, Araki, and not her husband, Dr. Kubo or his physician colleagues, would prove to be the first Japanese medical professional given equal consideration by Teusler.

Araki and Teusler also enjoyed a shared commitment to Christianity in nursing, though neither begrudged those students who chose to pursue other spiritual avenues within the institution. The school emphasized Christianity in nursing

30. AEC: Letter from Teusler to Wood. Aug. 22, 1908; Robbins and MacNaught, 59; AEC: Letter from Teusler to Wood. Jan. 27, 1909.
31. Robbins & MacNaught, 36, 33–34; AEC: Letter from Teusler to M. Mood. Aug. 7, 1902.
32. Azuma, 118; CUB: "A church in the capital of Japan: Being some account of the successful work of St. Luke's Hospital in the city of Tokyo." Rudolf Bolling Teusler. *The Spirit of Missions*. Dec. 1904. p. 1; Araki 1928, 1004; Tokiwa, 42.

education, and, in addition to the fundamentals of medicine, "Bible instruction forms a regular part of the training." Thus, as the medical missionaries reported proudly, "though several [of the nursing students] on entering were not baptized, all have now become Christians."[33]

It would make sense for graduates of Araki's school to be guaranteed placement at St. Luke's, but, in fact, neither Araki nor Teusler envisioned the institution as a finishing school for St. Luke's medical missionaries. Both medical professionals entertained the hope that, by sending well educated, Christian nurses throughout the country, both the religion and a dedication to medical charity would permeate Japan and Japanese beliefs. This was a more important task than merely creating a self-supporting institution, at least in terms of personnel. Thus, Araki maintained, her students would be "taught rather than trained and that the institution is really a college of nursing and not a training school for nursing to serve the interests of the hospital itself." By the end of their education, some three to four years later, the newly certified nurses would "exert a splendid influence in a practical way for Christianity."[34]

The spread of medical charity was important to Teusler and his staff, including Araki and Kubo, since it was this concept that Teusler believed to be key to Christianity and, more important, an idea that was foreign to Japan as well. What he did not count on was that, in addition to being purportedly foreign to Japan, it also seemed somewhat foreign to his countrymen. In order to serve as an example of Christian charity in Japan, Teusler determined that his hospital would provide care for those for whom care had been lacking, including those who had fallen through the cracks of previous medical missionary work in Japan. To the displeasure of much of his Board of Missions, he noted that "with our present equipment we are able to do practically nothing for the children, though out here the little ones, particularly among the poor, probably suffer more than many others." Overlooked by both native hospitals and medical missionary institutions, these children were "sent from one dispensary to another, plastered here, poulticed there, and carelessly treated throughout." In aiming to provide impoverished children with the care to which Teusler maintained they were entitled, he would have to argue with his home board by exacting payment for medical services from his fellow evangelists. When the hospital cared for the wife and child of a missionary in the Philippines, the Reverend Robb White, both the home board and the local board in the Philippines protested the costs, claiming that "since St. Luke's is a mission hospital and since Mr. and Mrs. White are our missionaries, the hospital may not reasonably be expected to render this service without cost." To John Wood, who was representing the home board, Teusler responded:

33. CUB: "A church in the capital of Japan: Being some account of the successful work of St. Luke's Hospital in the city of Tokyo." Rudolf Bolling Teusler. *The Spirit of Missions*. Dec. 1904. p. 1.

34. Araki 1928, 1006; AEC: Letter from Teusler to Wood. Oct. 3, 1908.

> You asked "whether the main charge of ¥72.00 (for Mr. White's account for hospital services whoever and whatever that is) might not reasonably be considered as fully covered by appropriation made by the Boards." To my mind undoubtedly no.
>
> The hospital is an institution doing a large charity work and with heavy running expenses. There is no endowment and it has to depend almost entirely on its own earnings to meet these expenses. During the year 1907 the total expenses of the hospital were a little under $16,000.00, (gold). Of this amount the Board paid $1,800.00 and the rest we had to earn.
>
> One of the chief ways we have of earning money is by taking in foreign patients. In 1907 the receipts from this Department amounted to $6,095.00. The regular charge for a private room is $3.00 a day. In a talk with the Bishop several years ago on this subject of the proper charge to be made [to] members of our own Mission, we decided it would be fair to charge the Mission the actual cost of taking care of the patient. In this way the hospital would suffer no loss and the Mission would get the hospital service at actual cost. This is the plan we have worked on for five years. When Miss Clarke of the Hankow District was in the hospital her account was rendered and paid according to this ruling.
>
> If I adopted the plan your Committee suggests the hospital would loose [*sic*] in actual money at least a thousand dollars a year and many questions would arise which it would be difficult to settle and out of which abuses would probably spring. Every body in the Tokyo and Kyoto Dioceses would have to be granted the same privilege of free board in the hospital whenever they have any ailment. This would also extend to all of our Missionaries passing through Japan. In addition to this as there is no regular arrangement in our other Mission hospitals for taking care of foreigners it would not be long before they would be sending their Missionaries from China and the Philippines up here for free board and lodging.

The rest of Teusler's missive is decidedly more pointed and even more vituperative:

> Putting all this aside I still fail to see what right your Committee has to think that an appropriation made to help out a Mission hospital amounting to about 1/8 of its total running expenses, is sufficient to fully cover a charge made for actual cost of food and lodging for two of the members of the Mission. We have another Department of the hospital for earning our money:— Exporting surgical instruments, etc., to China. We might be urged to sell these instruments to Dr. Jeffereys in Shanghai at cost, but it would hardly be fair to ask us to give them to him, would it? The proposition is exactly parallel. Our rooms for foreigners are merely a means of earning money for the hospital. The standard required for a hospital in Japan is much higher than in China and to meet the necessary additional expenses I have to resort to every way in my power to earn the money. . . .
>
> If we had sufficient endowment, of [*sic*] the Board gave us enough money to fully support such a large work I think we might take care of our Missionaries free of charge, though I question the wisdom of such an arrangement.[35]

35. Brent, 88; AEC: Letter from unknown author to Home Board. Jan. 16, 1909; AEC: Letter from Teusler to Wood. Feb. 15, 1909. Emphasis in original.

The fight for funds continued for months, with Teusler tenaciously refusing to permit a redefinition of "charity," which, while angering some of his counterparts elsewhere, allowed St. Luke's to grow "so steadily in the good will of the public that I am especially anxious just now for it to have no set back." Though headstrong, Teusler knew that he could not be so unyielding as to antagonize his compatriots and tried to appease them by appealing to their sense of superiority, noting that "a mission hospital in Japan certainly seems to require different handling from mission hospitals any where else, like every thing else in this 'Flowery Kingdom' which to our mind seems upside down." Moreover, though McKim informed Teusler that the Japanese government had "practically decided to give land for our hospital near the Red Cross hospital [*sic*], provided we only take in Japanese charity cases," this, too, Teusler refused, since—though "it show(s) there is something doing"—the condition "would cut us out of much of our income, limit our field of usefulness and in some ways injure our work."[36]

Teusler desired to maintain his charity work, particularly with the impoverished and young of Japan, as provided by the funds generated from caring for the wealthy, be they Japanese or foreign. To that end, despite the continued support and succor of Dr. Kubo and Ms. Araki, Teusler once again hired an American assistant, Dr. Theodore Bliss, a Cornell graduate, who, Teusler was pleased to discover, was as hard a worker as his Japanese staff and "well liked." Dr. Kubo continued to perform his job without the full accolades he deserved, though Teusler noted that the physician was "also very popular," and determined that he, the hospital, and the mission were "fortunate in having two such men." Indeed, after the fiasco that was Dr. Tinder, Teusler, the Hospital, and the mission were fortunate to have Dr. Bliss, the "steady hard worker" from Cornell, but Dr. Kubo had been a consistent and competent physician, able to weather the storms of a busy medical mission and a busy medical missionary boss, who finally had no choice but to acknowledge that Kubo "has earned golden opinions as to his ability and his character." Teusler considered Kubo "one of the finest Japanese I have ever known." Yet Teusler was lucky, as he knew that Dr. Kubo "will remain definately [*sic*] connected with the hospital, presumable [*sic*] for life, and will devote all of his time to our work alone." Similarly, Teusler was fortunate that Kubo was as dedicated an employee as he was a physician, since, "from the first of the year the hospital will pay him Yen 250 per month and all money he makes will be turned into the hospital, except some received for work he is doing for a life insurance company." It is hardly surprising that Dr. Kubo's salary at St. Luke's, regardless of whether he returned it to the hospital, was still less than the salaries of American employees. In 1910 St. Luke's newly arrived pharmacist made 1,500 dollars for the year, which was at least six dollars more than Dr. Kubo made that same year. Although this difference may seem scant, even taking into account inflation, the fact that an employee who had been with the hospital

36. AEC: Letter from Teusler to Wood. May 8, 1909; AEC: Letter from Teusler to Wood. Mar. 2, 1910.

essentially from its beginnings and whose position was more esteemed was making less than a recent hire in a less prestigious position is rather glaring. Yet because of his nationality, Dr. Kubo was regarded as the lesser of the two, at least in economic value.[37]

His wife also experienced similar relegation. Once chief nurse and principal of St. Luke's Nursing School, she soon was replaced by the American Alice C. St. John as principal of the school. St. John was well connected to the American Red Cross, and was seen as an asset to ensuring continued American instruction and philanthropic assistance, despite Araki's ability to ensure the school had acquired Japanese governmental recognition, and who, too, had endeavored rather successfully to acquire eleemosynary assistance.[38]

Araki, in addition to providing "able management" of the nursing school and enabling it to enter the Taishō period in "a flourishing condition," also ensured that both it and the hospital proper remembered the importance of the charity that Teusler fought so hard to maintain. Like her supervisor, Araki was committed to serving those whose livelihoods and neighborhoods meant that theirs was a life in Tokyo's slums—indeed, in the very environs of St. Luke's. Here, some of Japan's great epidemics preyed on the populace, claiming many in their youth. Along the banks of the Sumida River mortalities exhibiting symptoms of cholera and tuberculosis often surpassed other causes of death well past World War I.[39] It was the latter that troubled Araki the most. As she reported to the Sixth International Congress on Tuberculosis in Washington, DC, the disease, in all its myriad forms, was rampant in her country, and its prevalence was "much greater pro rata to the population than in America or Europe." Though the Japanese government calculated that among the lower class the number afflicted ranged "from 25 to 40 per cent," Araki noted that, in Japan, "among factory workers, milling hands, and those leading a laborious and exposed life, such as 'rickshaw pullers,' street peddlers, etc."—namely those living in the slums near her workplace—"the figures range from 55 to 70 per cent."[40] One of the participants of the international congress was more than aware of Araki's findings. Kitasato Shibasaburō, an honored speaker at the congress, noted that the mortality rate from pulmonary tuberculosis in Japan, increasing steadily since before the Sino-Japanese War, had reached 18 percent per 10,000 inhabitants throughout the country and across the economic spectrum. Though still considered a lower-class affliction, tuberculosis was beginning to cut swaths across Japan's military, and had

37. "Wants to Enlarge American Hospital"; AEC: Letter from Teusler to Kimber. Nov. 8, 1910; AEC: Letter from Teusler to Wood. Dec. 12, 1910; Langland, 179. The yen, in 1910, was valued at .498 of the dollar. Thus, Kubo made a total of $1,494 per annum from his work at St. Luke's.
38. Takahashi, 137–38; Noyes, 134; St. John, 486–87.
39. AEC: Report of St. Luke's Hospital to McKim. Aug., 1912, p. 4; Ishizuka 1981, 172; Ishizuka 1983, 8. These symptoms included diarrhea, enteritis, and nephritis in the case of cholera, and pulmonary and broncho-pneumonia symptoms in the case of tuberculosis. Although not pulmonary, other mortality causes common to tuberculosis and prevalent among the neighborhoods bordering the Sumida River included meningitis and various deformities, including those of the spine.
40. Araki 1908, 573.

not gone unnoticed by the nation's burgeoning life insurance companies: "Although the public conscience is well aroused as to the dangers of tuberculosis, no adequate instruction is given as to the proper modern measures for prevention and cure." Indeed, Araki noted, "The general poverty of the people prevents adequate curative measures from being taken by the individuals infected."[41] For so many of Japan's afflicted, government assistance—medical, educational, and social—was unknown.

Under the guidance of Teusler, Kubo, and Araki, St. Luke's became one of the few institutions to offer assistance to those suffering from tuberculosis, and to do so at little to no cost to the patients or their families. Not surprisingly, many government officials were grateful for the philanthropy. However, originally, the role of Christianity within the hospital was somewhat troubling to the same officials. In offering the affiliation of the government's Department of Communications, some ten thousand workers, and the necessary bureaucratic assistance and permission to build a hospital to serve them on condition that St. Luke's renounce its Christian affiliation, Prime Minister Katsura Tarō had hoped to employ Teusler's knowledge and assistance without his presumed religious association. Teusler, however, refused. Yet the wariness of Japan's government toward Christianity was actually shared by the American physician. As with his earlier spat with the native Christian church next door to the hospital, Teusler's relations with Japanese Christians, save for those in his employ, were rather strained. Even Sakai Tokutarō, known to his American friends and peers as Barnabas Tokutarō Sakai, a high-level Japanese government official, graduate of Hobart College and Harvard University, and a devout Christian, was considered unworthy of representing Christians. As Teusler sniffed to Wood, "It would be a waste of money to send Sakai to Edenburgh [*sic*] as a representative of the Church in Japan. He has never really been actively engaged in Mission work, is not a Priest and for the past several years has devoted himself almost entirely to Goverment [*sic*] and political work."[42] In dismissing Sakai, a highly placed government official, who could certainly prove a boon to the evangelization of Japan, Teusler made his prejudices clear. Teusler's distrust included not merely many Japanese Christians but also government officials, and a number of his fellow evangelists both in Japan and elsewhere. Though a devout Protestant, Teusler bristled at how his Mission failed to realize, as he did, that St. Luke's transcended mere missionary work. Indeed, neither McKim nor Wood, both considerable allies of Teusler and admirers of his work, saw the hospital as anything more than another aspect of the Episcopal Church's evangelical efforts. As McKim noted to Wood, when Teusler

41. Kitasato 1908, 2–3; Araki 1908, 573. As Anna C. Jammé, superintendent of nurses at St. Mary's Hospital Rochester, Minnesota, noted, Japan's Red Cross Hospital—purportedly independent, but actually connected to the government and presided over by director of nursing and colleague and friend of Princess Nashimotonomiya Itsuko, Hagiwara Take (whose name Jammé mistakenly reported as "Hagewara")—still used outmoded equipment in the tuberculosis ward as late as 1923: "All utensils, as basins and receptacles, instead of being white enamel, as we are accustomed to see, were of brass and highly polished" (Takahashi, 119; Jammé, 771).

42. Robbins and MacNaught, 75; AEC: Letter from Teusler to Wood. Mar. 2, 1910; AEC: Letter from Teusler to Wood. Apr. 13, 1910.

failed to cooperate with the home board, "I think that the doctor should be more generous and consider the evangelistic work as being equally important with that of St. Luke's." Wood concurred, and politely reminded Teusler "how easily some people get the impression that St. Luke's work is something apart from the Mission. I know you want to head off any such misapprehensions as that. Perhaps one of the best ways to do it is to be ready to give and take with the rest of the Mission when needs arise."[43]

Teusler's defensiveness might seem disparate and even odd, but, in truth, all his suspicion was cast upon those he feared would or could co-opt his work for their own—Japan's native Christians, Japan's government, and those within the Episcopal Church who believed that they should benefit from Teusler's charity. Teusler knew his worth, even if those around him did not. More important, he knew the worth of his work.

By the end of the Taishō period, however, Teusler would become more open to assistance by outsiders, and would begin to differentiate cooperation from co-optation, yet the Japanese government, it seemed, would have to make the first move. By 1914, the government had recognized how convenient St. Luke's was to the capital city, and, under Ōkuma, some of Japan's bureaucratic and intellectual elite forced a council with an eye towards granting "official recognition of the plan to build a new St. Luke's and [determining] the most satisfactory way in which assistance might be given by the Japanese." Assisted by Gotō Shinpei, Sakatani Yoshio, and Shibusawa Eiichi, the four men aimed to raise (though not necessarily personally donate) 200,000 yen (the equivalent of $100,000) for the hospital, since, as Ōkuma pointed out, "the past work of St. Luke's Hospital has already proven invaluable to our own people as well as to foreigners." Ōkuma claimed to be "pleading for your assistance in this great cause for suffering humanity, and for the advancement of medical science and learning both in the Occident and the Orient." The Taishō emperor answered his call with a gift of 50,000 yen. The commendation's worth was more than just financial, to both Teusler and Ōkuma. To the former, as recorded in the Mission bulletin, *The Spirit of Missions*, the gift "attracted attention throughout the length and breadth of Japan and will draw at once to St. Luke's the best of Japan's medical student and nurses. Any work or institution upon which the Emperor puts his stamp of approval secures the allegiance of the people." To Ōkuma, though his charitable interests certainly benefited in the same right, it once again meant he need not reduce his personal coffers.[44]

The coalition of government officials and Teusler also proved a boon to Japan's foreign policy. Like his colleagues in the YMCA, Teusler volunteered to assist Japan's mission in Siberia following World War I, but, more important, he also began to view St. Luke's as a true alliance of nations, even more so as the relations between Japan and America began to founder, the victim of fears of the Yellow Peril on the side of

43. AEC: Letter from McKim to Wood. Apr. 20, 1920; AEC: Letter from Wood to Teusler. June 21, 1920.
44. Robbins and MacNaught, 76–77; "Health," 675; "News of the Week," 1107.

Americans and the reaction to that fear on the side of the Japanese. Nevertheless, regardless of racism and distrust on both sides, with the abnegation of the 1907 Gentleman's Agreement, limiting Japanese immigration to the United States, Teusler persevered in maintaining work and relations of benefit to both nations. When representatives of the Rockefeller Foundation, including John D. Rockefeller Jr. himself, stopped in Tokyo en route to Beijing in 1921, Teusler invited them to tour his hospital, and accepted passage for himself and Dr. Kubo the following year to visit the Rockefeller-funded Peking Union Medical College, in order to "profit by innumerable suggestions for the plans of the new St. Luke's Hospital." Not satisfied to learn by example, Teusler bombarded Dr. George E. Vincent, then president of the foundation, with requests for assistance in founding Tokyo's public health program. Vincent, no friend of Japan or the Japanese government, was unmoved by the request to assist the nation and, as Gotō (then mayor of the city) claimed, "attract the attention of nearly 200 million people to a generous act of cooperation between Japanese and American citizens."[45]

Vincent's reticence was challenged by the Great Kantō earthquake of 1923. Though relations between the two nations often remained tense, the aftermath of the tragedy saw the Rockefeller Foundation reluctantly comply with Teusler's wishes, though, as medical historian John Farley claimed, even after the devastation wrought by the earthquake and the fires that ravaged the eastern seaboard immediately after it, "the Japanese seemed perfectly capable of organizing their own affairs. . . . One gains the impression that the Health Board was being taken for a very long ride."[46] What Farley failed to consider, however, was that, while Japanese science was, indeed, highly advanced, the nation still struggled against epidemics in the face of a government unwilling to invest fully in national public health. The issue, however, would remain moot for a few more years while the divisions between Kitasato's institute and that of the Japanese government continued.

Yet while Rockefeller Foundation funding foundered amid the divisions within the scientific and political bureaucracy, Teusler continued to work as a bastion of Japanese and American assistance—a fine alternative to pure American philanthropy, like the American Red Cross, to which many Japanese politicians and their constituents were increasingly averse to be beholden.[47] While grateful for the assistance, a large portion of the Japanese populace desired that Japan be considered capable of assisting itself, such that, once rebuilt, the nation could progress without interference. While at first glance this preference might seem "antiforeign," it began to make sense to Teusler, as it had to a handful of other foreign evangelists within larger organizations, though not necessarily to those leading the organizations themselves. "I cannot blame them very much," Teusler informed Wood. This

45. Robbins and MacNaught, 116–17; SSC: *In Memoriam: Rudolf Bolling Teusler*. His Excellency, Prince Iyesato Tokugawa; Stoddard, 293; Farley, 245–46.
46. Farley, 246.
47. AEC: Letter from Teusler to Wood. Feb. 16, 1924.

sense of self-sufficiency was important to a nation. Teusler's rejection of Western condescension is also apparent in his account of a dinner with a well-placed British resident of Yokohama who described the nature of the Japanese staff at the International Hospital in Kobe:

> He explained they had four British nurses and five Japanese women helpers, three of them trained nurses, and also explained, with characteristic British detachment and aloofness that 'of course we cannot permit the native nurses to give drugs or anything more than bathing the patient and serving them their food, . . . one can't put much confidence in these native nurses, can one?' I laughed, and replied that he had come to the wrong man, inasmuch as St. Luke's had about one hundred and twenty-five Japanese nurses, and only some four American nurses, not one of whom, so far as I knew, ever gave a dose of medicine from year's end to year's end. . . .
>
> My point is that the seven foreign doctors on the Staff of the International Hospital, together with the foreigners treated in the Hospital, and the nurses controlling it, almost without exception assume an air of superiority and conduct themselves in a way inimical to real friendship and understanding with the Japanese. The Hospital, with all of its services, is an exotic and will remain so, so long as they continue such a policy. . . . I believe, however, it should be run on lines more friendly to the Japanese, and more cooperative.[48]

In the wake of the earthquake, St. Luke's had become a symbol of Japanese resilience, and one that the government was far more willing to encourage. Gotō issued an official communication "as Home Minister and President of the Board of Reconstruction" in which he stated that he eagerly anticipated the hospital's restoration as well as that "of its service to the people of Japan. The needs of our suffering people are very great and the sooner you open your doors to receive them the greater will be their gratitude."[49] Though once again ravaged by fire in 1925, St. Luke's continued to serve the suffering people of Japan, be they victims of natural disasters or of diseases. And though gratitude continued and Japanese government support, even if usually only by means of lip service, remained firm, Teusler was willing to question his patrons in Japan for their continued disregard of the plight of the nation's infirm.[50]

48. AEC: Letter to Wood from Teusler. Jan. 18, 1927, pp. 2–3.
49. CUB: "Why St. Luke's Hospital Should Be Rebuilt." Dr. Rudolf B. Teusler.
50. As Teusler wrote to Wood:

> The whole problem of the care of lepers in Japan is very large, and the Government should be spurred to do better things for the lepers, and protect the rest of the community against them. I have talked with Professor Nagayo, the head of the Government Institute for Infectious Diseases, and one of the leading authorities on leprosy in Japan. He is an advocate of segregating the lepers on some island off the coast of Japan and already two or three such places have been tentatively selected. Sooner or later the Japanese Government will wake up, and do something about the miserable situation which now exists. Later if the opportunity comes our way to help in propaganda of this kind, or if it seems advisable later to try and develop in Kusatsu a small modern hospital to facilitate scientific treatment of lepers, and exemplify their proper hospital care, I will gladly do anything I can. (AEC: Letter to Wood from Teusler. Jan. 13, 1927, p. 2)

Though his commitment specifically to Japan's tubercular might seem more tenuous than that of his fellow medical missionaries in larger evangelical organizations like the YMCA or the Army, Teusler (and thus, St. Luke's) must nonetheless be credited for eventually realizing the necessity of employing Japanese medical professionals in positions of authority. As a moral entrepreneur, Teusler proved fairly successful at utilizing Japanese medical personnel, without facing such stricture from the Japanese government. Indeed, such men and women as Kubo and Araki were both fully capable of the work and were well aware of the conditions in their native land. Teusler's commitment to the health of Japan might not have been fixed solely on a single epidemic, but nor was it as self-serving as that of his compatriots. In contrast, William Merrell Vories melded Teusler's cooperation with Japanese medical professionals with an attempt to concentrate solely on one disease, and thus proved to surpass Teusler's work, and to do so outside Japan's capital.

William Merrell Vories

Unlike Teusler, Vories had not intended to become a medical missionary in Japan. In 1886, when he was seven years old, Vories' family had moved from Kansas to Arizona to facilitate his recovery from intestinal tuberculosis. Ten years later, and presumably cured of his disease, the family landed in Colorado, where Vories attended high school, eager to pursue architecture at Colorado College. An intelligent and confident youth, Vories joined his school's YMCA chapter, quickly becoming treasurer. Yet it was not until halfway through his education at Colorado College that his intended path shifted significantly. At the 1902 International Students Evangelical Movement Convention in Toronto, Vories was transfixed upon hearing Dr. John Mott speak of the importance of foreign evangelical work, a sentiment echoed by Mary Geraldine Taylor (née Guinness), the wife of Frederick Howard Taylor, a medical missionary based in China during the tumultuous Boxer Rebellion. Moved by their messages, Vories forsook his intended major and dedicated himself to philosophy, with the hope of becoming an evangelist in Asia.[51]

His faith was complemented by his devotion to the arts; in addition to the painting and drawing that led him to architecture originally, Vories was a gifted musician and composer, and an eager, though not particularly talented, poet. Now emboldened with a mission, the desire to fulfill it, and the gifts to do so, Vories believed that he had uncovered a universal truth:

51. OKS: "Omi Brotherhood and William Merrell Vories: Footsteps of the Omi Brotherhood Groups," pp. 1–2; Okumura, 14. Historian William H. Lyon claimed that Vories intestinal tuberculosis was both a misdiagnosis and undiscovered until soon after the turn of the twentieth century. He posits, instead, that the ailment continued to trouble him until the removal of his appendix, although, as he acknowledges, the likelihood of the disease being simple appendicitis was highly unlikely since the progress of appendicitis is far more rapid than Vories' case manifested (Lyon, 39).

One time a fool
Was sent to school
To learn some sense
And clear the dense
Delusion from
His cranium;
This is no lie:
That fool was I.[52]

No longer a fool, though still not much of a poet, Vories graduated in 1904, and within the next year the twenty-four-year-old was on his way to Japan to work as a high school English teacher under the auspices of the Young Men's Christian Association in Hachiman, a rural, small former castle town on the shores of Lake Biwa, once famous for its traveling merchants and its connection to Toyotomi Hidetsugu, the nephew and one-time heir of Toyotomi Hideyoshi, one of Japan's great unifiers.[53] Since the Meiji Restoration, however, the Ōmihachiman region had become somewhat more quiescent. Some three hundred miles from Tokyo, the town was closer to Kyoto, yet still far enough over land and water from even that city to feel a sense of isolation. Vories noted that his placement letter described "a Japanese government academy in an interior town, at the heart of a whole province in which no missionary yet resided." So desperately eager were the local government officials to remedy their isolation, both national and international, that Vories reported that the bureaucrats "would concede him (the English teacher) permission to teach Bible classes in his leisure time, so long as he refrained from mentioning religion in the class rooms." This suited Vories, since it meant that he "might earn [his] living by teaching, and at the same time inaugurate mission work in virgin soil." Unlike many of his colleagues in the association, Vories recognized that his situation was precarious, not merely because his position was at the mercy of the town government but because, even that late in the Meiji period, few men could survive as evangelists without a supplemental income source.[54]

To Vories, however, Hachiman seemed less than the sum of its parts, parts that were located far off the beaten path, seventeen hours by train from Tokyo: "At last—and a very long last it seemed—the train drew up at a desolate little station . . . Nothing of the town was in sight except a dozen or so shabby buildings clustered near by. . . . It seemed incredible that this could really be Hachiman—the Hachiman of my quest." Somewhat sobered by the discovery, Vories admitted that his arrival was inauspicious. "Here I was at last in the place of my dreams—and rather badly shaken in my enthusiasm for the great venture."[55]

52. Lyon, 41; Vories 1903, 5, 32.
53. Takeuchi et al., 29; Berry, 218.
54. OKD: "Vuo-rizu kinenkan goannai"; Fisher, 189; Vories 1925, 3.
55. Vories 1936, 1–2.

Confused, scared, and quite a bit homesick, Vories resolved not to give in to the "night-marish feeling of insufficiency, of foretasted defeat" that ate at him, and to continue on in his dream of "establishing . . . an ideal community on Christian principles," though, as he was warned by "Tokyo Americans," and as he imagined it, he was located "in the heart of the last determined stand of Buddhism, in its least enlightened manifestation." Yet perhaps the region was not so unenlightened as Vories had feared. After all, the school at which Vories was to teach had been established almost two years earlier, the brainchild of prefectural governor Nakai Hiroshi, a colleague of the pioneering Meiji minister of education Mori Arinori, in the hopes of promoting the same level of "wealth and power" that Nakai had observed when he visited England as both a student and a politician.[56] Nevertheless, to Vories in the first days after his arrival, it did, indeed, appear, as he had been warned, a desolate area, "cut off from surrounding parts by a girdle of mountains, isolated from foreign contact, conservative to a degree." Moreover, he had been advised that, though much of his new flock would remain strongly held in the grip of Buddhism, "the students and teachers of your school . . . being educated out of the superstitious forms of Buddhism,—which are all they have known,—will be either indifferently agnostic or openly opposed to all religion." Thus, even acknowledging the presumably progressive influence of the Meiji leadership meant only that those with whom Vories would have initial contact would be as intolerant of forms of Buddhism as they were of Christianity, preferring the nationalist value of Shinto. For foreign evangelists, the denial of all religion was far more difficult to counter than the embrace of a competing faith. The latter, presumably, required only education to correct ignorance; the former, however, demanded a method to overcome disbelief entirely.[57]

The town's greeting of Vories' February arrival seemed as cold as the weather, yet, as Vories would soon discover, a number of residents of Ōmihachiman would show themselves to be very pleased to engage the new teacher. At his encouragement, students arrived to interact with him, since "it was no small attraction that a real live American could be inspected at close range." Drawing upon his novelty, Vories offered the boys a chance to indulge the natural curiosity of youth, offering to show them "delectable foreign games—new and glamorous there (altho [*sic*] almost prehistoric at home)—such as *Dominoes*, *Flinch*, *Ping Pong*, and the like," as well as all of his "American furnishings and trinkets and a large and varied collection of views and picture post cards that gave intimate glimpses of that Promised Land of Japanese youth—America." Although he hoped to introduce the inquisitive students to another promised land, both Vories' loneliness and his intuition led him to realize that his task was to introduce America before he could heaven. Indeed, Vories was savvy. As historian Gregory Vanderbilt noted, in inviting the boys to his home, Vories would, by terms of his contract, be able to conduct religious study

56. Vories 1936, 7–8; "Tokushū: Shiga no rekishi 3," 4; Yokoyama, 55–56; Cobbing, 63–64.
57. Vories 1925, 4–5.

unimpeded, so long as the work was neither during school hours nor on school grounds. It also permitted the teacher to observe the students under more relaxed standards, and thus to conclude which students, regardless of their persona within the classroom, were the true leaders of the group. It was, therefore, to these students first that Vories put forth an invitation to pursue Bible study, his first foray into missionizing, before he turned to the sanatorium.[58]

Despite the ease by which Vories might have acquired disciples had he promoted his extracurricular group as one of English education, he determined that this could prove both misleading and difficult, particularly since his Japanese was nearly nonexistent and many of his students' knowledge of English was still basic. This was a distinction that few of his fellow association teachers made, often employing both language training and, eventually, physical activity and games as an (often unsuccessful) subterfuge by which to evangelize. Thus, with the assistance of a young Japanese Christian, Miyamoto Bunjirō, a graduate of the high school and now one of the instructors, Vories planned his first group as a slow progression of explanations of Bible passages, first in English by Vories, and then translated in Japanese by Miyamoto.[59] Although the head of the English department at the school demanded that he act as Vories' interpreter, the meeting went on unhindered by this slight change. As the number of attendants grew, Miyamoto, too, was allowed to act as interpreter when the original group became too numerous, and subgroups formed. Within eight months, the Bible study groups were attracting well over one hundred students, not counting the two-hundred-some students who attended Vories' groups at the two other institutions in which Vories taught weekly.[60]

Though interest was high, conversion was not. At first, the work seemed to many students a novelty. But Vories had the enthusiasm of youth, and his joy seemed infectious. As one man reported to him, some fifteen years after a chance encounter when the former was a college student who happened upon a YMCA conference at a rented Buddhist temple, "I could not understand much of what you said, but the way you talked to me made me feel that you had something which I did not have; and I was never afterward satisfied until I had found it." It was a sentiment shared by many of Vories' actual students. There was something terribly engaging about the man. Indeed, so eager was the teacher to convey his lessons that Vories opened

58. Vories 1925, 8–9; Vanderbilt, 27. Actually, Flinch, a card game, was younger than Vories' new acquaintances, having been invented not long after the turn of the twentieth century. Ping-pong, now more associated with Asian schoolchildren than American, was slightly older. While dominoes were considerably older than both games, the game existed in Asia in its current form over a decade before Vories' presumed introduction of it (Elliot Avedon, "Flinch" and "Dominoes"; Culin, 102).

59. Vories 1936, 18; Faris, 96; Curtis, 607.

60. Okumura, 4; Fisher 1914, 330; Vories 1925, 12. It was, of course, proper that the head of the English department act as interpreter, and to persist with Miyamoto as sole assistant would have been extremely rude. However, it is unclear for how long the department chair insisted on interpreting. He is not mentioned again in this regard in any of the sources I have encountered. I suspect that he gave up, eventually. Certainly, it is doubtful that he ever became a Christian.

his house to a few students, in addition to Miyamoto, as a proto-YMCA dormitory in the town.[61]

Emboldened by his success, Vories began to engage a disciple of Rev. Joseph Neesima, one of Japan's most famous converts, and together the two men established both an official YMCA building and a small church, using only the gentleman's charity for their foundation. Within this presumed bastion of Buddhism, Vories and his colleagues had begun to establish a small wellspring of Christianity. It was, he recorded in his diary, "a great privilege . . . But it costs much, much! No other teachers know of these . . . doings, or of the *bright side*, either. It costs blood and gray hairs; but it is *life worth living*!" Though Vories mentioned that the cost of the work was blood and aging, he failed to point out that the work cost him nothing economically, or, at least, it had not yet done. Nor (and more important) did it cost the home office anything. He proudly stated in 1925, "Not a cent for building, salary, or current expenses" of the little church in the town "has been given them from America."[62]

Evidence of the Buddhist animosity about which Vories had been forewarned seemed at first happily absent, and Vories' belief that "human nature is identical in Orient and Occident; that the recently acquired characteristics of races and nations are, like war paint and feathers and other clothing, only outward show" remained firmly intact. Yet, when, as Galen Fisher maintained, "the number of student converts aroused opposition," rumblings began in the local community. According to Vories, there were "two unfortunate elements" that led to conflict with this community:

> First, I was undoubtedly enthusiastic and active, and the Bible classes became unexpectedly popular and successful. This caused surprise and then consternation among the easy-going country priests of our community who feared loss of adherents and whose head temples in Kyoto began to fear loss of revenue. The local priests were incited to resistance and assisted in it by their superiors from Kyoto. Second, reports from my new friends, and then observations of my own, revealed a scandalously low standard of personal living and of community service on the part of the unfortunately low-grade priests who headed the local temples. Either directly or indirectly I was bound to condemn the local priesthood—even if I praised the ideals of their religions.

Indeed, Vories assured his readers, the first Buddhist officials with whom he had come into contact, a young priest and the head priest of his sect, were "men of good character and ability," and, he quickly noted, "they were not local men." While the superior priest differed philosophically from him, Vories nevertheless claimed that their character and ability was laudable as the younger priest was "well educated and fluent in English" and, more important, had informed Vories that "he felt

61. Vories 1936, 29, 22–23; Vories 1925, 16.
62. Vories 1925, 20, 23; Vories 1936, 27. Emphasis in original.

Buddhism to be decaying and inadequate to modern Japan, and that he personally hoped Christianity would become the standard of his Nation."[63]

However, no matter how positively Vories paints his consideration of his community (and of those people who did not subscribe to his beliefs), the work was disrupting some social relations. From his own varying accounts, Vories blames "a small group of the unruly element" among his students "whose chief enjoyment seemed to be to fight or to break discipline," as well as Buddhist priests who "did not come from the school" and who "instituted various forms of obstruction" (which then led to student unruliness) and who instigated "newspaper attacks . . . upon the character and motives of the new American teacher. Finally politicians were induced to make an issue of the school's appropriations from the provincial government being used to support a 'foreign' religious propagandist." Whoever was to blame originally, Vories claimed, the student bullies nevertheless perpetrated a "systematic and resourceful campaign of abuse and persecution, such as, I believe, the annals of modern missions in Japan have seldom, if ever, paralleled." Yet, even these students were reformed, and some so far as to become, like Watanabe, as described by one photo caption, a "Sunday School Superintendent and pillar of the church in his native town." Thus, it was the adults who continued persecuting Vories, culminating in the forced lapse of his contract with the school, since, as the principal admitted, the town "expected you to teach the Bible, but they did not expect anyone to believe." His first successes having come to ruin, Vories left his position in 1907 knowing that the town would remain closed to him, yet determined (albeit somewhat demoralized) to remain with his young flock.[64]

In hindsight, Vories' next move, to support his work through architecture, seems both wise and immediate. Both Galen M. Fisher, of the YMCA, and John T. Faris, of the Presbyterian Board, address the career change rather flippantly, as if it seemed to Vories the next obvious choice.[65] In truth, Vories' self-support faltered briefly, as did his faith, though only in himself. Instead of immediately searching for a new position, Vories benefited from the kindness of friends and strangers, both Japanese and American. After two years of self-support, and evidence that his evangelical work could be both self-supporting and expanding, was Vories able to earn and utilize philanthropy from America. Yet these foreign funds came, not from the association under which he had worked, but from men like one American businessman who, without visiting the town and without revealing his name for over two years, donated twenty-five dollars a month. Similarly, funds came from subscribers to Vories' newsletter, *Omi Mustard-Seed*, a self-published magazine that apprised foreign readers of the growth of Vories' independent Omi Mission, unconnected to

63. Vories 1936, 39–40; Fisher 1923, 189.
64. Vories 1925, 25–26, 34 and photo; Vories 1936, 42, 59; Okumura, 28.
65. Faris, 100; Fisher 1923, 189.

the various publications of either umbrella organizations like the association and the Army, or of entire religious sects.[66]

Once assured of continued subvention, Vories was free to explore options for continued organizational self-support, including the architecture he had previously abandoned. In fact, the necessity of further self-support had struck Vories a year earlier, suspecting that his teaching job could not last indefinitely. Either for sustenance or growth, he recorded in March 1906, "some lucrative side-issue for getting funds" was necessary "to be accumulating toward the *eventual Mission to Omi*." He had earlier abandoned architecture not merely because philosophy seemed more utilitarian for an evangelist but also because, as Vories later recalled, it was too easy to deny his call to serve abroad as an architect. As a future architect, Vories "had sought for excuses to stay at home," instead of attending his Colorado high school. He struggled against his inclination, and his planned career offered him the perfect excuse: "I determined that I would become an architect in America, make a large fortune, and send out half a dozen missionaries. That would be so much better for the Cause; and, more particularly, it would excuse me from going out!"[67]

Now architecture had to be rehabilitated. No longer an excuse, the occupation needed to become a more direct support of evangelical activity in the field. As Vories soon realized, architecture would support not only evangelical activity among his flock but also those throughout Japan. While providing funds for his work, Vories believed that his inchoate architectural firm could improve the nation's evangelical buildings, since, as he noted, "a good deal of uneconomical building had been done by various missions, and that some rather inconvenient buildings had cost over much, where the builders were at the mercy of native contractors." Thus, architecture would allow Vories to "serve other missions while earning support" for his own.[68]

Despite the education he lacked in both architecture and business, Vories proved a savvy businessman, in addition to being a natural architect. With the assistance of a former student, Yoshida Etsuzō, and young American architect Lester G. Chapin, Vories founded W. M. Vories and Company, Architects, an architectural firm with a solid basis in evangelical work, originally building mission offices and churches, and later including secular buildings both in town and across the nation.[69]

The architectural firm was far from the only business Vories would establish. Soon after the architectural firm received commissions, Vories realized that various equipment need not be imported from abroad, and began to build relationships with local suppliers, to the benefit of both groups. Within six years, Vories had established a network for building materials and interior goods. Yet, Vories' commercial successes were not merely pragmatic. Not surprising for a philosopher,

66. Vories 1925, 44; Vories 1936, 66–67.
67. Vories 1936, 66 (italics in original); Vories 1925, 45.
68. Vories 1925, 46.
69. OKS: Vories' Architectural Works; Vories 1936, 73; Lewis, 402.

Vories also based his business decisions on principles. As he admitted in one of his many memoirs of the growth of his evangelical community, "an additional stimulus was urging us to attempt a business venture." Vories' business savvy was meant to counter "the cynical attitude of our neighbors, who professed to believe that the principles of Christ which we were advocating, altho ideal in theory, were impossible to apply in a successful modern business."[70]

Even more than his architectural firm, Vories is often associated with another branch of his businesses, namely the Omi Sales Company, Ltd., which introduced and distributed Vories' so-called "healing cream," that very "well-known household remedy for little ills, like bruises, burns, and any inflammation—*Mentholatum*."[71] An 1893 invention of Wichita businessman Albert A. Hyde, Mentholatum, a combination of petroleum jelly, camphor, and menthol crystals, the "simple and really effective remedy for a score of little ills of the skin and mucous membrane" became popular in America soon after Hyde began selling it from his Yucca Company of soaps and shaving creams. By 1906, it became Hyde's sole product, making him a fortune, much of which he was inclined to tithe to various Protestant evangelical organizations, including the association and the Army.

Hyde was also given to assisting such organizations in more direct ways. Soon after meeting Hyde in Wichita, Vories convinced the businessman to give Omi Mission the exclusive rights to sell Mentholatum in Japan. By 1920, Mentholatum was distributed in Japan by the Omi Sales Company, Ltd., of the Omi Mission and would fund the work to which not only Vories but his entire organization dedicated their lives.[72]

One should not, of course, discount Vories' architectural firm, which funded the mission for some thirteen years before the commercial success of Mentholatum. Whereas the balm had already proved fiscally sound in America, there was no precedent for Vories' architectural success. After all, he was a self-professed "lone amateur" who could only count somewhat "more than ten years' study of architecture as a personal hobby" as his qualification. Nonetheless, in less than twenty years, his firm, having grown to thirty men, primarily Japanese, many of whom "trained wholly or chiefly in our offices" (although some also possessed degrees from Japanese and American universities), would be consistently commissioned by Japanese bureaucrats to build secular buildings in Japan. It was primarily this work that funded Vories' evangelization of the rural area across Lake Biwa, to the west, through literature and periodicals, railroad workers' YMCA branches, and, uniquely, his motorboat mission, *Galilee Maru*, whose sailors preached along the

70. Vories 1936, 76–77.
71. Vories 1925, 88.
72. Richmond et al., 255–56; Suzuki, 527; OKS: "Omi Brotherhood and William Merrell Vories." Suzuki points out that Mentholatum, though less expensive than a similar ointment (Tako no Suidashi, or Octopus Cupping Balm, invented by Machida Shin'osuke of the Meiji School of Pharmacy), was preferred by wealthier customers, whom Suzuki suspects were attracted by the presumed association of the former with America (Suzuki, 528).

shores of the large lake.[73] What Vories realized, as Teusler had eventually, was that, just as these works were for Japanese villagers, so, too, should they be primarily conducted by Japanese villagers. It was something that Galen Fisher discussed, even as the association had continued to reject it:

> Many a foreign missionary has insisted too long upon disbursing all funds granted for evangelism by his home board. No rule can be laid down as to just when he should let go of them, but some men have wasted their own strength and impaired their finer influence by failing to entrust funds more fully to Japanese colleagues. To be sure, some of the dollars might possibly appear to go further if the missionary were handling them, but it is very doubtful if they would carry so much of the love and power of Christ with them. I do not doubt that scores of Japanese [of] the largest caliber have been repelled from Christian service by the domineering spirit and close financial control of a few missionaries whose reputations have hurt the entire missionary body.[74]

Vories also recognized what many others, including Teusler, had not—namely, that the evangelization of Japan would be unsuccessful without equal emphasis on the nation's rural population as on its urban one. And, more important, he recognized that the evangelization of Japan had to be more important to the population of Japan than it was to Christians worldwide, but often was not. To Vories, this lacuna was "the weakest point in the missionary campaign in the Empire." It was a lacuna that Dr. Wilhelm Gundert, evangelist turned Japanese religious scholar, had attributed solely to "*the great gulf fixed between the missionary worker and those whom he ought to serve.*"[75]

By 1915, when Vories published his treatise, this gulf had come to include the spread of tuberculosis throughout the rural communities. As the early phase of industrialization ended, the nation's young, primarily female textile workers returned home, ill or as silent carriers, and spread the disease through a population that lacked resistance to what had previously been, as historian Mikiso Hane deemed it, "a relatively rare disease." Though Vories noted the "depredations of the 'white plague" soon after his arrival, and was particularly shocked by "the neglect of its victims in an avowed belief that it was 'as hopeless as leprosy'—then held absolutely incurable," his attempts to promote the need for medical mission assistance had remained unfulfilled.[76]

Vories' metaphor was not merely medical; the reference to leprosy also brought with it allusions to the New Testament, and to the belief that the faith of the patient together with both the tenderness and the faith of the physician could be curative. Certainly, Vories was not ignorant of the importance of medical science, but, in lieu of a scientific cure and, perhaps more important, in lieu of a sense of caring from the

73. OKS: "Omi Bortherhood and William Merrell Vories"; Vories 1925, 81; Okumura, 31.
74. Fisher 1923, 192–93.
75. Vories 1915, 1, 7 (italics in original); Gundert, 86.
76. Jannetta and Preston, 427, 432, 433; Hane, 191; Vories 1936, 95.

larger populace, the government, and even much of the Christian community, this was a rural need that he felt he could well fill. "For years," he noted, the Omi Mission marked its concern over "the terrific toll of tuberculosis in Japan," and had debated the merits of the establishment of "such fresh-air cures as we had seen in Colorado." (Though it is undeniable that Vories had seen such environments in Colorado, whether the majority of the Omi Mission had actually experienced this was doubtful. Still, that Vories spoke inclusively of his Mission and those who assisted him was certainly part of his personal success as an evangelist and as a leader.) Though late to the medical missionary world, Vories noted that, by the start of World War I, so few such missions had pursued this work, even after the passage and presumed enforcement of factory legislation, it was decided among Omi's leadership to undertake this new enterprise.[77]

There was a pragmatic need for tuberculosis care in Japan, but Vories was not a physician. Nor was he a dedicated amateur, as he might claim to be in architecture; indeed, he could not even be described as a medical dilettante. Thus, in his writings, particularly over time, Vories seemed to believe that he needed something more than his own credentials to justify his entrance into the medical mission sphere. In his 1925 memoir, he noted that his decision to undertake the work was assisted by the death of a young convert. By his next memoir, eleven years later, the incident had expanded from a sentence to a "rather romantic story" consisting of five pages in addition to a full-page portrait of the unfortunate young man. This young Buddhist priest, frustrated by the behavior of his superiors in his faith, turned to Vories, eventually embracing the Christianity that he witnessed his peers espousing happily. When he fell visibly ill with the scourge, he was moved into a little cabin on the mission's small plot of farmland, there to partake in the presumed curative powers of fresh air. Endō Kanryu, the infirm convert, had improved to the point that "he, and all of us, had thought him cured," only to have "over-exerted himself in the winter (which would not have occurred had we had a resident doctor and a real sanatorium) and a sudden cold had developed into pneumonia and brought on his death." In a very real sense, young Endō became a martyr to the mission's necessity for medical work. Before his death, Vories memorialized, Endō had "urged us to push forward our plan for the tuberculosis sanatorium, that others might share the joy he had found in Christ." For Endō, the sanatorium would first provide the mental health that his acceptance of Christianity and the Mission's continued acceptance of him had accorded to the former Buddhist priest. Even in his death, the work performed to assist Endō in recovering his physical health had proved a spiritual and mental salve. "No matter, he declared," recalled Vories, "whether we should be able to cure their bodies, if only they could have the peace and confidence which he had felt in the hour of death."[78]

77. Davies, 147; Aoki, 483.
78. Vories 1925, 77; Vories 1936, 95–99.

Vories knew that he could assist Japan's infirm in understanding the peace and confidence that he believed his faith could provide, but, though the importance of physical health had been minimized by Endō, and the lack of a cure for the disease remained disconcertingly obvious, a sanatorium and a medical mission nonetheless required a physician. Rather than seek out a foreign physician, whose acclimation and dedication to Japan could not be insured, Vories sought his medical professionals far closer to home. When the Omi Sanatorium opened in 1918, three years after Endō's death, it was staffed by Japanese professionals, all members of the growing Omi Mission. An image of the facilities' staff and volunteers in 1925, including physicians and nurses, pharmacists and laborers, revealed that all thirty-one men and women pictured were Japanese.[79]

Vories did, however, acquire from foreign sources the funds to establish the sanatorium and to care for its grounds. The main building, the Anna Danforth Tooker Building, was a memorial to the mother of the wife of a wealthy New York lawyer, while the cottages surrounding it, housing patients and other services, commemorated the lives of men and women half a world away. Yet, even with the considerable generosity of these individuals, the institution remained relatively small. Indeed, it did not aim to be a large home, whether hospital or hospice. In 1925, Vories proclaimed that, in addition to the dispensary, it "aims to provide only fifty beds for in-patients." It was not merely that the funds for further development were lacking; rather, Vories had no desire to build a larger institution. By 1936, in fact, the sanatorium had only gained another ten beds for inpatients. Yet, according to Vories, it remained "the first in Japan to have modern equipment and methods, and its effectiveness has been not alone in a very fine record of cures, but especially in influencing the Government in a widespread effort to combat the disease throughout the Empire." Certainly, in opening the year before the 1919 Tuberculosis Prevention Law, which mandated government construction of sanatoria at the local level, Omi Sanatorium had proved a trailblazer. Moreover, as long as local efforts to build similar institutions stalled in the face of bureaucratic and popular dissent, the sanatoriums at Omi remained uncommon As Vories (now Hitotsuyanagi, having adopted his wife's surname) proclaimed, Omi Sanatorium "has been practicing the most progressive methods of treatment with a strong emphasis on mental and spiritual health." Since its inception, it was "primarily interested in rendering a Christian service to those in need." Yet the "cure" of the Omi Sanatorium continued to be primarily based on "open-air" therapy, even after the introduction of bacillus Calmette-Guérin, the first, moderately successful antibiotic against TB, in Japan in 1925.[80]

79. Vanderbilt, 283; Yoshida, 124; Vories 1925, photograph between 80–81.

80. VKB: "Utsukushiku gogatsu" (5/25/1918). *Vuo-rizukinenbyōin 60nen tenbyō*, p. 7; "Heylman—Tooker"; Vories 1925, 77; Vories 1936, 98; VKB: "History." *Omi Sanatorium*. February, 1957; Johnston, 269, 259. Admittedly, BCG remained relatively unused in Japan until after 1940 (Johnston, 259).

Nevertheless, it was something where so often there had previously been nothing. And it did assist in the fulfillment of the platform of the Mission, specifically sections III, VI, and VII:

I. To preach the Gospel of Christ in the Province of Omi, Japan, without reference to denominations. There being no "Omi Mission Church," converts to be organized into self-supporting congregations of the denomination of their own choice.
II. To practise the complete unifying of the work and fellowship of Japanese and foreign workers.
III. To evangelize communities unoccupied by any Protestant Mission, and under no circumstances to overlap with the work of such Missions.
IV. To evangelize *Rural* communities, as the most conservative element of the nation, and the most probable source of leadership.
V. To seek, enlist, and train leaders and workers.
VI. To work for social reforms, including temperance, social purity, marriage customs, physical and sanitary betterment, and definite efforts for the neglected.
VII. To study and experiment with new methods of evangelization.

By working with a physically and psychologically isolated community, namely, the rural tubercular, the Omi Mission utilized new methods of evangelization through medical missionary work without overlapping with any preexisting foreign evangelical organizations. Given its success, it was no wonder that, of all of the mission's branches and departments—of which, in 1925, Vories counted seventeen—only the architectural department possessed a larger staff than the Omi Sanatorium. With an average staff of 6.5 people per department, the sanatorium required nearly three times that many. And, unlike the architectural department, "the Sanatorium is conducted on a non-profit basis." Staff gladly eked out a living primarily from donations, as the "patients pay only actual cost of their living."[81]

Their lives in the sanatorium involved "regular pastoral visitation and . . . frequent (religious) meetings," both as an evangelizing effort and for psychologically curative effect. Indeed, Vories intended to promote easy garden and farm labor as "a sort of 'graduate' institution" for "patients nearly cured, or quite 'cured' but not yet strong enough for full time work"—a rehabilitative effort to allow patients a return to normal working life. More importantly, however, these activities would serve as a response to what Vories' deemed the "Sanatorium Mondai," or problem of the sanatorium—the question of how the work could fail. Only by creating an "ideal Sanatorium" could the Sanatorium Mondai be solved. As Vories determined, the ideal sanatorium would be a "School of Health in which every pupil-patient has a full program of activities, made out of conference of the Staff, supervised, and adjusted periodically to suit the progress of each case." In spite of the

81. Vories 1925, I–III, 78.

hospital-setting, Vories insisted that, ideally, the institution "be kept Homelike, by a woman officer (or Superintendant) [*sic*] who knows and cares for each case as a personality." Notwithstanding the gendered dichotomy that designates feminine role to be that of a nurturer, Vories and his compatriots in the Omi Mission (later the Omi Brotherhood) could also conceive of a guiding role for women within the work of the sanatorium. Certainly, there was both a perception of woman as caretaker of the facility as a home, and caregiver of the patient as a child, thus lending the institution a sense of itself as a hospice, more than merely a hospital. And, indeed, it was an ideal, but the world of the Omi Mission was one of the most equitable of its time, allowing both Japanese Christians and women not only to rise in its ranks but also to serve within those ranks throughout the departments.[82]

That said, Omi Sanatorium remained somewhat infantilizing to its patients, as Vories also insisted that the motherly figure in charge limit the size of the institution to allow her only as many patients as she could "easily know in detail." She would explain "the entire system" to patients at the start, earning their trust. Finally, in addition to knowing about her wards, she would provide "proper food, sleep, rest periods, and exercise under supervision," as well as "some forms of occupations," like the farm, "to take patients' minds off themselves and provide interest." In the ideal institution, as in reality, to Vories, the insitution's "profit is less important." Yet the farm could also supplement the Mission's funds by acting as an "Independent Food Supply," which Vories had deemed "essential: not only to assure sufficient and proper food, but also to get it without exorbitant cost." The regulation of food was important in the Omi Sanatorium, which was both teetotalling and, obviously, wholly controlled.[83]

Although not necessarily Vories' ideal, the Omi Sanatorium was considered Japan's ideal institution by many who encountered it. According to Galen Fisher, the sanatorium was, in 1923, "recently declared, by the head of the largest government pulmonary hospital, to be the best in Japan." In the 1930 presentation of an honorary doctorate to Vories, Colorado College, in making note of all his accomplishments, singled out his sanatorium "which is the Japanese empire's standard for the treatment of tuberculosis." In 1957 Hitotsuyanagi proclaimed that in the thirty-nine years since its founding "the Sanatorium has grown in size and usefulness, and has won the favor of the public and the Imperial Household."[84]

Vories did in fact, earn the approbation of the emperor, but the circumstances surrounding the meeting and the reason for it were rather more complex. Vories was not granted an audience with the Shōwa emperor for his work with the sanatorium but rather because of his unique circumstances. After all, as a foreign national, he wed a Bryn Mawr–educated Christian woman, Hitotsuyanagi Makiko, the daughter of a viscount and member of the Japanese House of Peers. Lauded in

82. VKB: "Sanatorium Mondai." *Vuo-rizukinenbyōin 60nen tenbyō*, p. 11 Emphasis in original.
83. Ibid. Emphasis in original.
84. Fisher 1923, 189; Vories 1931, 3; VKB: "A Message from the Founder." *Omi Sanatorium*. Feb., 1957.

the foreign evangelical press as "a striking example of the superiority to race, rank, and worldly advantage which true Christian faith engenders and for which Omi Mission stands," the marriage would prove more controversial twenty years later. In 1941 Vories renounced his American citizenship and his status in Japan as a foreign national to naturalize as a Japanese citizen, taking the name Hitotsuyanagi Mereru. Unlike his native-born wife, Vories could and did become a citizen of his adopted homeland. During World War II, life proved difficult for the Vories family, as it had for their neighbors, though the persecution by the Japanese military police was lessened when the emperor's brother visited Vories' mission in Omi. Recruited by MacArthur to assist the Americans during the Occupation, Hitotsuyanagi met his emperor postwar as a loyal Japanese citizen, but also one whose position had proved highly unique.[85]

It is interesting, therefore, that, following the 1920 marriage, Japan's government did not assist or claim to assist the Omi Sanatorium. Though her parents had not approved of her choice of partner, Mrs. Vories was still a woman of means and influence. Nevertheless, both she and her husband preferred to continue their work and their fund-raising as far removed from Tokyo as was their dwelling. Vories noted in 1925, "The patronage of the Sanatorium is interesting." And it was. Though not his ideal, it was successful. "From all parts of Japan patients come. The reputation of the institution is nation-wide." As an evangelical method, it had not failed, as "not a few who came without a knowledge of Christ are baptized here and go back earnest advocates of the Gospel." Furthermore, without other foreign evangelists, without the Japanese government, in the quiet town of Omi, William Merrell Vories was succeeding in the battle against tuberculosis. A true moral entrepreneur, through his work, "finally the idea of the *cure* of tuberculosis by rational methods is gradually supplanting the old feeling of hopelessness toward this dread disease that is so prevalent in Japan."[86] Lacking a medical panacea, Vories had nonetheless found a spiritual one.

85. Fisher 1923, 191; Lyon, 43, 48.
86. Vories 1925, 80.

Afterword

"Let the Work Go On"

Where would Japan go from here? It need not start from scratch. After all, besides the assistance of the evangelical organizations, by 1915, Japan's government had recognized the need for public health care for the tubercular, founding its first sanatoriums, although it was seen as little more than a Band-Aid for a much larger problem that had spiraled out of control. Rather, the evangelists sparked what had been obvious to physicians and health bureaucrats—namely, the need for medical care of the infirmed.[1] If evangelists thought their efforts would fuel them through the remainder of the first half of the twentieth century, however, they were sadly mistaken.

If the 1904–1905 Russo-Japanese War was a watershed in Japanese political and foreign evangelical relations, the Second Sino-Japanese War and the subsequent Pacific War, unsurprisingly, marked a sea change. Having weathered the Great Kantō earthquake of 1923, a highpoint in donations to the nation, both missionary and lay, the road to war would alter the nature of the relationship between the two moral entrepreneurs, the Japanese government and the evangelical organizations, as much as it would the shape of the disease itself. Tuberculosis would run rampant during wartime, as it would in Europe, due both to the conditions in military camps, but also to the rise in heavy industrialization the war effort necessitated.[2] Even for the first years of the occupation, then, the disease would continue to plague a war-weary nation, with a death rate in 1947 of 1.9 per 1,000 citizens.[3] This should have led to a commensurate medical response, but the role of medical missionaries would come under fire in the 1930s and 1940s.

Even before becoming regarded as the enemy with the outbreak of hostilities between Japan and the United States, American missionaries often grew increasingly discomfited in a Japan that was at odds once more with China, a country where evangelical inroads often benefited from the confusing political landscape of the Republic which allowed for rather considerable proselytizing progress. By 1939, Japan's Shōwa government would cease to engage in the moral enterprise with

1. Johnston 1995, 195, 224.
2. Ibid., 102; Tsuneishi, 18; Mori, 566.
3. Mortality Statistics, 3.

foreign evangelists, promoting the removal of foreigners with the passage of the Religious Organizations Law. The law additionally severed economic ties between the Japanese churches of all denominations and foreigners performing any sort of missionary work.[4] Thereby the moral enterprise with foreign Protestant nondenominational medical missions would, ostensibly, be at an end. Things were not so pat, however. After all, in the decades since their entrance on the scene, foreign missionary groups had worked, in various ways, to indigenize. From attempts at the native policy of the Salvation Army (leading to the comic disembarkation in Tokyo wearing improper attire), to Teusler's entrusting hospital work to Japanese physicians, to merely attempting to be self-supporting domestically (as the Omi Brotherhood had achieved), levels of autochthonous involvement had seeped into each group.

For the Young Men's Christian Association, the move into Manchuria facilitated connections between the organizations across national borders, colonial or not. However, with the enactment of the Religious Organizations Law in 1941, the YMCA was forced to restructure itself under the auspices of the United Church of Christ in Japan (*Nippon Kirisuto Kyoudan*), with its chairman appointed by the United Church.[5] The UCCJ was seen as a "crowning achievement" of Japanese Christians, despite the fact that its ratification was thrust upon them. According to Shinohara Taira, a Seventh-Day Adventist seminarian in 1949, "Of constant fear to Japan's ruling clique was a widespread, disorganized body of public opinion, disseminating doctrines of universalism, pacifism, and resistance to the militarists and the emperor. . . . In short, they wanted the church in a position where they could control it."[6] The YMCA, then, with its reliance on foreign workers, despite its allegiance to the Japanese government, first solidified during the Russo-Japanese War, would fall victim to this control.

The Salvation Army, meanwhile, had increasingly come to rely on Japanese Christians to carry out quotidian tasks, both in the office and in the sanatoriums. Among the most highly regarded physician in the Salvation Army's medical mission was, as noted previously, Dr. Matsuda Sanya, a follower of Yamamuro, who pursued medicine to be, as he relayed, "a Christian doctor . . . [who] felt called to live especially for the poor and needy." His dedication to his craft would see his promotion to superintendent of Tokyo's largest sanatorium, private though it was, but also his subsequent death, in 1930, of the same disease whose suffering he sought to relieve.[7]

Matsuda's death paved the way for Dr. Iwasa Rin, Matsuda's pupil in medicine and Christ, to come into her own. Certainly one of the first female physicians to dedicate her life to medicine in Japan, Iwasa, too, sought to dedicate her life to care for the tubercular and she became "Dr. Matsuda's right-hand-man," with two hundred

4. Krämer, 204.
5. Y.M.C.A. shi, 72.
6. Shinohara, 12–13.
7. Harita, 364; Richards, 29, 27.

patients "under her care and fifty staff [who] took her directions." As Iwasa took up Matsuda's mantle, it was estimated that, in the population of some seventy million, one person perished from tuberculosis every five minutes.[8] An iconoclast as both a female physician and a Christian, an officer-wife in the Army related that "she must have been one of the first [female] doctors. She made it easier for Japanese girls to start working as doctors and nurses. As for our own Japanese women-officers, many just watched and took their lead from her." It was under her guidance that a second sanatorium was established, as Iwasa proved her business acumen alongside her medical know-how. As a fellow officer related, "The doctor was a first-class business woman . . . With the surplus of profit from the earlier sanatorium, the second could be put up. Almost everything eaten at the sanatorium was produced in the extensive grounds. Patients overjoyed at returning health worked with a will in the vegetable gardens and among the cows and pigs and chickens."[9] Though the sanatoriums would later be appropriated by the Shōwa government in 1939, under the auspices of the war effort, Iwasa was maintained as superintendent and chief medical officer. As one of Japan's leaders recalled, "No one did more than Lieut[enant] Colonel (Dr.) Iwasa to fan the glow of faith and hope among the loyal officers and soldiers in the 'liquidated' Salvation Army." Her public welfare efforts merited her the Medal of Honor with blue ribbon in 1944, and his continued patronage during the postwar years.[10]

Native command in the Salvation Army had been achieved, therefore, by 1926, and in the medical missionary world, it would follow soon thereafter. Nevertheless, the goal of complete financial self-support was more difficult. At the time native command under Yamamuro was achieved in 1926, the commander estimated that his charge was 75 percent self-supporting. In three years, it would be estimated at 100 percent, only to fall victim to the worldwide economic depression, again necessitating the use of funds from International Headquarters. For the next half a decade, international subsidies would hover around 8,000 pounds sterling per year, falling to half that from 1935 to 1937. Only in 1938, would the Army cease to receive any outside support.[11]

Nevertheless, an obvious link to foreigners, particularly with respect to the Army's ties to the British, tainted the work of the mission. Under Yamamuro, then, the organization worked to purge itself of so-called servitude to foreign interests. Yet when Yamamuro was forced to resign due to ill-health, he was succeeded by a dual command, split between Colonels Victor Rolfe and Sagawa Yasoo, the one and only time an arrangement of this kind has ever existed in the Army. So unpopular was this compromise that Army members at the International Headquarters in England urged Yamamuro to come out of retirement to take up the mantle of leadership once

---

8. Larsson, 120; Unsworth, 4.
9. Unsworth, 5, 6.
10. Misaki, 282–88; Unsworth, 7, 5.
11. Baggs, 301–4.

more so as to oversee the Army as the Japanese army pushed deeper into China. As the fifth general of the Salvation Army, George Lyndon Carpenter, lamented in 1940, "our circle is broken by events in the Far East."[12]

So too was it broken by Yamamuro's own mortality. Euphemistically promoted to glory in 1940, Yamamuro's death marked the end of the Salvation Army as an independent force within Japanese Christianity and medicine. The Army itself would be disbanded, first demoted to a "Salvation League," and then completely annulled, and its medical work would remain under the government's own auspices.[13]

Despite this eclipse, the postwar era would see a resurgence of the organization, and with it, an alteration of the medical work still performed by former Salvation Army physicians. As Dr. Nagasaki Taro, Chief Medical Officer of the Booth Memorial Hospital in Tokyo declared in 1970:

> Since the advent of anti-T.B. chemotherapy and surgical tuberculosis treatment, our sanatorium (Booth, on the site of the first Suginami Sanatorium) has been obliged to change its designation to that of a chest hospital . . .
>
> The change was mainly planned by Lieut.-Colonel (Dr.) Clifford Seamans, M.D., of the U.S.A. . . . Medical staff and nurses working in the Suginami Sanatorium were prepared to undertake non-tuberculosis medical and surgical care of patients with other forms of chest disease . . .
>
> It was becoming unnecessary to run two Salvation Army sanatoria here in Japan, and after careful discussion among the administrative staff at both centres it was recommended to Territorial Headquarters that Suginami Sanatorium should function as a hospital for chest diseases and eventually Kiyose (Sei Shin) Sanatorium become a geriatric hospital.[14]

St. Luke's Hospital, under the guidance of Dr. Teusler and the auspices of the American Episcopal Church, which had endured complete destruction during 1923's Great Kantō earthquake, saw a rebuilding by 1933 and an expansion of Japanese staff, such that, by 1934, of the 390 personnel working at the hospital, only four doctors (of fifty-seven) were American.[15] Nevertheless, 1934 also witnessed Teusler's death on August 10, in the very hospital he helped revitalize. His final wish, expressed to his Japanese physician, was to "let the work go on."[16]

Teusler was in luck. Due to the work performed at St Luke's and the nature of the performers, the hospital was largely unaffected by the Religious Organizations Law, and was able to continue ministering to the ill, if not to the foreign population. Facing a name change to the Greater East Asia Central Hospital, the hospital's work persisted unabated, and proved so successful that, in his monograph on Tsukiji Fish Market, a stone's throw from the hospital, historian Theodore Bestor notes that the

12. Ibid., 316, 329.
13. Rightmire, 161; Baggs, 329–30.
14. Richards, 138–39.
15. Lyon, 6; "Handbooks on the Mission," 56, 59.
16. Robbins & MacNaught, 204.

presence of the hospital itself may have saved the neighborhood from the American firebombing that had destroyed the rest of downtown Tokyo near the end of the war.[17]

In a somewhat ironic twist of fate, St. Luke's had truly come to embody what US ambassador to Japan Joseph C. Grew had deemed in 1935 "a mighty testimonial, a lasting monument to Japanese-American cooperation and friendship," and what Japanese Foreign Minister Count Uchida Yasuya deemed "an important link in the cordial relations between Japan and the United States."[18] Thus, it was hardly surprising that, a month after the end of the war, as contemporary physician Hinohara Shigeaki recalled, "General Douglas MacArthur announced the requisition of St Luke's for 10 years."[19] In a sense, and without volition, St. Luke's survived by being indoctrinated into a cross-cultural relationship with the American government long after it had proven its utility to the Japanese.

Like Teusler's St. Luke's Hospital, the Omi Brotherhood soldiered on as best it could during the war. Unlike St. Luke's, though, it continued to be led by an American. In truth, to call William Merrell Vories an American is a bit of a misnomer. As noted above, in January 1941, Vories became naturalized as a Japanese citizen under the name Hitotsuyanagi Mereru. Doing so required a demonstration of obeisance in a Shinto ceremony. Vories performed what he deemed a merely political, irreligious act. Eleven months later, Japan was at war with Hitotsuyanagi's birth nation.[20]

It would be foolish to believe, however, that Omi was the work of one man, American or Japanese. After all, for years, Vories had lauded the efforts of his new compatriots involved in his endeavors, particularly in the establishment of the sanatorium, an architectural firm, and a manufacturing plant, in which Mentholatum was processed. By 1933, Vories was supported by some two hundred workers.[21] Even as the mission was pressed by the Japanese government to diversify its holdings in order to remain both independent and solvent, Vories persisted in his belief that his was a cross-cultural mission. As he wrote in 1937, "the principle of *international* cooperation . . . is one of our central ideals. . . . It has become our conviction that it is impossible to establish an authentic demonstration of the Kingdom of God in our day in any single nation." To that end, Vories demanded that his mission employ "at least four Nationalities which are most closely thrown together politically and industrially in the Pacific basin—Japanese, Americans, Chinese, and Koreans."[22]

In spite of this, or perhaps because of this, Japan's Shōwa government had no problem shuttering branches of his mission, save for the distribution of

17. Jaffe, xxxii; Bestor, 116–17.
18. "Tomorrow in the Orient."
19. Hinohara, 102; Otake.
20. Lyon, 40; Okumura, 35.
21. Okumura, 53; Vories 1937, 84, 102.
22. Vories 1937, 109–10.

Mentholatum.[23] After all, Mentholatum had come to permeate Japan's public sphere such that when Ozu Yasujirou, master of cinema, discussed what was necessary to take to the front in China, he noted the primacy of a "notebook, knife, and mentholatum."[24]

Still, like its founder, the Brotherhood would survive the war, though the former only managed to do so through primarily sequestering himself in Karuizawa, far from Omihachiman. From there, he was unable to see how the Imperial Japanese Army requisitioned the sanatorium as a field hospital, practically destroying its facilities.[25]

As historian William Lyon notes, in what has become one of the surprising stories of occupation in Japan, Vories witnessed his own rebirth as an agent of international conciliation liaison between Japan's imperial family and the Supreme Commander of the Allied Powers, General Douglas MacArthur, who had requisitioned St. Luke's Hospital for American use. Unlike St. Luke's, MacArthur would return the Omi Sanatorium to its original owners. By 1959, the sanatorium would have 180 beds, several acres of land, thirty-seven buildings, and treat "hundreds of patients annually for only the cost of their food . . . To it come health authorities from all over the Far East, modeling their institutions on its architecture and methods of treating Japan's age-old killer."[26]

Vories would continue to work with MacArthur to establish Japan's new government structure, and, despite at times shaky relations between the two men, would, in true Vories fashion, thank the general in characteristically, if rather naively overblown poetry, proclaiming him "the first conqueror in history dared/employ the super-bomb of LOVE." For the moral entrepreneur Vories, then, the end of the war, in spite of all that had led up to it, manifested that

> Love conquers all,
> However late its victory;
> Invincible, eternal is its rise.
> Love is of Life,
> Love is of GOD.[27]

23. Lyon, 48.
24. Bordwell, 167.
25. Lyon, 49.
26. Ibid., 49; C. Hall, 96.
27. Lyon, 58.

Conclusions

Cui Bono?

Tuberculosis in Japan existed long before the arrival of the first medical missionaries, and it would remain after them as well. In that it would take a public health intervention in the aftermath of war to address this lacuna adequately, this is the story of the something that did not happen, or at least, did not happen in the time frame one might have expected. Still, the epidemic during the period from the 1880s until the 1920s proved salient because of the historical questions it answered and some of the theoretical light it shed. Through the actions of the government, scientists, evangelical leaders, and the tubercular themselves, we discovered how a nation defined itself and its obligations to its subjects, and how evangelical organizations sought to utilize, as much as to assist, those in their care. In the process, we considered the following: how Protestantism allowed some of the disease's victims to withstand societal stigma, and how its proponents viewed their obligation to their fellow man; how concepts of public health changed when faced with a disease with no known cure, and how many of the attempts to respond to the disease fell victim to partisan politics and personality disputes; how gender affected national, societal, and religious rights, and how disease affected perceptions of gendered behavior. Finally, we considered how the value of human life was parsed and differentiated, particularly vis-à-vis utility to the nation. Thus, moral entrepreneurs used people as political and soteriological currency—the lives of patients of tuberculosis worth less than their souls. Some did so more deftly than others.

For so much of this work, as with historical studies in general, the question that seems to guide our study is cui bono—to whose benefit? How do the actions of politicians, scientists, and evangelical leaders serve themselves, and how do these actions serve others? And to what extent does an unfortunate, yet seemingly expendable group, the tubercular, get to exercise their own actions within the overarching machinations and manipulations of the other three?

Let us begin with the tubercular. The victims of social stigma as much as of the disease, Japan's tubercular comprised a wide swathe of society—poets, bureaucrats, and soldiers—but the disease became most strongly identified with its numerous victims in the textile mills. Young, impoverished workers, primarily female, caught and spread the disease in droves. Cui bono? First and foremost among beneficiaries was the nation, as determined by Japan's politicians. Presumably assisted, as subjects, by the benefits they wrought, to what extent could these women and girls have exercised agency and altered their situations? The need of women to support families and their relative lack of technical skills had led just as many to the brothels, rarely far from the factories. It was a double bind.

Yet it was the factories and the conditions therein with which tuberculosis became associated. Analyses along these lines have been made by physicians, sociologists, and historians—Hosoi Wakizō, Ishihara Osamu, Janet Hunter, E. Patricia Tsurumi, Sharon Sievers, and Mikiso Hane. As they questioned what recourse these females had. As subjects, they had little or none. Suffrage was, of course, limited. Most males remained unable to vote until the end of the Taishō period, to say nothing of the women. As workers, again they had scarce recourse. The opportunities for labor disputes and unionization were limited; on the rare occasions that such disputes came to a head, a mediator could be encouraged to participate, but these men were outsiders. Even sympathetic labor leaders could not maintain a presence in the factory as labor organizers. There could be no real representation, only advocacy, and only when it suited the advocates. And who would step up as advocates?[1]

National politics remained tied to industry. As the basis for the goals of developing a modern military-industrial complex, many of Japan's politicians pandered to bureaucrats, and vice versa. For research scientists who pursued science in its own right, not as a national bulwark or tool for teaching Japan's future elite, the priorities of the politicians did not always match up to their own. As we have seen, most notably in the case of Kitasato Shibasaburō, the resultant friction rarely permitted either side to fulfill its objectives entirely. More importantly, politicizing science, and making it a victim of partisan and personality clashes, failed to benefit those who looked to medical science or politically driven public health to ameliorate their conditions.

Public health was privatized, the realm of families and villages. But misconceptions about illness prevailed, even after the acceptance of germ theory. Within these misconceptions, stigmas about illness and the infirmed blossomed. Not merely contained in the literary works of the day, these stigmas often proved as hurtful as the disease which they claimed to illustrate.

Thus, the tubercular were placed in the custody of people too often ruled by misconceptions and fear. Secrecy, hatred, and dread kept proper care from being administered. Few experienced the care and divine healing that Kagawa Toyohiko claimed to have received when, suffering from tuberculosis, he felt "an ecstatic consciousness of God; a feeling that God was inside me and all around me. . . . I coughed up a cupful of clotted blood. I could breathe again. The fever was reduced. I forgot to die." When visited by his theological teacher, Dr. Myers, during his next episode a

1. Kishimoto, 48.

little over a month later, the same love radiated. Whereas previously, "people didn't like to get close to me because of my terrible disease, so I was very lonesome." With Myers' visit, however, the two men "stayed in that cottage about four days. We slept in the same bed. I asked if he wasn't afraid of me. 'Your disease is contagious,' he said, 'but love is more contagious.'"[2]

Yet love was not the only weapon in the foreign evangelists' arsenal. Acceptance, assistance, assuagement, and a promise of salvation rounded out their cache. But sometimes this was not enough to garner the support of a new population. Evangelists seemed to hit a point of diminishing returns and conversion rates plateaued without a novel approach. For many, but not for all, medical missions provided the innovation with which to counter the trend as well as the social utility, which was an essential component of moral entrepreneurship.

One of the first Protestant evangelical organizations to arrive in Japan, the YMCA had attracted Japanese followers even before its official entry into Japan in 1889. However, because it was an organization in a foreign country, unlike unaffiliated evangelists who had arrived earlier, it was answerable not only to Japan's government, but the American board who headed the YMCA. At times this was constricting, since the goals of each were not always complementary, but it also granted it a sense of legitimacy in Japan, a nation that was interested in revising its international position. This meant that a few of the nation's political and bureaucratic elite were open to working with the YMCA (or allowing it to work for them), in the hopes that it would raise international opinions of the new nation.

The leadership of the YMCA in Japan, American men, similarly believed in the importance of good relations with the influential elite of Japan. Though they longed to add Japanese politicians among the ranks of their followers, they were almost equally happy winning their support if not their souls. Careful not to antagonize Japan's leadership, the YMCA quickly fell into the less controversial role of assisting soldiers both on the front lines and those convalescing at home, providing university students with housing and entertainment, and, eventually, offering similar entertainment to the urban middle class, all of which benefited Japan's government, and did so in the least offensive way possible.

Although a few among the leadership of Japan's YMCA assisted the working class, mostly these men sought to create favorable relations within the factory, and, since they worked at the behest of the factory owners, were hardly of a rabblerousing inclination. It was, of course, hard to ignore Japan's tuberculosis epidemic, but such medical missionary work was abandoned by the YMCA in favor of more rewarding work, both in terms of political prestige and fundraising, although not in the number of converts won.

For both the Japanese government and the YMCA, theirs was a utilitarian arrangement masked as a symbiotic relationship. Both sides assumed that it had the

---

2. Kagawa 1998, 16–17.

more powerful position in the relationship. Both assumed that the other was less aware of the utility of the relationship.

But it was never merely a two-sided relationship.

Although it had not originally intended to do so, the Salvation Army presented itself in stark contrast to the YMCA, not just in Japan, but around the world. It was a newer institution, but one that based itself on old organizational models. Where the YMCA had been a true association (a rather loosely bound conglomeration of like-minded Protestants), the Army had established itself as just that—an army. It had a clear set of regulations and goals, as well as a distinct chain of command, at the top of which was the Booth family, installed not only as its founders but also as its generals and commanders, seemingly in perpetuity. This monopoly of the Booth family could have easily been an organizational weakness, but, in Japan, it proved a boon to the Army. For starters, it gave Japan's leaders a specific commander of the organization with whom to communicate and to work, if need be. Where the YMCA's leadership was constantly in flux, the Army, at least at the top, was stable.

Moreover, due to the influence of William Booth, the paterfamilias and founder of the Army, the organization began as an evangelical force within the city slums of England, and kept this emphasis on the urban lower classes as it spread internationally. Due to the power and influence of his wife, Catherine, the Army became one of the only truly coed evangelical groups at the turn of the twentieth century. In employing women among its officer corps, the Army also ensured that it would be more aware of the plight of women in the countries in which it worked. The Army also was keenly aware of the importance of medical missionary work in general, and of tuberculosis care in particular, as this was a disease with which both William and Catherine Booth had first-hand experience.

Perhaps one of the biggest differences between the Army and other evangelical organizations like the YMCA was the Army's emphasis on what it called its "native policy." Unlike other groups in Japan, the Army prided itself on its officers' willingness to live like and among the Japanese subjects with whom it sought to interact. In addition, it allowed Japanese subjects not only to join the Army, but to advance to positions of leadership. (Nevertheless, they did generally have to speak English to reach the better positions.) Whereas the YMCA had Japanese members in more auxiliary positions or, rarely, in cooperative leadership positions, assisting a foreign member, the Army in Japan was rather quickly led by its most famous convert, Yamamuro Gunpei. This, then, brings up the second requisite for successful moral entrepreneurship in cross-cultural circumstances, namely, that it is culturally adaptive and involves the instrumental participation of locals.

Because of its stronger ties to the Japanese urban working class, it had less of a fear of angering prominent Japanese political and bureaucratic elites than did the YMCA. This was both good and bad. The YMCA had garnered powerful friends (though not converts), but little respect. The Army, on the other hand, often personally annoyed the leadership of the countries in which it spread, but its efforts were viewed as earnest. Before the Army's medical mission in Japan, it was predominantly known for driving prohibition and for assisting Japanese prostitutes to escape such a life. Needless to say, neither was terribly successful but both still managed to exasperate some powerful politicians. But the Salvation Army always stayed within the legal bounds established by the nation in which it worked, recognizing the sovereignty of these nations as part of the native policy. Thus, rather than changing Japan, the Army worked with individuals within Japan and within its social mores and customs, which allowed the Army to work without seriously antagonizing the leadership, even if it failed to win friends in higher places.

Still, what it lacked in political and bureaucratic friendships, it made up for in imperial admiration. Nearing the end of his reign, Emperor Meiji had an audience with General William Booth, an unprecedented event. Although the meeting was short, it legitimized the Army's work in Japan to the rest of the world, and earned the Army the respect of Japan's royal family. (In fact, Meiji later claimed that the meeting was one of the two most memorable of his career, the second being with President Ulysses S. Grant.) At the meeting, Booth was reported to have broached the subject of a tuberculosis sanatorium, to the funding of which both Emperor Meiji and, later, Japan's royal family would donate. Fundraising was slow going. The YMCA, with its philanthropic friends, had an easier time raising funds, but the Army managed to scrimp and save enough to establish its first sanatorium under the care of Dr. Matsuda, on the outskirts of Tokyo, by 1924.[3]

Once tuberculin, Robert Koch's presumed remedy, had proved a bust as a cure, what could one do in a sanatorium? Actually, convalescing proved helpful. So too did the fact that a sanatorium quarantined the diseased. But most importantly, the sanatorium gave the sick a place to recover from societal stigmas. Matsuda also started a small farm on the sanatorium grounds, in which patients would work. This gave meaning to an existence otherwise measured only in time on a sickbed. Without a magic bullet, the sanatorium still allowed the patients to live in a healthy place, physically and mentally. In some ways, at this time, that the mere idea of caring for these people existed was as significant as the actual care they received.

The most interesting thing about the relationship between the Japanese government and the foreign evangelical groups is the extent to which they involved themselves in constant maneuvering, an enterprise based not on money or souls, but seemingly on morals. The very nature of the relationships—between the government and the YMCA, the government and the Army, and the YMCA and the Army—was a negotiation of appearances. How to make one's own group appear to hold the moral high ground by providing cross-cultural social utility, while still maintaining the relationship—namely, how to keep doing well without angering the other party. And in these relationships, the victims of tuberculosis often became

3. Harita, 364.

a focal point, essentially currency between moral entrepreneurs. Where souls had been the previous currency, now there was trade in individuals.

But individuals also assisted. From the larger organizations, a few evangelists broke off to form their own medical missions. When work was performed on a more atomized level, by individuals and for individuals, the Japanese government was less likely to interfere, and the evangelists were less likely to negotiate terms. Working in Japan's capital, Rudolf Teusler had a more difficult time performing work uninterrupted, but he also was not unaided. With a network of foreign and, increasingly, Japanese contacts, both medical and governmental, Teusler traded full autonomy for assistance. He traded specialization for general practice. Neither exchange seemed to trouble him, and his staff knew that, in working at his institution, they, too, were aligning themselves not only with Teusler's mission writ large, but also with his quotidian mission. As a moral entrepreneur, of course, Teusler succeeded. After all, the fact that St. Luke's exists to this day is part of the testament to his success.

Yet it was William Merrell Vories who had the most success at his sanatorium on Lake Biwa. Vories had become self-sufficient in a way no other foreign evangelical group had, and his Omi Mission was staffed by a group of native Japanese Christians to the point that it seems silly to identify it as foreign at all. Yet, with Vories at the helm, it was, which allowed it a liminal status vis-à-vis Japan's government, as did its location and the number of its adherents. The Omi Mission did not extend to Tokyo; it barely crossed the then relatively remote lake on which it was located. The patients at the sanatorium were few, and were isolated from the rest of the villages from which they came, and from which they remained quarantined. And, like the Salvation Army, the Mission had no desire to work outside the law or mores of the society in which its members and their families lived. Save for the peccadillo which resulted in his losing his position at the high school soon after his arrival, Vories did little to annoy the local politicians, let alone the national ones.

Like Kagawa's Dr. Myers, Vories treated his charges with love, as did those who staffed the sanatorium for him. And though, for most, it was better to be loved than despised or feared, the rapport between physician and patient remained an unbalanced relationship. If the physician was caretaker, the tubercular was child. Vories' ideal sanatorium was built upon these archetypes. And, though it was hardly a novel relationship, it seemed the best attention that the patients could have expected. More significant, it was merely a redefinition of the stigmas that plagued them elsewhere. Christianity, it seemed, for all its love, was not free from stigmatizing the victims of the epidemics, albeit more subtly. It merely tarred them as incapable of independent salvation. The tubercular men and women alone could not ensure the salvation of their souls or their lives, remaining dependent upon the medical missionaries who, in caring for them with loving kindness, could facilitate both.

Perhaps it was a small price to pay—survival but with loss of control—and perhaps it was a false dichotomy, for who, in the face of illness, really controls his own life? But it remained disconcertingly antithetical to the sense of empowerment that the evangelists claimed Christianity could offer. What Christianity could rightly claim to offer, in the case of the medical missionaries, was a modicum of public health, an authoritative presence to ensure future control of infection in the absence of governmental work. Whether Christian care of the tubercular was the "ideal care" was irrelevant when it was the only care available.

Why was there no governmental care for so long? Why did there need to be, a public official might have wondered? If the Christians could hold the illness at bay in absence of a certain cure, why waste the funds? Why bother when it remained beyond the realm of the military? If the question of who benefited ruled the pragmatism and the utilitarianism of Japan's government, it was not an unknown question to many foreign evangelists either. Salvation, be it of souls or lives, was a large part of the mission, but it remained only a part. Evangelical enterprises were just that—and required capital and official approbation to continue the work of salvation, no matter how beneficial that work seemed or was. Though many evangelists were well intentioned, they worked within a larger system, and that system was peopled by those who, like the evangelists, needed to perpetuate it. Whether many of them understood this consequence, a question that might have been better in keeping with their doctrine was not cui bono, but who deserves to benefit?

Bibliography

Archives

Columbia University Burke Theological Library (CUB)
John T. Gulick papers, Bancroft Library (JTG)
Kautz Family YMCA Archives (KFA)
Kitasato Kenkyūjo—Kitasato kinenshitsu (KKS)
Kitasato Memorial Medical Library (KMM)
Kitasato Museum (KM)
National Archives of Japan (NA)
National Diet Library of Japan (NDL)
Ōkuma Monjo (OM)
Ōmikyōdaisha (OKS)
Online Archive of California (OAC)
Small Special Collections, University of Virginia (SSC)
The Archives of the Episcopal Church (AEC)
The National Council of YMCAs of Japan (NCY)
The Salvation Army National Archives and Research Center (SANA)
The Salvation Army Research Room Archives, Tokyo (SAR)
Vuo-rizu Kinenbyōin (VKB)
Waseda University Archives (WUA)

Publications

Abe, Ikuo. "Muscular Christianity in Japan: The Growth of a Hybrid," edited by John J. MacAloon. *Muscular Christianity and the Colonial and Post-colonial World*. Routledge, 2008.

Abe, Yoshiya. "From Prohibition to Toleration: Japanese Government View Regarding Christianity, 1854–1873." *Japanese Journal of Religious Studies*, vol. 5, no. 2–3, pp. 107–38.

Abrams, Jeanne A. "'Spitting Is Dangerous, Indecent, and against the Law!': Legislating Health Behavior during the American Tuberculosis Crusade." *Journal of the History of Medicine and Allied Sciences*, vol. 68, no. 3, July 2013, pp. 416–50.

Addison, James Thayer. "Religious Life in Japan." *The Harvard Theological Review*, vol. 18, no. 4, Oct. 1925, pp. 321–56.

秋元巳太郎. 『日本における救世軍七十年史』. 第一巻. 東京: 救世軍出版供給部, 1965. [Akimoto Midarō. *Nihon ni okeru kyūseigun shichijūnenshi*. Dai 1 cho. Tokyo, Kyūseigun shuppan kyōkyūbu, 1965.]

秋元巳太郎. 『日本における救世軍七十年史』. 第二巻. 東京: 救世軍出版供給部, 1965. [Akimoto Midarō. *Nihon ni okeru kyūseigun shichijūnenshi*. Dai 2 cho. Tokyo, Kyūseigun shuppan kyōkyūbu, 1965.]

Alden, Percy. "Social Problems in Japan." *Public Opinion: A Comprehensive Summary of the Press Throughout the World on All Important Current Topics*, vol. XXV, July 1898–December 1898. New York, The Public Opinion Company, Publishers, 1898.

"*Among the Industrial Workers (Ways and Means): A Hand Book for Associations in Industrial Fields*." The International Committee of Young Men's Christian Associations, 1916.

Amundson, Ron. *Darwin's Laboratory: Evolutionary Theory and Natural History in the Pacific*. Edited by Roy M. MacLeod and Philip F. Rehbock. U of Hawai'i Press, 1994.

Anderson, Benedict. *Imagined Communities: Reflections on the Origin and Spread of Nationalism*. Verso, 1983.

Anesaki, Masahira. "History of Public Health in Modern Japan: The Road to Becoming the Healthiest Nation in the World." *Public Health in Asia and the Pacific: Historical and Comparative Perspectives*, edited by Milton J. Lewis and Kerrie L. MacPherson. Routledge, 2008.

Aoki, K. "Epidemic of Tuberculosis in Meiji and Taisho Eras in Japan and Excess Deaths from Tuberculosis in Females." *Kekkaku*, vol. 70, no. 8, Aug. 1995, pp. 483–90.

青木正和. 『結核の歴史: 日本社会との関わり—その過去, 現在, 未来』. 東京: 講談社, 2003. [Aoki Masakazu. *Kekkaku no rekishi: nihon shakai tono kakawari—sono kako, genzai, mirai*. Tokyo, Kōdansha, 2003.]

Appel, Joseph H. *The Business Biography of John Wanamaker: Founder and Builder, America's Merchant Pioneer from 1861 to 1922; with Glimpses of Rodman Wanamaker and Thomas B. Wanamaker*. New York, Macmillan, 1930.

Araki, Iyo. "Nursing in Japan: Its Origins and Development." *The American Journal of Nursing*, vol. 28, no. 10, Oct. 1928, pp. 1003–06.

Araki, Iyo. "Tuberculosis in Tokyo and Vicinity." *Transactions of the Sixth International Congress on Tuberculosis: Washington, September 28 to October 5, 1908*. Vol. 3. William F. Fell Company, 1908.

"Association News & Notes." *Record of Christian Work*, vol. 24, no. 4, Apr. 1905, p. 248.

"Attitude of the Japanese People towards Christianity." *The Christian Movement in Japan Seventh Annual Issue 1909*.

Aydin, Cemil. *The Politics of Anti-Westernism in Asia: Visions of World Order in Pan-Islamic and Pan-Asian Thought*. Columbia UP, 2007.

吾妻知美. "ナイチンゲールの看護の本質はどのように伝えられたか." 『教授学の探究』. 第23号 (2006年1月31日), pp. 111–21. [Azuma Tomomi. "Naichinge-ru no kango no honshitsu ha donoyōni tsutaeraretaka." *Kyōjugaku no tankyū*, dai 23 gō (2006 nen 1 gatsu 31 nichi), pp. 111–21.]

Bacon, John. "Medical Report." 63rd *Annual Report of the Inspectors of the State Penitentiary for the Eastern District of Pennsylvania*. Philadelphia, 1892.

Baelz, Erwin. *Awakening Japan: The Diary of a German Doctor*. Edited by Toku Baelz. Translated by Eden and Cedar Paul. Viking Press, 1932.

Baggs, Albert Edward. *Social Evangel as Nationalism: A Study of the Salvation Army in Japan, 1895–1940*. State U of New York at Buffalo, 1966. 407 pgs. UM. 66–12, 103.

Baldensperger, Fernand. "Introduction." *American Reconstruction: 1865–1870*. Da Capo Press, 1969.

Banno, Junji, and Ohno Kenichi. "The Flexible Structure of Politics in Meiji Japan." Research Paper 07. The Developmental Leadership Program, Apr. 2010. http://www.dlprog.org/ftp/download/Public%20Folder/1%20Research%20Papers/The%20Flexible%20Structure%20of%20Politics%20in%20Meiji%20Japan.pdf.

Barnes, David S. *The Making of a Social Disease: Tuberculosis in Nineteenth-Century France*. U of California P, 1995.

Barr, Alan P., ed. "Agnosticism." *The Major Prose of Thomas Henry Huxley*. U of Georgia P, 1997.

Barrows, John Henry. *A World-Pilgrimage*. Edited by Mary Eleanor Barrows. Chicago, A. C. McClurg and Company, 1897.

Barshay, Andrew E. *State and Intellectual in Imperial Japan: The Public Man in Crisis*. U of California P, 1988.

Bartholomew, James. *The Formation of Science in Japan: Building a Research Tradition*. Yale UP, 1989.

Bartholomew, James R. "Japanese Nobel Candidates in the First Half of the Twentieth Century." Osiris. 2nd Series, Vol. 13—Beyond Joseph Needham: Science, Technology, and Medicine in East and Southeast Asia, 1998, pp. 238–84.

Bartholomew, James R. "Towards a History of Christian Scientists in Japan." *Xavier's Legacies: Catholicism in Modern Japanese Culture*, edited by Kevin M. Doak. UBC Press, 2011.

Bashkirtseff, Marie. *Marie Bashkirtseff: The Journal of a Young Artist, 1860–1884*. Translated by Mary J. Serrano. New York, Cassell, 1889.

Bay, Alexander R. "Beriberi, Military Medicine, and Medical Authority in Prewar Japan." *Japan Review*, vol. 20, 2008, pp. 111–56.

Becker, Harold S. *Outsiders: Studies in the Sociology of Deviance*. Free Press of Glencoe, 1963.

Begbie, Harold. *The Life of General William Booth: The Founder of the Salvation Army*. Vol. 1. New York, Macmillan, 1920.

Bennett, David Malcolm. *The General: William Booth, Volume 1—The Evangelist*. Xulon Press, 2003.

Benthall, Jonathan. "The Red Cross and Red Crescent Movement and Islamic Societies, with Special Reference to Jordan." *British Journal of Middle Eastern Studies*, vol. 24, no. 2, Nov. 1997, pp. 157–77.

Berry, Mary Elizabeth. *Hideyoshi*. Harvard UP, 1989.

Besant, Walter, Sir. *London in the Nineteenth Century*. London, A. & C. Black, 1909.

Best, Ernest E. *Christian Faith and Cultural Crisis, the Japanese Case*. Leiden, E. J. Brill, 1966.

Best, Gary Dean. "Financing a Foreign War: Jacob H. Schiff and Japan, 1904–05." *American Jewish Historical Quarterly*, vol. 61, no. 4, June 1972, pp. 313–24.

Bestor, Theodore. *Tsukiji: The Fish Market at the Center of the World*. U of California P, 2004.

Bibel, David J., and T. H. Chen. "Diagnosis of Plague: An Analysis of the Yersin-Kitasato Controversy." *Bacteriological Reviews*, vol. 40, no. 3, Sept. 1976, pp. 633–51.

Bikle, George B., Jr. *The New Jerusalem: Aspects of Utopianism in the Thought of Kagawa Toyohiko*. U of Arizona P, 1976.

Birnie, Arthur. *An Economic History of Europe, 1760–1930*. Routledge, 1930.

Booth, Bramwell. *Echoes and Memories*. London, Salvationist Publishing and Supplies, 1925.

Booth, William. *Essential Selections from the Writings of General William Booth*. Kessinger Publishing, 2005.

Booth, William. *In Darkest England and the Way Out*. London, The Salvation Army, 1890.

Booth Tucker, Frederick. *The Life of Catherine Booth: The Mother of the Salvation Army*. Vol. 1. London, Simpkin, Marshall, Hamilton, Kent & Co., 1912.

Bordwell, David. *Ozu and the Poetics of Cinema*. U of Michigan Publishing, 2004.

Bowers, John Z. *When the Twain Meet: The Rise of Western Medicine in Japan*. Johns Hopkins UP, 1980.

Bradt, Charles Edwin, William Robert King, and Herbert Ware Reherd. *Around the World: Studies and Stories of Presbyterian Foreign Missions*. Missionary Press, 1912.

Brent, Charles H. "Among the Philippine Mountain Tops." *The Spirit of Missions: An Illustrated Monthly Review of Christian Missions*, vol. 74, no. 2, Feb. 1909, pp. 88–94.

Briggs, Charles A. "The Salvation Army." *The North American Review*, vol. 159, no. 457, Dec. 1894, pp. 697–710.

Browne, Junius Henri. *The Great Metropolis; A Mirror of New York*. Hartford, American Publishing, 1869.

Bryder, Linda. "'Wonderlands of Buttercup, Clover and Daisies': Tuberculosis and the Open-Air School Movement in Britain, 1907–39." *In the Name of the Child: Health and Welfare, 1880–1940*, edited by Roger Cooter. Routledge, 1992.

Buckley, Sarah Craig. "The Training School for Nurses." *Life and Light for Women*, vol. 18, no. 2, Feb. 1888. Boston, Woman's Boards of Missions, 1888.

Bullard, Henry. *A Missionary's Memories*. London, Salvationist Publishing and Supplies, 1946.

Bullivant, Stephen. "Son of God or 'Red Son-of-a-Bitch'? John Steinbeck, Woody Guthrie and Left-Wing Folk Christology." *Journal for Faith, Spirituality and Social Change*, vol. 1, no. 2, May 2008, pp. 243–54.

Bureau for Social Work. *Social Work in Japan*. Tokyo, Home Department, Japanese Government, 1922.

Burkman, Thomas W. "The Urakami Incidents and the Struggle for Religious Toleration in Early Meiji Japan." *Japan's Hidden Christians, 1549–1999*, vol. 2, edited by Stephen R. Turnbull. London, Taylor & Francis, 2000.

Burns, Susan L. "Contemplating Places: The Hospital as Modern Experience in Meiji Japan." *New Directions in the Study of Meiji Japan*, edited by Helen Hardacre with Adam L. Kern. Leiden, Brill, 1997.

Burton, Sir Richard Francis. *Supplemental Nights to the Book of the Thousand Nights and a Night, with Notes Anthropological and Explanatory*. Benares, Kamashastra Society, 1887.

Butler, Glentworth Reeve. *The Diagnostics of Internal Medicine: A Clinical Treatise upon the Recognised Principles of Medical Diagnosis, Prepared for the Use of Students and Practitioners of Medicine*. D. Appleton and Company, 1901.

Calman, Donald. *The Nature and Origins of Japanese Imperialism: A Reinterpretation of the Great Crisis of 1873*. Routledge, 1992.

Cary, Otis. *A History of Christianity in Japan: Protestant Missions*. F. H. Revell, 1909a.

Cary, Otis. *A History of Christianity in Japan: Roman Catholic and Greek Orthodox Missions*. F. H. Revell, 1909b.

Cassell's History of the Russo-Japanese War. Volume I. London, Cassell, 1905.

Chakraborty, A. K. “Estimating Mortality from Tuberculous Meningitis in a Community: Use of Available Epidemiological Parameters in the Indian Context.” *Indian Journal of Tuberculosis*, vol. 47, 2000, pp. 9–12.

Chamberlain, Basil Hall. *Things Japanese: Being Notes on Various Subjects Connected with Japan for the Use of Travellers and Others*. London, Kelly & Walsh, 1905.

Checkland, Olive. *Humanitarianism and the Emperor's Japan, 1877–1977*. St. Martin's Press, 1994.

The Christian Movement in Its Relation to the New Life in Japan. Edited by Daniel Crosby Greene. Tokyo, The Methodist Publishing House, 1905.

The Christian Movement in Japan: Seventh Annual Edition 1909. Edited by Ernest W. Clement and Galen M. Fisher. Tokyo, The Methodist Publishing House, 1909.

Chung, Yuehtsen Juliette. *Struggle for National Survival: Chinese Eugenics in a Transnational Context, 1896–1945*. Routledge, 2002.

“The Church and the World: Missions.” *The Biblical World*, vol. 44, July–Dec. 1914. U of Chicago P, 1914.

The Churchman's Year Book & American Church Almanac, 1920. Vol. XC. R. L. Polk, 1920.

Clark, Robert E. D. *The Christian Stake in Science*. Paternoster Press, 1967.

Clement, Ernest Wilson. *Christianity in Modern Japan*. American Baptist Publication Society, 1905.

Clodd, Edward. *Thomas Henry Huxley*. Dodd, Mead and Company, 1902.

Cobbing, Andrew. *The Japanese Discovery of Victorian Britain: Early Travel Encounters in the Far West*. Surrey, UK, Japan Library, 1998.

Condliffe, J. B. “John Merle Davis: In Memoriam.” *Pacific Affairs*, vol. 34, no. 1, Spring 1961, pp. 66–71.

Coutts, Frederick. *No Discharge in This War*. London, Hodder & Stoughton, 1974.

Coutts, John J. *The Salvationists*. London, Mowbrays, 1977.

Crow, Carl. *Japan and America: A Contrast*. Robert M. McBride, 1916.

Culin, Stewart. *Korean Games: With Notes on the Corresponding Games of China and Japan*. U of Pennsylvania, 1895.

Curtis, Pierson. “Moving Mountains in Japan: The Story of the Founding of the Omi Mission in an Unoccupied Province.” *The Missionary Review of the World*, vol. 37, no. 8/vol. 27, no. 8, Aug. 1914, pp. 606–12.

“第10表　全国の人口階級別市町村数, 人口及び人口の割合 (大正9年～平成12年).” 『日本の人口ー国勢調最終報告書 (平成12年資料編)』. 東京: 総務省, 2005. http://www.e-stat.go.jp/SG1/estat/ListE.do?bid=000000030587&cycode=0 [“Dai 10 hyō zenkoku no jinkō kaikyūbetsu shichōsonsū, jinkō oyobi jinkō no wariai (taishō 9 nen–heisei 12 nen). *Nihon no jinkō—kokusei chōsa saishū hōkokusho (heisei 12 nen shiryō hen)*. Tokyo, Sōmushō tōkei kyoku, 2005.]

Daniel, Thomas M. *Captain of Death: The Story of Tuberculosis*. U of Rochester P, 1997.

Dannenberg, Arthur M., Jr. *Pathogenesis of Human Pulmonary Tuberculosis: Insights from the Rabbit Model*. ASM Press, 2006.

Davidann, Jon Thares. *A World of Crisis and Progress: The American YMCA in Japan, 1890–1930*. London, Associated University Presses, 1998.

Davies, T. Wytton. “Bible Leprosy.” *Old and New Testament Student*, vol. 11, no. 3, Sept. 1890, pp. 142–52.

Davis, Jerome Dean. *Rev. Joseph Hardy Neesima: A Maker of New Japan*. New York, Fleming H. Revell Company, 1894.

Davison, Charles. "The Japanese Earthquake of 1 September 1923." *The Geographical Journal*, vol. 65, no. 1, Jan. 1925, pp. 41–61.

Dazai Jun. "Food and Wealth." Translated by R. J. Kirby. *Transactions of the Asiatic Society of Japan*. Yokohama, The Asiatic Society of Japan, 1907.

De Bary, Wm. Theodore. "Sagehood as a Secular and Spiritual Ideal in Tokugawa Neo-Confucianism." *Principle and Practicality: Essays in Neo-Confucianism and Practical Learning*, edited by Wm. Theodore de Bary and Irene Bloom. Columbia UP, 1979.

De Lange, William. *A History of Japanese Journalism: Japan's Press Club as the Last Obstacle to a Mature Press*. Richmond, Surrey, UK, Japan Library, 1998.

Denison, Charles. "The Limitations to the Eradication of Tuberculosis." *American Medicine*, vol. 12, no. 4, July 1906, pp. 24–28.

Dewey, John. *Essays on China, Japan, and the War, 1918–1919*. The Middle Works of John Dewey, 1899–1924, Volume 11, edited by Jo Ann Boydston. Southern Illinois UP, 1988.

Dohi, Akio. "The First Generation: Christian Leaders in the First Period." *A History of Japanese Theology*, edited by Furuya Yasuo. Wm. B. Eerdmans Publishing Company, 2001.

Dore, R. P. "The Modernizer as a Special Case: Japanese Factory Legislation, 1882–1911." *Comparative Studies in Society and History*, vol. 11, no. 4, Oct. 1969, pp. 433–50.

Dormandy, Thomas. *The White Death: A History of Tuberculosis*. London, Hambledon and London, 2001.

Douglas, Mary. *Leviticus as Literature*. Oxford, UK, Oxford UP, 1999.

Draper, Gideon F. "Missionary Obituaries 1931–32." *The Japan Christian Year Book Continuing the Japan Mission Year Book Being the Thirtieth Issue of The Christian Movement in Japan and Formosa*, edited by Willis C. Lamott. Tokyo, Kyo Bun Kwan, 1932.

Dubos, René, and Jean Dubos. *The White Plague: Tuberculosis, Man, and Society*. Rutgers UP, 1987.

Eddy, Sherwood. *The Students of Asia*. Student Volunteer Movement for Foreign Missions, 1915.

"EDWARD HOWARD HOUSE." *New York Times*, 25 Jan. 1902.

"Electric Lighting in Japan." *The Electric World*, vol. 16, no. 9, 30 Aug. 1890, p. 164.

Eliade, Mircea. *Patterns in Comparative Religion*. Translated by Rosemary Sheed. U of Nebraska P, 1996.

Eller, Paul H. *History of Evangelical Missions*. Evangelical Press, 1942.

Elliott Avedon Virtual Museum of Games at the University of Waterloo. "Flinch" and "Dominoes." 8 Mar. 2010, http://gamesmuseum.uwaterloo.ca/VirtualExhibits/CardGames/Flinch/index.html; 4 Feb. 2010, http://gamesmuseum.uwaterloo.ca/VirtualExhibits/Dominoes/index.html.

Faison, Elyssa. *Managing Women: Disciplining Labor in Modern Japan*. U of California P, 2007.

Falk, Avner. *A Psychoanalytic History of the Jews*. Fairleigh Dickinson UP, 1996.

Faris, John T., D.D. *The Book of Faith in God*. George H. Doran Company, 1915.

Farley, John. *To Cast Out Disease: A History of the International Health Division of the Rockefeller Foundation (1913–1951)*. Oxford, UK, Oxford UP, 2004.

Farrar, Frederic W. "The Salvation Army." *Harper's Monthly*, vol. 82, May 1891, pp. 897–906.

Faust, Allen K. "Tuberculosis and Anti-tuberculosis Work in Japan." *Journal of the Outdoor Life*, vol. X, no. 12, Dec. 1913, pp. 353–57.

"First Census of the Japanese Empire Gives Its Total Population as 77,005,112." *New York Times*, 2 Mar. 1921, p. 10.

Fisher, Galen. *Creative Forces in Japan*. The Missionary Education Movement of the United States and Canada, 1923.

Fisher, Galen M. "Prospecting in Rural Japan." *The North American Student*, vol. 2, no. 7, Apr. 1914, pp. 329–33.

Foster, Michael, and Thomas Henry Huxley. *Michael Foster and Thomas Henry Huxley, Correspondence, 1865–1895*, edited by W. F. Bynum and Caroline Overy (*Medical History*, Supplement No. 28). London, The Wellcome Trust Centre for the History of Medicine at UCL, 2009.

Fowler, Edward. *The Rhetoric of Confession: Shishosetsu in Early Twentieth-Century Japanese Fiction*. U of California P, 1992.

Frank, Ronald. "General Provision." *History of Law in Japan since 1868*, edited by Wilhelm Röhl. Leiden, Brill, 2005.

Franklin, James H. "John Lincoln Dearing." *Missions: An International Baptist Monthly Magazine*, vol. 8, no. 1, Jan. 1917.

French, Paul. *Carl Crow—A Tough Old China Hand: The Life, Times, and Adventures of an American in Shanghai*. Hong Kong UP, 2006.

Frühstück, Sabine. *Colonizing Sex: Sexology and Social Control in Modern Japan*. U of California P, 2003.

Fujio, Ikado. "The Origin of the Social Status of Protestant Christianity in Japan: Chapter III The Emergence of the White-Collar Class (1891–1905)." *Contemporary Religions in Japan*, vol. 2, no. 2, June 1961, pp. 30–68.

福田真人. "佳人と天才の病: 結核のロマン化." 『疫病の時代』. Ed. 酒井しづ. 東京: 大修館書店, 1999. [Fukuda Mahito. "Kajin to tensai no yamai: kekkaku no romanka." *Ekibyō no jidai*, edited by Sakai Shizu. Tokyo, Taishukanshoten, 1999.]

福田真人. 『結核という文化: 病の比較文化史』. 東京: 中公新書, 2001. [Fukuda Mahito. *Kekkaku toiu bunka: yamai no hikakubunkashi*. Tokyo, Chūkōshinsho, 2001.]

福田真人. 『北里柴三郎: 熱と誠があれば』. 東京: ミネルヴァ書房, 2008. [Fukuda Mahito. *Kitasato Shibasaburō: Netsu to makoto ga areba*. Tokyo, Mineruva shobō, 2008.]

Fukuda, Mahito H. "Public Health in Modern Japan: From Regimen to Hygiene." *The History of Public Health and the Modern State*, edited by Dorothy Porter. Amsterdam, Editions Rodopi B. V., 1994.

Fukuzawa, Yukichi. *Autobiography*. Translated by Eiichi Kiyooka. Columbia UP, 1966.

Furukawa, Y. *Japanese Medicine*. Translated by John Ruhräh. Paul B. Hoeber, 1934.

Garon, Sheldon. *Molding Japanese Minds: The State in Everyday Life*. Princeton UP, 1997.

Garon, Sheldon. "State and Family in Modern Japan: A Historical Perspective." *Economy and Society*, vol. 39, no. 3, Aug. 2010, pp. 317–36.

Garon, Sheldon. *The State and Labor in Modern Japan*. U of California P, 1987.

Garon, Sheldon. "The World's Oldest Debate? Prostitution and the State in Imperial Japan, 1900–1945." *The American Historical Review*, vol. 98, no. 3, June 1993, pp. 710–32.

"General Missionary Intelligence: Japan—Korea, A Hospital for the Poor." *The Missionary Review of the World*, vol. 34, no. 12, Dec. 1911, pp. 951–54.

Gill, Tom. *Men of Uncertainty: The Social Organization of Day Laborers in Contemporary Japan*. State U of New York P, 2001.

Gleason, George. *What Shall I Think of Japan?* New York, Macmillan, 1921.

Gluck, Carol. "Thinking with the Past: History Writing in Modern Japan." *Sources of Japanese Tradition, Volume Two: 1600–2000*. 2nd edition. Compiled by Wm. Theodore de Bary, Carol Gluck, and Arthur E. Tiedemann. Columbia UP, 2005.

Goldstein, Sanford, and Seishi Shinoda. "Notes (Sad Toys)." *Romaji Diary and Sad Toys*. Tuttle Publishing, 1985.

Gordon, Rev. Marquis Lafayette. *An American Missionary in Japan*. Boston, Houghton, Mifflin and Company, 1892.

Greene, Daniel Crosby. *The Christian Movement in its Relation to the New Life in Japan*. 2nd issue. Yokohama, Fukuin Printing, 1904.

Greene, Daniel Crosby. "Conditions under Which Missionary World Has Been Carried On since 1883." *Proceedings of the General Conference of Protestant Missionaries in Japan, Held in Tokyo October 24–31, 1900*. Tokyo, Methodist Publishing House, 1901.

Grew, Joseph C. Preface. *Dr. Rudolf Bolling Teusler: An Adventure in Christianity*, by Howard Chandler Robbins and George K. MacNaught. Charles Scribner's Sons, 1942.

Grierson, Robert. "The Medical Situation." *The Christian Movement in Japan, Korea and Formosa: A Year Book of Christian Work*, 22nd issue, edited by D. C. Holtom. Tokyo, Federation of Christian Missions Japan, 1924, 379–92.

Griffis, William Elliot. *Dux Christus: An Outline Study of Japan*. New York, Macmillan, 1904.

Griffis, William Elliot. *Hepburn of Japan and His Wife and Helpmates: A Life Story of Toil for Christ*. Westminster Press, 1913.

Griffith, J. P. Crozer. *The Diseases of Infants and Children*. Vol. 1. W. B. Saunders Company, 1919.

Grosset, Jacques. "Guest Commentary—*Mycobacterium tuberculosis* in the Extracellular Compartment: An Underestimated Adversary." *Antimicrobial Agents and Chemotherapy*, vol. 47, no. 3, Mar. 2003, pp. 833–36.

Gulick, John Thomas. "Christianity and the Evolution of Rational Life: A Statement Made on Solicitation of the Late George H. Romanes." *Bibliotheca Sacra*, vol. 53, edited by G. Frederick Wright and Z. Swift Holbrook. Oberlin, Bibliotheca Sacra Company, 1896.

Gulick, Sidney L. *Working Women of Japan*. Missionary Education Movement of the United States and Canada, 1915.

Gulick, Sidney L. *The White Peril in the Far East: An Interpretation of the Significance of the Russo-Japanese War*. Fleming H. Revell Company, 1905.

Gundert, Wilhelm. *Japanische religiongeschichte; die Religionen der Japaner und Koreaner in geschichtlichem Abriss*. Tokyo, Japanisch-deutsches Kulturinsitut, 1935.

Grundfossen, Peter D. *A Study of the Arguments for and against the Factory Act of 1833 Used by Members of Parliament in the House of Commons*. MST Thesis at Porland State University, July 30, 1965.

Haak, Ronald O. "The Zesty, Structured World of a Weaver." *Journal of Asian and African Studies*, vol. 10, no. 1–2, 1975, pp. 42–50.

Hagin, Fred Eugene. *The Cross in Japan: A Study of Achievement and Opportunity*. Fleming H. Revell Company, 1914.

Hall, Clarence W. *Adventurers for God*. Harper & Brothers, 1959.

Hall, M. Penelope. *The Social Services of Modern England*. Routledge and Kegan Paul, 1952.

"Handbooks on the Missions of the Episcopal Church. Japan." The National Council of the Protestant Episcopal Church, 1934.

Hane, Mikiso. *Peasants, Rebels, and Outcastes: The Underside of Modern Japan*. Pantheon Books, 1982.

Hara, Kimi. "Challenges to Education for Girls and Women in Modern Japan: Past and Present." *Japanese Women: New Feminist Perspectives on the Past, Present, and Future*, edited by Kumiko Fujimura-Fanselow and Atsuko Kameda. The Feminist Press at the City U of New York, 1995.

Hardacre, Helen. *Lay Buddhism in Contemporary Japan: Reiyukai Kyodan*. Princeton UP, 1984.

Harita, Nozomi. "Matsuda, Sanya (1870–1930)." *Historical Dictionary of the Salvation Army*. Edited by Major John G. Merritt. Scarecrow Press, 2006.

橋本龍太郎. 『紡織人事の話』. 大阪: 工場世界社, 1931. [Hashimoto Ryūtarō. *Bōshoku jinji no hanashi*. Osaka, Kōjōsekaisha, 1931.]

Havens, Thomas R. H. "Comte, Mill, and the Thought of Nishi Amane in Meiji Japan." *The Journal of Asian Studies*, vol. 27, no. 2, Feb. 1968, pp. 217–28.

"HEALING THE HEATHEN SICK; BISHOP STEVENS ON MEDICAL MISSIONS IN CHINA, JAPAN, AND MEXICO." *New York Times*, 10 Jan. 1881.

"Health." *The Survey*, vol. 33, no. 25, 20 Mar. 1915, p. 675.

"HEATHEN CRUELTY AND FANATICISM; Missionaries Tell of Harrowing Conditions in Eastern Lands. CRIME OF INDIAN WIDOWHOOD Twenty-Seven Million Women Accursed of the Gods and of Men—Degradation of Blind Girls in China—Christian Literature." *New York Times*, 1 May 1900.

Herschel, William J. *Nature*, vol. 51, no. 1308, pp. 77–78.

"Heylman—Tooker." *New York Times*, 5 Oct. 1922.

Hijiya-Kirschnereit, Irmela. *Rituals of Self-Revelation: Shishōsetsu as Literary Genre and Socio-cultural Phenomenon*. Harvard University Asia Center, 1996.

日野原茂明. 『戦争といのちと聖路加国際病院ものがたり』. 東京: 初学間, 2015. [Hinohara Shigeaki. *Sensou to inochi to Seirukabyouin monogatari*. Tokyo: Shogakukan, 2015.]

平山洋. 『諭吉の流儀:「福翁自伝」を読む』. 東京: PHP研究所, 2009. [Hirayama Yō. *Yukichi no ryūgi: fukuō jiden wo yomu*. Tokyo, PHP kenkyūjo, 2009.]

Hitchcock, Alfred M. *Over Japan Way*. Henry Holt and Company, 1917.

Holmes, T. "Psychosocial and Psychophysiological Studies of Tuberculosis." *Physiological Correlates of Psychological Disorders*, edited by R. Roessler and N. Greenfeld. U of Wisconsin Press, 1962.

Hornbeck, Stanley K. "Review." *The American Political Science Review*, vol. 11, no. 4, Nov. 1917, pp. 774–77.

細井和喜蔵. 『女工哀史』. 東京: 岩波書店, 1988. [Hosoi Wakizō. *Jokō aishi*. Tokyo, Iwanamishoten, 1988.]

House, Edward. H. *Yone Santo: A Child of Japan*. Chicago, Bedford, Clarke & Co., 1888.

Howes, John F. "Japanese Christianity and the State: From Jesuit Confrontation/Competition to Uchimura's Noninstitutional Movement/Protestantism." *Indigenous Responses to Western Christianity*, edited by Steven Kaplan. New York UP, 1995.

Huffman, James L. *Creating a Public: People and Press in Meiji Japan*. U of Hawaiʻi Press, 1997.

Huffman, James L. “Edward Howard House: In the Service of Meiji Japan.” *Pacific Historical Review*, vol. 56, no. 2, May 1987, pp. 231–58.

Huffman, James L. *A Yankee in Meiji Japan: The Crusading Journalist Edward H. House.* Rowman & Littlefield, 2003.

Humphreys, Mary Guy. “Trade Unions in Japan.” *The Century Illustrated Monthly Magazine*, vol. LXI, Nov. 1900 to Apr. 1901. The Century Co., 1901.

Hunter, Janet. “Gendering the Labor Market: Evidence from the Interwar Textile Industry.” *Gendering Modern Japanese History*, edited by Barbara Molony and Kathleen Uno. Harvard UP, 2005.

Huffman, James L. “Textile Factories, Tuberculosis and the Quality of Life in Industrializing Japan.” Working Paper No. 4/92. London School of Economics & Political Science, Working Papers in Economic History, June 1992.

Hutcheon, Linda, and Michael Hutcheon. *Opera: Desire, Disease, Death.* U of Nebraska Press, 1996.

Hutchinson, John F. *Champions of Charity: War and the Rise of the Red Cross.* Westview Press, 1996.

Huxley, Thomas H. “Agnosticism.” *Christianity and Agnosticism: A Controversy.* New York, D. Appleton and Company, 1889.

Huxley, Thomas H., F. R. S. *Social Diseases and Worse Remedies: Letters to the “Times” on Mr. Booth's Scheme.* London, Macmillan, 1891.

Iijima, Wataru. “Colonial Medicine and Malaria Eradication in Okinawa in the Twentieth Century: From the Colonial Model to the United States Model.” *Disease, Colonialism, and the State: Malaria in Modern East Asian History*, edited by Ka-che Yip. Hong Kong UP, 2009.

Ikawa, Hiroshi. “The Development of the Prewar Local Autonomy System (1909–1929).” *Historical Development of Japanese Local Governance*, vol. 3. Tokyo, Council of Local Authorities for International Relations (CLAIR), 2010.

Ikegami, Naoki. “Japan.” *Comparative Health Policy in the Asia-Pacific*, edited by Robin Gauld. Berkshire, UK, Open UP, 2005.

Imbrie, William. “An Interview with Count Katsura.” *The Christian Movement in Its Relation to the New Life in Japan*, 2nd issue, edited by Daniel Crosby Greene. Yokohama, The Fukuin Printing Co., Ltd., 1904.

Imperial University of Japan (Teikoku Daigaku). The Calendar for the Year 1890–91. Tokyo, Imperial University of Japan, 1891.

“An International Hospital for Japan: Memorial to the Trustees of the Carnegie Endowment.” *Some Roads Towards Peace: A Report to the Trustees of the Endowment on Observations Made in China and Japan in 1912*, edited by Charles W. Eliot. The Carnegie Endowment for International Peace, 1913.

International Labour Office. *Industrial Labour in Japan*, vol. 5. Edited by Janet Hunter. Routledge, 2000.

Ion, A. Hamish. *The Cross in the Dark Valley: The Canadian Protestant Missionary Movement in the Japanese Empire, 1931–1945.* Wilfrid Laurier UP, 1999.

Ion, A. Hamish. *The Cross and the Rising Sun: The British Protestant Missionary Movement in Japan, Korea, and Taiwan, 1865–1945.* Wilfrid Laurier UP, 1993.

敬子 五十子. “明治期における「看護」の問題: 仰臥の医師、近藤常次郎をめぐって.” 『尚美学園大学総合政策研究紀要』1: 19–34. [Irako Keiko. “Nursing in the Meiji

Era: The Contribution of Tsunejiro Kondo." *Bulletin of Policy and Management, Shobi-Gakuen University*, vol. 1, pp. 19–34.]
Ise, Masaomi. "Entrepreneur Ichizaemon Morimura." *Japan Close-Up*, Aug. 2007, pp. 20–24.
Ishida, Takeshi. "The Meaning of 'Independence' in the Thought of Uchimura Kanzō." *Culture and Religion in Japanese-American Relations: Essays on Uchimura Kanzō, 1861–1930*, edited by Ray A. Moore. Center for Japanese Studies, U of Michigan, 1981.
石原修.『女工と結核』. 東京: 光生館, 1970. [Ishihara Osamu. *Jokō to kekkaku*. Tokyo, Kōseikan, 1970.]
Ishii, Noriko Kawamura. *American Women Missionaries at Kobe College, 1873–1909: New Dimensions in Gender*. Routledge, 2004.
Ishikawa, Takuboku. *Romaji Diary and Sad Toys*. Translated by Sanford Goldstein and Seishi Shinoda. Tuttle Publishing, 1985.
Ishizuka, Hiromichi. "The Early History of the Control of Water-Borne Diseases in Tokyo." *Project on Technology Transfer, Transformation, and Development: The Japanese Experience*. Tokyo, The United Nations University, 1983.
Ishizuka, Hiromichi. "The Slum Dwellings and the Urban Renewal Scheme in Tokyo, 1868–1923." *The Developing Economies*, vol. 19, Issue 2, 1981, pp. 169–193.
Ito, Araki. "Tuberculosis in Tokyo and Vicinity." *Transactions of the Sixth International Congress on Tuberculosis. Washington, September 28 to October 5, 1908*. W. F. Fell Company, 1908.
Ito, Ken K. "The Family and the Nation in Tokutomi Roka's *Hototogisu*." *Harvard Journal of Asiatic Studies*, vol. 60, no. 2, Dec. 2000, pp. 489–536.
Jaffe, Richard, ed. *Selected Works of D.T. Suzuki*. Vol. I, Zen. U of California Press, 2014.
Jammé, Anna C. "Nursing Education in Japan." *The American Journal of Nursing*, vol. 23, no. 9, June 1923, pp. 767–73.
Jannetta, Ann Bowman. "From Physician to Bureaucrat: The Case of Nagayo Sensai." *New Directions in the Study of Meiji Japan*, edited by Helen Hardacre with Adam L. Kern. Leiden, Brill, 1997.
Jannetta Ann Bowman, and Samuel H. Preston. "Two Centuries of Mortality Change in Central Japan: The Evidence from a Temple Death Register." *Population Studies*, vol. 45, no. 3, 1991, pp. 417–36.
"Japan in 1909." *The British Medical Journal*, vol. 1, no. 2681, 18 May 1912, pp. 1139–40.
"JAPANESE WAR CASUALTIES; Suppressed Statistics Come to Public Knowledge Via Berlin." *New York Times*, 10 Sept. 1911.
"Japan's Factory Law." *Grey River Argus*, 17 Jan. 1911.
Johnston, William. "A Genealogy of Tubercular Diseases in Japan." *Social History of Medicine*, vol. 7, no. 2, 1994, pp. 247–67.
Johnston, William. *The Modern Epidemic: A History of Tuberculosis in Japan*. Council on East Asian Studies, Harvard University, 1995.
Kafka, Franz. "Letters to Felice." *The Basic Kafka*. Translated by James Stern and Elizabeth Duckworth. Washington Square Press, 1979.
Kagawa, Toyohiko. *Christ and Japan*. Translated by William Axling. Friendship Press, 1934.
Kagawa, Toyohiko. *Living Out Christ's Love: Selected Writings of Toyohiko Kagawa*. Edited by Keith Beasley-Topliffe. Upper Room Books, 1998.
Kagawa, Toyohiko. *Meditations on the Cross*. Willet, Clark & Co., 1935.

籠山京. "解説: 女工と結核." 『女工と結核』. 第5巻. 東京: 光生館, 1970. [Kagoyama Takashi. "Kaisetsu: jokō to kekkaku." In Ishihara. *Jōko to kekkaku*. vol. 5. Tokyo, Kōseikan, 1970.]

梶井基次郎. 『梶井基次郎全集』. 全4巻. 東京: 筑摩文庫, 1999. [Kajii Motojirō. *Kajii Motojirō zenshū*. Zen3kan. Tokyo, Chikuma Shobō, 1999.]

鹿子木敏範. 『北里柴三郎回顧』. 熊本: 肥後医育記念館, 1978. [Kanogoki Toshinori. *Kitasato Shibasaburō kaiko*. Kumamoto: Higoiikunenkan, 1978.]

柄谷公人. 『意味という病』. 東京: 講談社, 1989. [Karatani Kōjin. *Imi toiu yamai*. Tokyo, Kōdansha, 1989.]

Karatani, Kōjin. *Origins of Modern Japanese Literature*. Translated by Brett de Bary. Duke UP, 1993.

Kasza, Gregory J. *The State and the Mass Media in Japan, 1918–1945*. U of California Press, 1988.

片岡寛光. 『国民リーダー大隈重信』. 東京: 冨山房インターナショナル, 2009. [Kataoka Hiromitsu. *Kokumin ri-da-ōkuma shigenobu*. Tokyo, Fuzanbō Inta-nashonaru, 2009.]

Kawakami, Kiyoshi Karl. *The Political Ideas of Modern Japan: An Interpretation*. U of Iowa Press, 1903.

川俣馨一. 『日本赤十字社発達史』. 東京：日本赤十字社発達史発行所, 1909. [Kawamata Keiichi. *Nihon Sekijujisha hattatsushi*. Tokyo, Nihon Sekijujisha Hattatsushi Hakkōjo, 1909.]

Kayne, George Gregory, Walter Pagel, and Laurence O'Shaughnessy. *Pulmonary Tuberculosis: Pathology, Diagnosis, Management and Prevention*. London, Oxford UP, 1939.

Keene, Donald. *Dawn to the West: Japanese Literature of the Modern Era*. Vol 1. "Fiction." Holt, Rinehart and Winston, 1984.

Keene, Donald. *Emperor of Japan: Meiji and His World, 1852–1912*. Columbia UP, 2002.

Keyes, Ralph. *Euphemania: Our Love Affair with Euphemisms*. Little, Brown and Company, 2010.

桐生操. 『知っておきたい—世界の悪人・暴君・独裁者』. 東京: 西東社, 2008. [Kiryū Misao. *Shitteokitai—Sekai no akunin, bōkun, dokusaisha*. Tokyo, Seitōsha, 2008.]

Kishimoto, Eitaro. "The Characteristics of Labour-Management Relations in Japan and Their Historical Formation." *Kyoto University Economic Review*, vol. 35, no. 2, Oct. 1965, pp. 33–55.

Kitasato, Shibasaburō. "The Behavior of Native Japanese Cattle in Regard to Tuberculosis (Perlsucht)." *Collected Papers of Shibasaburo Kitasato*. Tokyo: Kitasato Institute & Kitasato University, 1977a.

Kitasato, Shibasaburō. "Tuberculosis and its Prevention in Japan: Special Lecture Prepared for the International Congress on Tuberculosis. Washington, September 28 to October 12, 1908." *Transactions of the Sixth International Congress on Tuberculosis, Volume 8: A Series of Public Lectures*. William F. Fell Company, 1908.

Kitasato, Shibasaburō. "Ueber das Verhalten der einheimischen japanischen Rinder zur Tuberculose (Perlsucht)." *Collected Papers of Shibasaburo Kitasato*. Tokyo, Kitasato Institute & Kitasato University, 1977b.

Knibbs, G. H., C.M.G. *Official Year Book of the Commonwealth of Australia, Containing Authoritative Statistics for the Period 1901–1918 and Corrected Statistics for the Period 1788 to 1900*. Melbourne, Commonwealth Bureau of Census and Statistics, 1919.

Koch, Robert. "The Aetiology of Tuberculosis. An Address Delivered by Dr. Robert Koch before the Physiological Society of Berlin." Translated by W. D. Oakley. *Canada Medical and Surgical Journal*, June 1882, pp. 649–55.

小松良夫. 『結核: 日本近代史の裏側』. 大阪: 清風堂書店, 2000. [Komatsu Yoshio. *Kekkaku: Nihon kindaishi no uragawa*. Osaka, Seifudōshoten, 2000.]

Konishi, Sho. "Translation and Conversion Beyond Western Modernity: Tolstoian Religion in Meiji Japan." *Converting Cultures: Religion, Ideology and Transformations of Modernity*, edited by Dennis Washburn and A. Kevin Reinhart. Leiden, Brill, 2007.

Kosuge, N. Margaret. "The 'Non-religious' Red Cross Emblem and Japan." *International Review of the Red Cross*, no. 849, Mar. 2003, pp. 75–93.

Kowner, Rotem. "Becoming an Honorary Civilized Nation: Remaking Japan's Military Image during the Russo-Japanese War, 1904–1905." *The Historian*, vol. 64, issue 1, Sept. 2001, pp. 19–38.

Krämer, Hans Martin. "Beyond the Dark Valley: Reinterpreting Christian Reactions to the 1939 Religious Organizations Law." *Japanese Journal of Religious Studies*, vol. 38, no. 1, 2011.

Kublin, Hyman. *Asian Revolutionary: The Life of Sen Katayama*. Princeton UP, 1964.

Kuriyama, Shigehisa. "Between Mind and Eye: Japanese Anatomy in the Eighteenth Century." *Paths to Asian Medical Knowledge*, edited by Charles Leslie and Allan Young. U of California Press, 1992.

Lambroza, Shlomo. "The Tsarist Government and the Pogroms of 1903–06." *Modern Judaism*, vol. 7, no. 3, Oct. 1987, pp. 287–96.

Langland, James, M.A., ed. "Approximate Value of Foreign Coins." *The Chicago Daily News Almanac and Year-Book for 1911*, vol. 27. The Chicago Daily News Company, 1910.

Larsson, Flora. *My Best Men Are Women*. The Salvation Army, 1974.

League of Nations. *International Labor Conference: First Annual Meeting (October 29, 1919–November 29, 1919)*. Washington, DC, Government Printing Office, 1920.

Lebra, Joyce C. *Ōkuma Shigenobu: Statesman of Meiji Japan*. Canberra, Australian National UP, 1973.

Lee, Kyoungae. "Uchimura's View of Atonement in *Kyūanroku* (*The Search for Peace*)." *Living for Jesus and Japan: The Social and Theological Thought of Uchimura Kanzō*, edited by Shibuya Hiroshi and Chiba Shin. William B. Eerdmans, 2013.

Lee, Robert. "Service to Christ and Country: Uchimura's Search for Meaning." *Culture and Religion in Japanese-American Relations: Essays on Uchimura Kanzō, 1861–1930*, edited by Ray A. Moore. Center for Japanese Studies, The U of Michigan, 1981.

Lenoir, Timothy. "Laboratories, Medicine and Public Life in Germany, 1830–1849: Ideological Roots of the Institutional Revolution." *The Laboratory Revolution in Medicine*, edited by Andrew Cunningham and Perry Williams. Cambridge, UK, Cambridge UP, 2002.

Lewis, Alice G. "Japan Notes: A Visit to Omi Mission." *The Friend*, vol. 95, no. 34, 23 Feb. 1922, p. 402.

Linton, Derek S. *Emil von Behring: Infectious Disease, Immunology, Serum Therapy*. American Philosophical Society, 2005.

Liu, Shiyung. "The Ripples of Rivalry: The Spread of Modern Medicine from Japan to Its Colonies." *East Asian Science, Technology and Society: An International Journal*, vol. 2, 2008, pp. 47–71.

"Local News." *The Westfield Leader*. 12 Mar. 1929.

Loch, C. S. *An Examination of "General" Booth's Social Scheme: Adopted by the Council of the London Charity Organisation Society*. 2nd edition. London, Swan, Sonnenschein & Co., 1890.

Longford, Joseph H. *Japan of the Japanese*. Charles Scribner's Sons, 1912.

Loomis, H., Rev. "Christian Work among Japanese Soldiers." *The Missionary Review of the World*, edited by Rev. Arthur T. Pierson, vol. 28 (or 18 in the "new series"), no. 2, Feb. 1905.

Lord, Herbert A. *A Man Set Apart (Gunpei Yamamuro, O.F.)*. The Salvation Army, 1970.

Ludvigsson, J. F., J. Wahlstrom, J. Grunewald, A. Ekbom, and S.M. Montgomery. "Coeliac Disease and Risk of Tuberculosis: A Population Based Cohort Study." *Thorax*, vol. 62, 2007, pp. 23–28.

Lyon, William H. "An American in Japan: William Merrell Vories (Hitotsuyanagi), 1905–1964." 同志社アメリカ研究第39号, 2003, pp. 37–60.

Mackie, Vera. *Creating Socialist Women in Japan: Gender, Labour and Activism, 1900–1937*. Cambridge, UK, Cambridge UP, 1997.

Maeda, Ai. "Their Time as Children: A Study of Higuchi Ichiyō's *Growing Up (Takekurabe)*." Translated by Edward Fowler. *Text and the City: Essays on Japanese Modernity*, edited by James A. Fujii. Duke UP, 2004.

Maegawa, Masayuki. "Formation et déformation de l'idée de politique sociale à la fin de l'ère Meiji." *Zibun*, no. 37, 2003/2004, pp. 105–27.

Marshall, Byron K. *Capitalism and Nationalism in Prewar Japan: The Ideology of the Business Elite, 1868–1941*. Stanford UP, 1967.

Maruyama, Masao. "Theory and Psychology of Ultra-nationalism." *Thought and Behaviour in Modern Japanese Politics*. Translated by Ivan Morris. Oxford, UK, Oxford UP, 1963.

Mass, William, and Andrew Robertson. "From Textiles to Automobiles: Mechanical and Organizational Innovation in the Toyoda Enterprises, 1895–1933." *Business and Economic History*, vol. 25, no. 2, Winter 1996, pp. 1–37.

Mathews, Basil. *John R. Mott, World Citizen*. Harper & Brothers, 1934.

Matsumoto, Sheila. "Women in Factories." *Women in Changing Japan*, edited by Joyce Lebra, Joy Paulson, and Elizabeth Powers. Stanford UP, 1978.

Matsuoka, Asa. "Labor Conditions of Women and Children." *Bulletin of the United States Bureau of Labor Statistics*, no. 558, Nov. 1931.

McCaul, Ethel, R. R. C. *Under the Care of the Japanese War Office*. London, Cassell, 1904.

McDannell, Colleen. *Picturing Faith: Photography and the Great Depression*. Yale UP, 2004.

McLaren, W. W. Review. *The American Political Science Review*, vol. 12, no. 2, May 1918, pp. 322–24.

Mclean, Archibald. *The History of the Foreign Christian Missionary Society*. Fleming H. Revell Company, 1919.

Mechanic, David. *Medical Sociology: A Selective View*. Toronto, Collier-Macmillan, 1968.

"Medicine in the Far East." *The Journal of the American Medical Association*, vol. 33, 11 Nov. 1899, pp. 1238–39.

Meikeljohn, A. "Industrial Health—Meeting the Challenge." *British Journal of Industrial Medicine*, vol. 16, no. 1, Jan. 1959, pp. 1–10.

Minami, Ryoshin. "The Turning Point in the Japanese Economy." *The Quarterly Journal of Economics*, vol. 82, no. 3, Aug. 1968, pp. 380–402.

御崎夕子. "明治女医の基礎資料." 『日本医学雑誌』, vol. 54, no. 3, 2008. [Misaki Yūko. "Meiji joi no kisoshiryou." *Nihon ishigaku zasshi*, vol. 54, no. 3, 2008.]

三田村徳二郎. "胤道の世界道徳." 『思いでの青山胤道先生』. 熊谷謙二編. 東京: 青山先生誕生百年際準備委員会, 1959. [Mitamura Tokujirō. "Tanemichi no sekai dōtoku." *Omoide no aoyama tanemichi sensei*, edited by Kumagai Kenji. Tokyo, Aoyama Sensei Tanjō hyakunensai junbi iinkai, 1959.]

三谷種吉. 『基督教百話』. 東京: 基督教書類會社, 1923. [Mitani Tanekichi. *Kirisutokyō Hyakuwa*. Tokyo, Kirisutokyō shoruikaisha, 1923.]

Mitman, Gregg. "Geographies of Hope: Mining the Frontiers of Health in Denver and Beyond, 1870–1965." *Osiris*, vol. 19, 2nd series, 2004, pp. 93–111.

Miyahira, Nozomu. "Christian Theology under Feudalism, Nationalism and Democracy in Japan." *Christian Theology in Asia*, edited by Sebastian C. H. Kim. Cambridge, UK: Cambridge UP, 2008.

Miyajima, Mikinosuke. *Robert Koch and Shibasaburo Kitasato*. Geneva, Sonor, 1931.

Miyamori, Asatarō. *A Life of Mr. Yukichi Fukuzawa*. Revised by E. H. Vickers. Tokyo, Maruzen Kabushiki Kaisha, 1902.

Miyazaki, Shigeki. "The Martens Clause and International Humanitarian Law." *Études et essais sur le droit international humanitaire et sur les principles de la Croix-Rouge, en l'honneur de Jean Pictet,* edited by Christophe Swinarski. Geneva, le Comité international de la Croix-Rouge, 1984, 443–44.

Mjagkij, Nina. "The Negro Service Committee and African-American Soldiers." *Politics and Progress: American Society and the State since 1865*, edited by Andrew Edmund Kersten and Kriste Lindenmeyer. Westport, Praeger Publishers, 2001.

Molony, Barbara. "Activism among Women in the Taishō Cotton Textile Industry." *Recreating Japanese Women, 1600–1945*, edited by Gail Lee Bernstein. U of California Press, 1991.

Molyneux, J. F., with James A. Lowson. "Notes on the Bubonic Plague, Hongkong Epidemic, 1894, with Professor Kitasato's Preliminary Notice." *The Australasian Medical Gazette: The Journal of the Australasian Branches of the British Medical Association*, vol. 18, Jan. to Dec. 1899. Sydney, New South Wales Branch of the British Medical Association, 1899.

Monbushō. "Part IV: Higher Education." *Education in Japan*. Tokyo, The Department of Education, 1904.

Mori, Toru. "Recent Trends in Tuberculosis, Japan." *Emerging Infectious Diseases*, vol. 6, no. 6, Nov.–Dec. 2000.

Morley, Patricia. *The Mountain Is Moving: Japanese Women's Lives*. U of British Columbia P, 1999.

Morris, J. *Makers of Japan*. London, Methuen, 1906.

Morse, Edward S. *Japan Day by Day*. Vol II. Houghton Mifflin, 1917.

Morse, Richard C. *My Life with Young Men: Fifty Years in the Young Men's Christian Association*. The International Committee of Young Men's Christian Associations, 1918.

Mortality Statistics of Tuberculosis by Prefecture, Each City and County, Health Center and Individual Cities, Towns and Villages, 1947. Tokyo, Department of Statistics and Investigation, Welfare Minister's Secretariat, Dec. 1949.

Murphy, U. G. *The Social Evil in Japan and Allied Subjects, with Statistics, Social Evil Test Cases, and Progress of the Anti-brothel Movement*. Methodist Publishing House, 1908.

Murray, Nicholas. *Kafka*. Yale UP, 2004.

Najita, Tetsuo. *Japan: The Intellectual Foundations of Modern Japanese Politics*. U of Chicago P, 1974.

Najita, Tetsuo, and H. D. Harootunian. "Japan's Revolt against the West." *Modern Japanese Thought*, edited by Bob Tadashi Wakabayashi. Cambridge, UK, Cambridge UP, 1998.

中川右介. 『歌舞伎座物語明治の名優と興行師たちの奮闘史』. 東京: PHP研究所, 2010. [Nakagawa Yūsuke. *Kabukiza monogatari: meiji no meiyū to kogyōshitachi no funtōshi*. Tokyo, PHP kenkyūjo, 2010.]

中村徳吉. 『聖路加国際病院創設者: ルドルフ・ボリング・トイスラー小伝』. 東京: 聖路加国際病院, 1968. [Nakamura Tokukichi. *Seirukakokusaibyōin sōsetsusha: rudorufu boringu toisura-shouden*. Tokyo, Seirukakokusaibyōin, 1968.]

中瀬安清. "北里柴三郎資料館49—北里柴三郎博士のライフワーク: 結核の予防, 撲滅." [Nakase Yasukiyo. "Kitasato Shibasaburō shiryōkan 49—Kitasato Shibasaburō hakushi no raifuwa-ku: kekkaku no yobō, bokumetsu." *The Kitasato*, no. 49, Winter 2006, pp. 7–9.]

Nakayama, Kazuhisa. "The Characteristics of the Japanese Labour Law and Its Problems." *Waseda Bulletin of Comparative Law*, vol. 14, 1993, pp. 1–9.

National Science Foundation's Government-University-Industry Research Roundtable. *The Academic Research Enterprise within the Industrialized Nations: Comparative Perspectives, Report of a Symposium*. National Academies Press, 1990.

Nelson, Jack E. "Moral Entrepreneuring in Japan: A Labeling Theory Analysis of the Salvation Army's Efforts." *Review of Religious Research*, vol. 40, no. 1, Sept. 1998, pp. 35–54.

"News of the Week." *Medical Record: Weekly Journal of Medicine and Surgery*, vol. 99, 25 June 1921, pp. 1106–8.

Nimura, Kazuo. *The Ashio Riot of 1907: A Social History of Mining in Japan*. Translated by Terry Boardman and Andrew Gordon. Duke UP, 1997.

Nolte, Sharon H., and Sally Ann Hastings. "The Meiji State's Policy Toward Women, 1890–1910." *Recreating Japanese Women, 1600–1945*, edited by Gail Lee Bernstein. U of California P, 1991.

Notehelfer, F. G. *American Samurai: Captain L.L. Janes and Japan*. Princeton UP, 1985.

"Notes, News and Gleanings." *Journal of Outdoor Life: The Anti-tuberculosis Magazine*, vol. 14, no. 3, Mar. 1917, pp. 88–98.

Noyes, Clara D. "The Red Cross." *The American Journal of Nursing*, vol. 20, no. 2, Nov. 1919, pp. 134–38.

Oberländer, Christian. "The Rise of Western 'Scientific Medicine in Japan: Bacteriology and Beriberi." *Building a Modern Japan: Science, Technology, and Medicine in the Meiji Era and Beyond*, edited by Morris Low. Palgrave Macmillan, 2005.

"Obituary." *The British Medical Journal*, vol. 2, no. 3844, Sept. 8, 1934, p. 496.

"Obituary Notes." *The Publishers' Weekly*, vol. LXI, no. 4, Whole No. 1565, 25 Jan. 1902, p. 96.

Odell, Joseph H. "The New Spirit of the New Army: The Men behind the Men Who Fight the Huns." *The Outlook*, 12 Dec. 1917, pp. 604–9.

Ogyū, Sorai. *Master Sorai's Responsals: An Annotated Translation of* Sorai Sensei Tōmonsho. Translated Samuel Hideo Yamashita. U of Hawai'i P, 1994.

Ohara, Shin. "The Thought of Uchimura Kanzō and Its Relevance to Contemporary American Religion." *Culture and Religion in Japanese-American Relations: Essays on Uchimura Kanzō, 1861–1930*, edited by Ray A. Moore. Center for Japanese Studies, The U of Michigan, 1981.

Ohno, Kenichi. *The Economic Development of Japan: The Path Travelled by Japan as a Developing Country*. Tokyo, GRIPS Development Forum, 2006.

Ohnuki-Tierney, Emiko. *Illness and Culture in Contemporary Japan: An Anthropological View*. Cambridge, UK, Cambridge UP, 1984.

Ohtsu, Makoto, with Tomio Imanari. *Inside Japanese Business: A Narrative History, 1960–2000*. M. E. Sharpe, 2002.

奥村直彦. W・メレル・ヴォーリズ（一柳米来留）: 近江に「神の国」を. 近江八幡: 近江兄弟社湖声社, 2006. [Okumura Naohiko. *W. mereru vo-rizu (hitotsuyanagi mereru): Ōmi ni "kami no kuni" wo*. Ōmihachiman: Ōmikyōdaishakogoesha, 2006.]

大隈重信. 『大隈重信のことば』. 高野善一編者. 東京: 稲言社, 1964. [Ōkuma Shigenobu. *Ōkuma Shigenobu no kotoba*. Takano Zenichi hensha. Tokyo, Tōgensha, 1964.]

Ōkuma Shigenobu. "A Summary of the History of Japan." *Fifty Years of New Japan (Kaikoku Gojūnen Shi)*, compiled by Shigenobu Ōkuma, translated by Marcus B. Huish, vol. 1. London, Smith, Elder, & Col, 1909.

Ōmori Fusakichi. "The Sakura-jima Eruptions and Earthquakes, I–III." *Bulletin of the Imperial Earthquake Investigation Committee*, vol. 8, 1914, pp. 1–231. (Part I also published in 『東洋学芸雑誌』486号.)

Orchard, Dorothy J. "An Analysis of Japan's Cheap Labor." *Political Science Quarterly*, vol. 44, no. 2, June 1929, pp. 215–58.

Osler, William. "Introduction: The Evolution of Internal Medicine." *Modern Medicine: Its Theory and Practice*, edited by William Osler and Thomas McCrae, vol. 1. Lea Brothers & Co., 1907.

Otake, Tomoko. "Shigeaki Hinohara: Doctor of reforms." *Japan Times*, 8 Jan. 2006.

Otis, Edward O., M.D. *Tuberculosis: Its Cause, Cure and Prevention*. Thomas Y. Crowell Company, 1914.

Ozaki, Yukio. *The Autobiography of Ozaki Yukio: The Struggle for Constitutional Government in Japan*. Translated by Fujiko Hara. Princeton UP, 2001.

小澤三郎. 『日本プロテスタント史研究』. 東京: 東海大学出版会, 1964. [Ozawa Saburō. *Nihon purotesutantoshi kenkyū*. Tokyo, Tōkaidaigakushuppankai, 1964.]

Palmer, Henry Spencer. *Letters for the Land of the Rising Sun*. Yokohama, The "Japan Mail" Office, 1894.

Park, Yong-Shin. "Protestant Individualism in the Course of Modern Japanese Transformation: A Study in the Ideological Structure of Uchimura Kanzō." MA Thesis, U of California, Berkeley, 1969.

Parker, F. Calvin. *The Southern Baptist Mission in Japan, 1889–1989*. University Press of America, 1991.

"The Past Year and the Present Outlook in Japan from a Japanese Point of View." *The Missionary Herald: Containing the Proceedings of the American Board of Commissioners for Foreign Missions with a View of Other Benevolent Operations, for the Year 1896*. Boston, Press of Samuel Usher, 1896.

Phelps, G. S. "Young Men's Christian Association." *The Christian Movement in Japan, Korea and Formosa: A Year Book of Christian Work*, 22nd issue, edited by D. C. Holtom. Tokyo, Federation of Christian Missions Japan, 1924, 307–10.

Pieters, Albertus. *Mission Problems in Japan: Theoretical and Practical*. Board of Publication of the Reformed Church in America, 1912.

Plesset, Isabel R. *Noguchi and His Patrons*. Associated University Presses, 1980.

Pooley, Andrew Melville. *Japan at the Cross Roads.* London, G. Allen & Unwin, 1917.
Pope, Alton S. "The Role of the Sanatorium in Tuberculosis Control." *The Milbank Memorial Fund Quarterly*, vol. 16, no. 4, Oct. 1938, pp. 327–37.
Porter, Roy. *The Greatest Benefit to Mankind: A Medical History of Humanity.* W. W. Norton, 1997.
Pospielovsky, Dimitry. *The Orthodox Church in the History of Russia.* St. Vladimir's Seminary Press, 1998.
Prang, Margaret. *A Heart at Leisure from Itself: Caroline Macdonald of Japan.* U of British Columbia P, 1997.
Price, George Moses. "Administration of Labor Laws and Factory Inspection in Certain European Countries." *Bulletin of the United States Bureau of Labor Statistics*, no. 142, 27 Feb. 1914.
"Proceedings of the International Commercial Congress, Seventh Day's Session." *Official Proceedings of the International Commercial Congress: A Conference of all Nations for the Extension of Commercial Intercourse*, edited by William Mill Butler. Philadelphia, Press of the Philadelphia Commercial Museum, 1899.
Putney, Clifford. *Muscular Christianity: Manhood and Sports in Protestant America, 1880–1920.* Harvard UP, 2003.
Pyle, Kenneth B. *The New Generation in Meiji Japan: Problems of Cultural Identity, 1885–1895.* Stanford UP, 1969.
Railton, George Scott. *General William Booth: Founder of the Salvation Army.* George H. Doran Company, 1912.
Ramseyer, J. Mark. "Indentured Prostitution in Imperial Japan: Credible Commitments in the Commercial Sex Industry." *The Journal of Law, Economics, & Organization*, vol. 7, no. 1, 1991, pp. 89–116.
Ramseyer, J. Mark. *Odd Markets in Japanese History: Law and Economic Growth.* Cambridge, UK, Cambridge UP, 1996.
Ramsmeyer, J. Mark, and Frances McCall Rosenbluth. *The Politics of Oligarchy: Institutional Choice in Imperial Japan.* Cambridge, UK, Cambridge UP, 1998.
Ransome, Stafford. *Japan in Transition: A Comparative Study of the Progress Policy, and Methods of the Japanese Since Their War with China.* New York, Harper & Brothers Publishers, 1899.
Reischauer, Haru Matsukata. *Samurai and Silk: A Japanese and American Heritage.* Harvard UP, 1986.
Richards, Miriam. *It Began with Andrews: The Saga of a Medical Mission.* London, Salvationist Publishing and Supplies, Ltd., 1971.
Richmond, Lesley, Julie Stevenson, and Alison Turton, eds. *The Pharmaceutical Industry: A Guide to Historical Records.* Hants, UK, Ashgate Publishing, 2003.
Rightmire, R. David. *Salvationist Samurai: Gunpei Yamamuro and the Rise of the Salvation Army in Japan.* Scarecrow Press, 1997.
Robbins, Howard Chandler, and George K. MacNaught. *Dr. Rudolf Bolling Teusler: An Adventure in Christianity.* Charles Scribner's Sons, 1942.
Roberts, Michael J. D. "Charity Disestablished? The Origins of the Charity Organisation Society Revisited, 1868–1871." *The Journal of Ecclesiastical History*, vol. 54, issue 1, 2003, pp. 40–61.
Robinson, Charles Henry. *History of Christian Missions.* Charles Scribner's Sons, 1915.

Rogala, Joseph. *A Collector's Guide to Books on Japan in English: An Annotated List of over 2500 Titles with Subject Index*. Surrey, Japan Library, 2001. (Also listed as: Rogala, Jozef. *A Collector's Guide to Books on Japan in English: A Select List of over 2500 Titles/Compiled and Annotated by Joseph Rogala).*

Röhl, Wilhelm. "Social Law." *History of Law in Japan since 1868*, edited by Wilhelm Röhl. Leiden, Brill, 2005.

Ruxton, Ian. *The Correspondence of Sir Ernest Satow, British Minister in Japan, 1895–1900: Volume One*. Fukuoka, Researchers with Notes (Lulu Press/Kyushu Institute of Technology), 2005.

Ryan, Frank. *The Forgotten Plague: How the Battle Against Tuberculosis Was Won—and Lost*. Little, Brown and Company, 1992.

Ryder, Stephen Willis. "A Historical-Educational Study of the Japan Mission of the Reformed Church in America." PhD Dissertation, Columbia University, 1935.

St. John, Alice C. "The Open Forum—Japan." *The American Journal of Nursing*, vol. 27, no. 6, June 1927, pp. 486–87.

Sakura O. "Similarities and Varieties: A Brief Sketch on the Reception of Darwinism and Sociobiology in Japan." *Biology and Philosophy*, vol. 13, no. 3, July 1998, pp. 341–57.

Salkin, David. "Tuberculosis as a Cause of Upper Lobe Bronchiectasis." *California Medicine*, vol. 73, no. 6, pp. 577–80.

Salmon, D. E. "Reliability of the Evidence Obtained in the Study of Contagia." *Science*, vol. 2, no. 29, 24 Aug. 1883, pp. 2–3.

Sasakuba, Yakichi. "The Church of Christ in Japan." *The Christian Movement in the Japanese Empire Including Korea and Formosa: A Year Book for 1916*, edited by John Lincoln Bearing. 14th Annual Edition. Tokyo, Conference of Federated Missions Japan, 1916.

Sasamori, U., and W. de L. Kingsbury. "South Japan Conference of the Report of Committee on Summer Institute." *Official Minutes and Year Book, South Japan Mission Conference*. Tokyo, The Methodist Publishing House, 1907.

Sato, Hiroshi. *Democracy and the Japanese Government*. Columbia University, 1920.

佐藤尚子 & 大林正明. 『日中比較教育史』. 横浜: 春風社, 2002. [Satō Hisako & Ōbayashi Masaaki. *Nicchū hikaku kyōikushi*. Yokohama, Shunpūsha, 2002.]

Satofuka, Fumihiko. "Towards Fusion: Technology and Tradition in Japan." *Culture and Technology in Modern Japan*, edited by Ian Inkster and Fumihiko Satofuka. London, I.B. Tauris, 2000.

Saunders, Kenneth J. "Glimpses of the Religious Life of New Japan." *The Journal of Religion*, vol. 2, no. 1, Jan. 1922, pp. 70–80.

Saunders, Kenneth J. "Toyohiko Kagawa: The St. Francis of Japan." *Pacific Affairs*, vol. 4, no. 4, Apr. 1931, pp. 308–17.

Sawayanagi, Masataro. "The Spirit of Japanese Education." *Japan to America: A Symposium of Papers by Political Leaders and Representative Citizens of Japan on Conditions in Japan and on the Relations between Japan and the United States*, edited by Naoichi Masaoka. G. P. Putnam's Sons, 1915.

Saxonhouse, Gary R. "Country Girls and Communication among Competitors in the Japanese Cotton-Spinning Industry." *Japanese Industrialization and Its Social Consequences*, edited by Hugh Patrick. U of California Press, 1976.

Scalapino, Robert A. *Democracy and Party Movement in Pre-war Japan: The Failure of the First Attempt*. U of California P, 1953.

Scheiner, Irwin. *Christian Converts and Social Protest in Meiji Japan*. U of California P, 1970.

Scheiner, Irwin. "Christian Samurai and Samurai Values." *Modern Japanese Leadership: Transition and Change*, edited by Bernard S. Silberman and Harry D. Harootunian. U of Arizona P, 1966.

Schwantes, Robert S. "I. Christianity Versus Science: A Conflict of Ideas in Meiji Japan." *The Far Eastern Quarterly*, vol. 12, no. 2, Feb. 1953, pp. 123–32.

Schwartz, Eugene G., ed. *American Students Organize: Founding the National Student Association after World War II: An Anthology and Sourcebook*. American Council on Education/Praeger Publishers, 2006.

Seaman, Louis Livingston. *The Real Triumph of Japan: The Conquest of the Silent Foe*. D. Appleton and Company, 1906.

Searle, J. D. "Faith and Action." *The Expository Times: International Journal of Biblical Studies, Theology and Ministry*, vol. 84, 1973, p. 187.

社団法人北里研究所北里柴三郎記念室.『生誕150年記念:北里柴三郎』. 東京: 社団法人北里研究所, 2003. [Shadanhōmin Kitasato Kenkyūjo Kitasato Shibasaburōkinenshitsu. *Seitan 150 nen kinen: Kitasato Shibasaburō*. Tokyom Shadanhōmin Kitasato Kenkyūjo, 2003.]

Sherman, Irwin W. *The Power of Plagues*. ASM Press, 2006.

Shibusawa, Keizō. *Japanese Society in the Meiji Era*. Tokyo, Obunsha, 1958.

しまようこ.『「フェミニズム」という命の思想』. 東京: 文芸社, 2005. [Shima Yōko. *"Feminizumu" to iu inochi no shisō*. Tokyo, Bungeisha, 2005.]

Shimao, Eikoh. "Darwinism in Japan, 1877–1927." *Annals of Science*, vol. 38, no. 1, Jan. 1981, pp. 93–102.

Shinohara, Taira. "United Church of Christ in Japan." *The Ministry*, vol. 22, no. 2, Feb. 1949.

Sievers, Sharon L. *Flowers in Salt: The Beginnings of Feminist Consciousness in Modern Japan*. Stanford UP, 1983.

"Signs of the Times." *The Missionary Review of the World*, vol. 26, no. 6, June 1913, pp. 401–6.

Smethurst, Richard J. "Fukai Eigo and the Development of Japanese Monetary Policy." *New Directions in the Study of Meiji Japan*, edited by Helen Hardacre, with Adam L. Kern. Leiden, Brill, 1997.

Smiles, Samuel. *Self-Help; with Illustrations of Character and Conduct*. Harper & Brothers, Publishers, 1860.

Snedden, David. "Open-Air Schools." *The Boston Medical and Surgical Journal*, vol. 165, no. 17, 26 Oct. 1911, pp. 629–30.

Social Problems in Solution (Papers Read by Salvation Army Officials at the International Social Council). London, Salvation Army Press, 1921.

Societe des Nations. *La Cooperation Intellectuelle*, vol. 1, issue 1, 1929.

Sontag, Susan. *Illness as Metaphor; and AIDS and Its Metaphors*. Picador, 1990.

Sorensen, André. *The Making of Urban Japan: Cities and Planning from Edo to the Twenty-First Century*. Routledge, 2002.

Speer, Robert. "Missionary Progress during the Past Year." *The Sabbath Recorder*, vol. 78, no. 4, 25 Jan. 1915, pp. 116–18.

Steinbeck, John. *The Grapes of Wrath*. London, Penguin, 2006.

Steslicke, William E. *Doctors in Politics: The Political Life of the Japan Medical Association*. Praeger Publishers, 1973.

Stirewalt, A. J. "In Memoriam." *The Japan Christian Yearbook 1956: A Survey of the Christian Movement in Japan during 1955*, edited by Alden E. Matthews and John H. Skillman. Friendship Press, 1956.

Stoddard, Lothrop. "Japanese Question in California, Annals of the American Academy." *Selected Articles on Immigration*. Compiled by Edith M. Phelps. The H. W. Wilson Company, 1920.

Stolberg, Eva-Maria. "Review: *The Russo-Japanese War in Cultural Perspective, 1904–1905*, eds. David Wells and Sandra Wilson." *Russian Review*, vol. 60, no. 3, July 2001, pp. 443–44.

Stolberg, Eva-Maria. "Review: *Shamanism and Christianity: Native Encounters with Russian Orthodox Missions in Siberia and Alaska, 1820–1917* by Andrei A. Znamenski." *Russian Review*, vol. 60, no. 2, Apr. 2001, pp. 287–88.

Stone, Alan. "The Japanese Muckrakers." *The Journal of Japanese Studies*, vol. 1, no. 2, Spring 1975, pp. 385–407.

砂川幸雄. 『北里柴三郎の生涯: 第1回ノーベル賞候補』. 東京: NTT出版, 2003. [Sunagawa Yukio. *Kitasato Shibasaburō no shōgai: dai1kai no-beru shōhōko*. Tokyo, NTT Shuppan, 2003.]

Suzuki, Akihito. "Illness Experience and Therapeutic Choice: Evidence from Modern Japan." *Social Science History*, vol. 32, no. 4, Winter 2008, pp. 515–34.

Swain, Shurlee. "In These Days of Female Evangelists and Hallelujah Lasses: Women Preachers and the Redefinition of Gender Roles in the Churches in Late Nineteenth-Century Australia." *The Journal of Religious History*, vol. 26, no. 1, Feb. 2002, pp. 65–77.

Sweetland, Monroe. "The New Democracy in Social Welfare." *The Antioch Review*, vol. 3, no. 3, Autumn 1943, pp. 418–24.

Tai, Kuo-hui. "Confucianism and Japanese Modernization: A Study of Shibusawa Eiichi." *Japanese Business: Cultural Perspectives*, edited by Subhash Durlabhji and Norton E. Marks. State U of New York Press, 1993.

Taira, Koji. "Factory Labour and the Industrial Revolution in Japan." *The Economic Emergence of Modern Japan*, edited by Yamamura Kozo. Cambridge, UK, Cambridge UP, 1997.

Taira, Koji. "Factory Legislation and Management Modernization during Japan's Industrialization, 1886–1916." *The Business History Review*, vol. 44, no. 1, Japanese Entrepreneurship, Spring 1970, pp. 84–109.

Taiz, Lillian. "Applying the Devil's Works in a Holy Cause: Working-Class Popular Culture and the Salvation Army in the United States, 1879–1900." *Religion and American Culture: A Journal of Interpretation*, vol. 7, no. 2, Summer 1997, pp. 195–223.

Takahashi, Aya. *The Development of the Japanese Nursing Profession*. London, RoutledgeCurzon, 2004.

Takai, Toshio. *Watashi no "Jokō aishi"*. Tokyo, Sōdo Bunka, 1980.

Takano, Fusatarō. "Proposed Factory Act in Japan." *American Federationist*, vol. IV, no. 11, Jan. 1898, pp. 250–52.

Takeuchi, Yukiko, Noralene Uy, and Rajib Shaw. "Community-Based Water Management Practices in Japan." *Water Communities*, edited by Rajib Shaw and Danai Thaitakoo. Emerald Group Publishing, 2010.

Tanaka, Stefan. *Japan's Orient: Rendering Pasts into History*. U of California P, 1993.

Tanaka, Yukiko. *Women Writers of Meiji and Taishō Japan: Their Lives, Works and Critical Reception, 1868–1926*. McFarland & Company, 2000.

Tang, John P. "Public- versus Private-Led Industrialization in Meiji Japan, 1868–1912." Feb. 2008. http://emlab.berkeley.edu/users/webfac/cromer/e211_sp08/tang.pdf.

Taylor, Sandra C. "The Ineffectual Voice: Japan Missionaries and American Foreign Policy, 1870–1941." *The Pacific Historical Review*, vol. 53, no. 1, Feb. 1984, pp. 20–38.

Teusler, Rudolph B. "Clinical Medicine and Public Health in Japan." *The Japan Christian Year Book Continuing The Japan Mission Year Book*, edited by Willis C. Lamott, issue 30. Tokyo, Kyo Bun Kwan, 1932.

The Spirit of Missions. *A Church Hospital in the Capital of Japan: Being Some Account of the Successful Work of St. Luke's Hospital in the City of Tokyo*. The Domestic and Foreign Missionary Society of the Protestant Episcopal Church in the United States, 1904.

Thomas, Julia Adeney. *Reconfiguring Modernity: Concepts of Nature in Japanese Political Ideology*. U of California P, 2001.

Thompson, Alexander Mattock. *Japan for a Week (Britain for Ever!)*. London, J. Lane, 1911.

Tobimatsu, Jingo. *Hannah Riddell: Known in Japan as "The Mother of Lepers"*. Kumamoto, Kaishun Hospital, 1937.

常葉惠子. "病院と大学の関わりから." 『聖路加国際病院の100年』. 東京: 聖路加国際病院, 2002. [Tokiwa Keiko. "Byōin to daigaku no kakawarikara." *Seirokakokusaibyōin no hyakunen*. Tokyo, Seirokakokusaibyōin, 2002.]

特集「滋賀の歴史3」. いきいきニュースーレター第10号（平成1411月11日), pp. 3–5. ["Tokushū: Shiga no rekishi 3." *Ikiiki nyu-su-reta-*. Dai 10 gō, 11 Nov. 2002, pp. 3–5.]

Tokutomi, Roka. *Hototogisu* (translated as *Nami-ko: A Realistic Novel*). Translated by Sakae Shioya and E. F. Edgett. Herbert B. Turner, 1904.

徳富蘇峰. 『蘇峰自伝』. 東京: 中央公論者, 1935. [Tokutomi Sohō. *Sohō jiden*. Tokyo, Chūō Kōronsha, 1935.]

Tomes, Nancy. *The Gospel of Germs: Men, Women, and the Microbe in American Life*. Harvard UP, 1998.

Tomes, Nancy. "Moralizing the Microbe: The Germ Theory and the Moral Construction of Behavior in the Late-Nineteenth Century Anti-tuberculosis Movement." *Morality and Health*, edited by Allan M. Brandt and Paul Rozin. Routledge, 1997.

Tomida, Hiroko. "The Association of New Women and Its Contribution to the Japanese Women's Movement." *Japan Forum*, vol. 17, no. 1, 2005, pp. 49–68.

"Tomorrow in the Orient: The Future of a Medical Mission in Japan." The American Council of St. Luke's International Medical Center of Tokyo, 1935.

筑波昭. 『津山三十人殺し—村の秀才青年はなぜ凶行に及んだか』. 東京: 草思社, 1981. [Tsukuba Akira. *Tsuyama san-jūnin goroshi—mura no shūsai seinen ha naze kyōkō ni oyondaka*. Tokyo, Sōshisha, 1981.]

常石敬一. 『結核と日本人: 医療政策検証する』. 東京: 岩波書店, 2011. [Tsuneishi Keiichi. *Kekkaku to Nihonjin: iryou seisaku wo kenshou suru*. Tokyo, Iwanami Shoten, 2011.]

Tsurumi, E. Patricia. *Factory Girls: Women in the Thread Mills of Meiji Japan*. Princeton UP, 1990.

Tsurumi, E. Patricia. "Whose History Is It Anyway? And Other Questions Historians Should Be Asking. In This Case about the Cotton and Silk Thread Factory Women of Meiji Japan." *Japan Review*, vol. 6, 1995, pp. 17–36.

Tucker, John A. "Japanese Views of Nature and the Environment." *Nature across Cultures: Views of Nature and the Environment in Non-Western Cultures*, edited by Helaine Selin. Springer, 2003.

Tucker, Henry St. George. "A Great Christian." *Dr. Rudolf Bolling Teusler: An Adventure in Christianity*, by Howard Chandler Robbins and George K. MacNaught. Charles Scribner's Sons, 1942.

Uchimura, Kanzō. *How I Became a Christian: Out of My Diary*. Tokyo, Keiseisha, 1895.

University of Chicago Alumni Council. *Alumni Directory of the University of Chicago 1861–1906*. U of Chicago P, 1906.

Unoura, Hiroshi. "Hiroyuki Kato: A Social Darwinist Approach to the Emperorship in Modern Japan." 『経済と経営』, vol. 29, no. 2, Sept. 1998, pp. 209–28.

Unsworth, Madge. *Great Was the Company*. London, Salvationist Publishing and Supplies, 1963.

Uyehara, George Etsujiro. *The Political Development of Japan, 1867–1909*. E. P. Dutton & Co., 1910.

Vanderbilt, Gregory Allen. "'The Kingdom of God Is Like a Mustard Seed:' Evangelizing Modernity between the United States and Japan, 1905–1948." PhD Dissertation. University of California, Los Angeles, 2005.

van der Sprenkel, Otto B. "Max Weber on China." *History and Theory*, vol. 3, no. 3, 1964, pp. 348–70.

Vittinghoff, Natascha. *Die Anfänge des Journalismus in China (1860–1911)*. Wiesbaden, Harrassowitz, 2002.

Vories, Wm. Merrell. *College Memories and Other Rimes*. Colorado College, 1903.

Vories, Wm. Merrell. *The Evangelization of Rural Japan*. Tokyo, Kyōbunkan, 1915.

Vories, William Merrell. "Let No Man Despise Thy Youth." *Colorado College Publication*, no. 177, May 1931, pp. 3–16.

Vories, Wm. Merrell. *A Mustard-Seed in Japan*. 5th ed., Omi-Hachiman: Omi Mission, 1925.

Vories, Wm. Merrell. *The Omi Brotherhood in Nippon*. 3rd ed., Omi-Hachiman: The Omi Brotherhood Book Department, 1936.

Walker, Pamela J. "A Chaste and Fervid Eloquence: Catherine Booth and the Ministry of Women in the Salvation Army." *Women Preachers and Prophets through Two Millennia of Christianity*, edited by Beverly Mayne Kienzle and Pamela J. Walker. U of California P, 1998, 288–302.

Walker, Pamela J. *Pulling the Devil's Kingdom Down: The Salvation Army in Victorian Britain*. U of California P, 2001.

Walkowitz, Judith R. *City of Dreadful Delight: Narratives of Sexual Danger in Late-Victorian London*. U of Chicago P, 1992.

"Wants to Enlarge American Hospital: Dr. R. B. Teusler Is Here from Tokio to Get Added Support for St. Luke's." *New York Times*, 7 June 1913.

Watanabe, Keiko. "Hatsuko Yuasa and Kieko Yamamuro: Two Meiji Era Christian Women with *Samurai* Spirit." *Essays 2007*. Nagoya, Nagoya Women's Studies Research Group, 2007, pp. 76–86.

渡辺正雄.『日本人と近代科学: 西洋への対応と課題』. 東京: 岩波新書, 1976. [Watanabe Masao. *Nihonjin to kindai kagaku: seiyōheno taiō to kadai*. Tokyo: Iwanamishinsho, 1976.]

Waters, Neil Leroy. "A Political History of the Kawasaki Region: 1860–1890." PhD Dissertation, University of Hawai'i, 1978.

Wells, David, and Sandra Wilson. Introduction. *The Russo-Japanese War in Cultural Perspective, 1904–05*, edited by David Wells and Sandra Wilson. St. Martin's Press, 1999.

White, Paul. *Thomas Huxley: Making the "Man of Science."* Cambridge, UK, Cambridge UP, 2003.

Whitney, Willis Norton. "Notes on the History of Medical Progress in Japan." *Transactions of the Asiatic Society of Japan*, vol. 12, part 4. Yokohama, R. Meiklejohn & Co., July 1885, pp. 245–470.

Wittelsey, Sarah Scovill, and Arthur Twining Hadley. "Massachusetts Labor Legislation, an Historical and Critical Study." *The Annals of the American Academy of Political and Social Science*, vol. 17, Supplement 15, Jan. 1901, pp. 1–157.

Wilson, H. Schütz. "Marie Bashkirtseff." *The Gentleman's Magazine: Volume CCLXXX—January to June 1896*, edited by Sylvanus Urban. London, Chatto & Windus, 1896.

Wilson, P. W. *General Evangeline Booth of the Salvation Army*. The Salvation Army, 1948.

Witte, Sergei. *The Memoirs of Count Witte*. Edited and translated by Sidney Harcave. M. E. Sharpe, 1990.

Woodall, Ann M. *What Price the Poor? William Booth, Karl Marx and the London Residuum*. Aldershot, UK, Ashgate Publishing, 2005.

Woodman, E. R., Rev. "Ten Years of an Episcopate in Japan." *The Sacramento Missionary*, 19 Mar. 1903, pp. 85–96.

Worboys, Michael. "From Heredity to Infection: Tuberculosis, 1870–1890." *Heredity and Infection: The History of Disease Transmission*, edited by Jean-Paul Gaudillière and Ilana Löwy. Routledge, 2001.

Wright, Robert A. "The Canadian Protestant Tradition 1914–1945." *The Canadian Protestant Experience, 1760–1990*, edited by George A. Rawlyk. McGill-Queen's UP, 1990.

Xing Jun. *Baptized in the Fire of Revolution: The American Social Gospel and the YMCA in China: 1919–1937*. Associated University Presses, 1996.

Yakhontoff, Victor. *Eyes on Japan*. Coward-McCann, 1936.

Yamakawa, Kikue. "Record of the Generations of Women (*Onna nidai nikki*)." *Sources of East Asian Tradition: The Modern Period*, vol. 2, edited by William Theodore De Bary and Brett De Bary. Columbia UP, 2008.

Yamamoto, Saburo, and Yamamoto Toshiko. "Historical Review of BCG Vaccine in Japan." *Japanese Journal of Infectious Diseases*, vol. 60, 2007, pp. 331–36.

山室軍平.『ブース大将伝』. 東京: 救世軍日本本営, 1906. [Yamamuro Gunpei. *Būsu Taishō den*. Tokyo, Kyūseigun Nihon Honei, 1906.]

山室軍平.『平民之福音』. 東京: 救世軍日本本営, 1901. [Yamamuro Gunpei. *Heimin no fukuin*. Tokyo, Kyūseigun Nihon Honei, 1901.]

山内みな. "六千人の女のその「東京モスリン」."『女のはたらき. ドキュメント女の百年: 3. 編集解説もろさわようこ』. 東京: 平凡社, 1978. [Yamanouchi Mina. "Rokusennin no onna no sono 'Tōkyō Mosurin.'" *Onna no hataraki*, vol. 3 of *Dokyumento onna no hyakunen*, edited by Morosawa Yōko. Tokyo, Heibonsha, 1978.]

"Y.M.C.A. AIMS TO AID SOLDIERS OF INDUSTRY; Will Provide Social Centres for the Men Engaged in War Work." *New York Times*, 11 Mar. 1918.

Y.M.C.A.史学会編集委員会.『新編日本Y.M.C.A史：日本Y.M.C.A.同盟結成100周年記念』. 東京：日本YMCA同盟日本YMCA史刊行委員会、2003. [YM.C.A. shi gakkai henshū iinkai. *Shinpen nihon Y.M.C.A.shi: Nihon Y.M.C.A. doumei kessei 100 shūnen kinen*. Tokyo, Nihon Y.M.C.A. doumei nihon Y.M.C.A. shi kankou iinkai, 2003.]

横手慎二.『日露戦争史』. 東京: 中央公論新社, 2005. [Yokote Shinji. *Nichiro sensōshi*. Tokyo, Chuokoron-Shinsha, 2005.]

Yokoyama, Toshio. "Even a Sardine's Head Becomes Holy: The Role of Household Encyclopedias in Sustaining Civilisation in Pre-industrial Japan." *Sansai: An Environmental Journal for the Global Community*, vol. 1, 2006, pp. 41–57.

吉田悦蔵.『近江の兄弟』. 東京: 春秋社, 1926. [Yoshida Etsuzō. *Ōmi no kyōdai*. Tokyo, Shunjūsha, 1926.]

Index

www.ingramcontent.com/pod-product-compliance
Ingram Content Group UK Ltd.
Pitfield, Milton Keynes, MK11 3LW, UK
UKHW021837100926
8556IPUK00004B/394

9 789888 52814